CLINICAL NEUROPSYCHOLOGY OF EMOTION

Clinical Neuropsychology of Emotion

Yana Suchy

THE GUILFORD PRESS
New York London

A Division of Guilford Publications, Inc.
72 Spring Street, New York, NY 10012
www.guilford.com

Printed in the United States of America

This book is printed on acid-free paper.

Last digit is print number: 9 8 7 6 5 4 3 2 1

Library of Congress Cataloging-in-Publication Data

Suchy, Yana.
Clinical neuropsychology of emotion / Yana Suchy.
p. ; cm.
Includes bibliographical references and index.
ISBN 978-1-60918-072-0 (hardcover: alk. paper)
1. Emotions. 2. Neuropsychology. 3. Clinical neuropsychology. I. Title.
[DNLM: 1. Emotions—physiology. 2. Models, Neurological. 3. Motivation—physiology. 4. Neuropsychology—methods. 5. Stress, Psychological. WL 103]
QP401.S843 2011
612.8′232—dc22

2010040305

Rodičům,
s láskou a vděčností

(To my parents, with love and gratitude)

About the Author

Yana Suchy, PhD, is Associate Professor of Psychology and Clinical Neuropsychology Program Director in the Department of Psychology at the University of Utah. Her professional responsibilities include graduate training, research, and clinical neuropsychological practice. Dr. Suchy's research focuses on understanding the interface among executive, affective, and motor processes, with the long-term goal of developing new methods for detecting subtle, preclinical deficits in executive and emotional control. In line with her research interests, she feels strongly about the need to integrate assessment of affective processes into everyday neuropsychological clinical practice. She serves on the editorial boards of the *Journal of the International Neuropsychological Society* and *The Clinical Neuropsychologist*, and as an ad hoc reviewer for a number of other journals. Dr. Suchy has published widely in a variety of peer-reviewed journals and neuropsychology textbooks and presents regularly at national and international meetings.

Contents

About This Book 1

PART I. Historical Origins: Emotions and Personality from Antiquity to the 20th Century 7

CHAPTER 1. Traditional Models and Theories of Emotions and Personality 9

CHAPTER 2. Early Neuroatomic Models of Emotional Processing 23

PART II. Anatomy of an Emotional Event: From Emotional Trigger to Emotion Regulation 43

CHAPTER 3. The Trigger Mechanism and the Detection of Emotionally Salient Stimuli 45

CHAPTER 4. Reflexive Emotional Responses 70

CHAPTER 5. Awareness and Understanding of an Emotional Experience 94

CHAPTER 6. Emotional Communication 111

CHAPTER 7. Emotion Regulation 135

PART III. Emotions, Affective Styles, and Motivation: How Emotions Shape Who We Are and What We Do 155

CHAPTER 8. Mood and Motivation 159

CHAPTER 9. Motivation and Sensitivity to Incentives 176

CHAPTER 10. Stress and Motivation 204

PART IV. A Glimpse at Tomorrow from an Interdisciplinary Perspective 221

CHAPTER 11. Temperament, Personality, and Heritability of Individual Differences in Executive Functioning 223
with Paula G. Williams

CHAPTER 12. Stress Regulation, Executive Functioning, and Physical and Mental Health 235
with Paula G. Williams

CHAPTER 13. Future Directions for Clinical Neuropsychology of Emotion 247

APPENDIX A. Affective Deficits, Symptoms, and Syndromes Associated with Select Clinical Populations 253

APPENDIX B. Disorders and Populations Associated with Select Affective Deficits, Symptoms, or Syndromes 260

APPENDIX C. Select Measures for Assessment of Affective Deficits, Symptoms, or Syndromes 263

References 265

Index 353

CLINICAL NEUROPSYCHOLOGY OF EMOTION

About This Book

THE IMPETUS

Over the past 30 years, clinical neuropsychology has witnessed a tremendous growth and maturation, both as a science as a clinical profession. The handful of tests available to clinical neuropsychologists in the late 1970s and early 1980s has exploded into a broad array of theoretically and psychometrically sophisticated instruments. The 1990s, the Decade of the Brain, further propelled neuropsychology along its already impressive trajectory. Methodology for studying brain–behavior relationships has evolved well beyond the study of naturalistic human lesions and animal ablations, supplementing the older practices with modern structural and functional imaging techniques. Our understanding of cognitive domains and subdomains has also expanded: No longer is the "frontal lobe syndrome" considered a unitary construct, and the relationships among complex and overlapping processes such as mental speed, attention, and working memory are beginning to be understood. With better methods and better understanding of the brain, clinical neuropsychology has arrived as a mature and sophisticated clinical specialty.

Against the backdrop of this exponential growth, the neuropsychology of emotion represents a popular but poorly defined area that has yet to become fully integrated into the practice of clinical neuropsychology. Casual conversations with clinical neuropsychologists will reveal many different views on the subject matter. For some, the neuropsychology of emotion represents the study of deficits in affective communication and behavioral control resulting from brain disease or brain injury. For others, the neuropsychology of emotion translates into the neuropsychology of psychopathology—that is, the study of neurocognitive profiles associated with schizophrenia, major depression, obsessive–compulsive disorder, and so on. And for others yet, the neuropsychology of emotion is synonymous with affective neuroscience, offering fascinating academic inquiries into the workings of the brain, but with little clinical applicability.

The impetus for this book was the desire to take the widely varied topics and levels of analysis that comprise the neuropsychology of emotion and extract from them the knowledge and techniques that are clinically relevant, with the hope of moving toward a clinically applicable integration (i.e., *clinical* neuropsychology of emotion) that our profession could utilize, foster, and begin to call its own.

THE AIMS

The aims of this book are fivefold: (1) to propose clinically meaningful domains of emotional processing; (2) demonstrate the clinical utility of each domain; (3) demonstrate that emotions and cognitions are much more closely intertwined than was historically thought; (4) explore the interdisciplinary future of the *clinical* neuropsychology of emotion; and (5) provide an easy reference for clinical neuropsychologists when questions about emotional processing arise. Table 1 illustrates how these aims are addressed throughout the book.

THE OVERALL ORGANIZATION

This book is organized into four parts. Part I provides a historical perspective, both on how emotions have been conceptualized since antiquity through the 20th century, and how the neuroanatomy of emotion came to be understood. Part II reviews emotional processes that comprise a single emotional event, from the initial bottom-up trigger of an emotional response (Chapter 3) through the ultimate top-down process of emotion regulation (Chapter 7). Next, Part III moves beyond the level of a single event to examine how patterns of emotional responses come together to *motivate* behavior. Lastly, Part IV looks toward the future, demonstrating the interdisciplinary relevance of clinical neuropsychology of emotion, and

TABLE 1. Where/How the Book's Aims Are Addressed

Aims	General chapter sections	Specific chapter sections	Chapters
1. Domains of emotional processing	Theoretical Background	Defining the Constructs Neuroanatomic Substrates	3–10
2. Clinical utility of each domain	Integrating Theory and Practice	Assessment Everyday Functioning Clinical Signs and Syndromes Clinical Populations	3–10
3. Relationship between emotions and cognition	Theoretical Background	Interplay with Cognition	3–12
4. Interdisciplinary future of *clinical* neuropsychology of emotion	N/A	N/A	11–12
5. Resources for clinicians	N/A	N/A	Appendices A, B, and C

forging linkages to behavioral medicine, personality theory, and human genetics.

Arguably, Parts II and III have the more immediate relevance for the practicing neuropsychologist. So as to facilitate the utility of these book portions as a reference, each chapter is organized in the same fashion, beginning with a *Theoretical Background* section and followed by a section entitled *Integrating Theory and Practice*, in which clinical syndromes, clinical populations, and various assessment implications are discussed. Appendices are provided at the end of the book, and these cross-reference populations and syndromes across all book chapters for an easy reference. Figure 1 illustrates this overall organizational structure.

HOW TO READ THIS BOOK

One could argue that there are two kinds of people: readers and skimmers. Readers don't like to be rushed; they like to pause and reflect, and don't mind being taken by the hand and led through a story. Skimmers, on the other hand, are a take-charge kind of people. When picking up a book they may skip straight to the end, likely glossing over passages that meander or don't move a story along at a fast enough pace.

There are arguably advantages and disadvantages to either approach: In other words, there is no right or wrong way. Recognizing that not every-

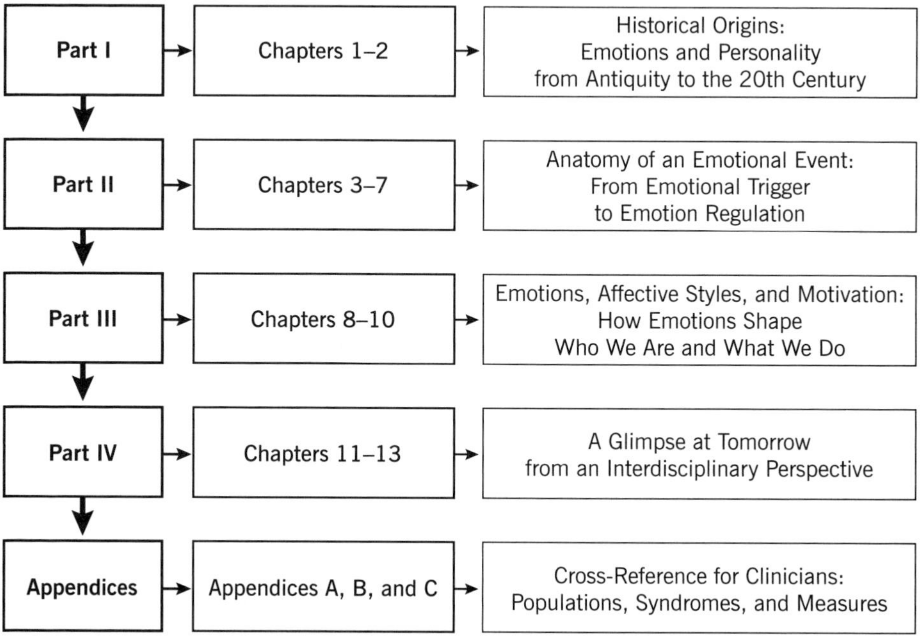

FIGURE 1. The overall organization of the book.

one will use this book in the same manner, care was taken to accommodate both the skimmers and the readers in the audience. Figure 2 illustrates two approaches to how this book could be used.

For the readers (i.e., the top-down approach): This book was written with the expectation that it would be read sequentially, from the start to the finish. It begins with a historical section, inviting the reader to reflect upon whence we came, indulging a bit in the "story of history" beyond the simple names and dates. It then moves on to a description of progressively more complex aspects of emotional processing, going beyond the basic facts, providing the reader with real-life examples and analogies, as well as opportunities to *feel* the constructs at hand. To facilitate review of the materials, appendices are provided at the end that cross-reference syndromes, populations, and assessment instruments across Parts II and III of the book.

For the skimmers (i.e., the bottom-up approach): To facilitate skimming or using the book primarily as a reference tool, ample headings and consistent organization of chapter sections (particularly in Parts II and III) have been provided. Additionally, appendices are provided at the end of the book, allowing the user to "fast-forward" to chapters that contain a desired topic.

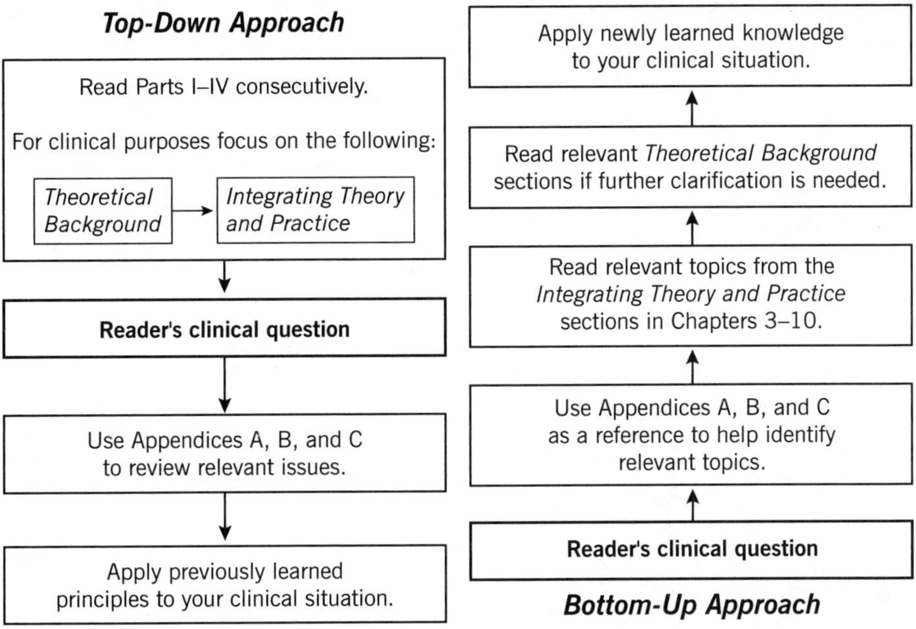

FIGURE 2. Two approaches for using this book. The *top-down approach* is intended for "readers" (i.e., individuals who will read the book consecutively from start to finish). Readers may return to the book when encountering a clinical question in their practice, at which point they may use the appendices to direct them to the relevant sections of the book for a review. The *bottom-up approach* is intended for "skimmers" (i.e., those individuals who will use the book primarily as a reference). Skimmers may pick up the book when they encounter a clinical question in their practice, at which point they may wish to direct their attention to the appendices first, and then proceed to additional relevant sections of the book as needed.

PART I

Historical Origins

Emotions and Personality from Antiquity to the 20th Century

INTRODUCTION TO PART I

The word *emotion* dates back to 1579, when it was adapted from the French *émouvoir*, "to stir up" (Merriam-Webster, 2004),[1] although the earliest precursors of the word likely date back to the very origins of language. Children as young as 2 years of age describe basic emotions spontaneously and without any need for formal instruction (Widen, 2005), and even Koko the signing gorilla is famed to have used signs for "sorry" and "sad" (De La O, 2005). Despite the ubiquity of emotions in everyday life, the worthiness of emotions has traditionally been questioned. For example, in ancient China, it was believed that excesses of emotions cause damage to the *qi*, which in turn damages vital organs; and in the Western World, from Plato to the Middle Ages, emotions were viewed as unhealthy, immoral, and inferior to reason. Even William Shakespeare, whose writings are chockful of "passion," cautioned against emotional excesses: Ten of Shakespeare's characters suffered death due to experiencing strong emotions, 18 characters fainted due to emotional upsets, and death as a possible consequence of strong emotions was mentioned in dialogue 29 times (Heaton, 2006).

Fast forward another few centuries, and, oh, how have times changed! In today's Western society, the question "*How did that make you feel?*" is daily uttered from the lips of countless psychotherapists, and the clients' typical responses—"*I think it wasn't fair,*" or "*I think I should have done something*"—are simply viewed as *un*acceptable. "*No, no, no,*" protest the bewildered psychotherapists, "*How did that make you FEEL?*", their words a testament to a new era in which emotions are not only encouraged, but, at least in some situations, *preferred* over reason.

In recent decades, the interest in emotions has evolved further yet, capturing the imagination of not only psychologists and neuroscientists, but also researches in such unlikely fields as the economics, ecology, and computer science. This growing interest in emotions from even the "hard" sciences reflects the increasing recognition that emotions may not only be good for us, but also that they may be less separate from cognition than has traditionally been thought. These latter views are evidenced by such apparent oxymorons as "emotional intelligence" and "emotional reasoning." In light of these emerging and changing attitudes, the next two chapters review the history of philosophical, psychological, and neuroanatomic models of emotions.

NOTE

1. The word *emotion* replaced the older word *passion.*

CHAPTER 1

Traditional Models and Theories of Emotions and Personality

EARLY PHILOSOPHIC MODELS

The underpinnings of human emotional experiences and temperamental styles have intrigued thinkers for millennia. It wasn't lost on ancient man (or woman) that most of us are characterized by distinct and fairly stable ways of responding to the world, not only behaviorally but emotionally as well. In times past, without the benefit of microscopes, psychophysiological measurements, neuroimaging devices, and statistical methodologies, ancient thinkers and philosophers interested in understanding emotions and temperaments were left to rely on naked-eye observations of the world. Their theories and models consisted of a good dose of imagination, literary savvy, and poetic hyperbole, combined with an even larger, albeit understandable, dose of biopsychosocial naiveté. In unpredictable ways, these past fancies of imagination have not only found a secure place in the language, arts, and literature of today's Western world, but have also imposed influences on Western medicine and psychology as recently as a century ago.

Ancient Greece and the Doctrine of the Four Humors

In Ancient Greece, philosophy and medicine went hand in hand. Ancient Greek philosophers were in the business of trying to understand not only what the world around them was made of; or where the living forces of plants, animals, and humans came from; or why, and whether, sadness or happiness mattered—but also how all these principles came together to create a physically and emotionally healthy person. The Greek philosophers' interest in health was no coincidence, since, in addition to serving as the principle theoreticians of medicine, they were also the medical *practitioners*, responsible for examining, diagnosing, and treating their fellow citizens. Around 400 B.C.E., one such practicing physician was the Greek philosopher Hippocrates (ca. 460–ca. 370 B.C.E.). Among the central themes of his writings is the theory of the four humors.

According to this theory, the human body consisted of four basic elements: blood, phlegm, black bile, and yellow bile (Arikha, 2007). These elements corresponded to four basic substances that were presumed to make up the world (see Table 1.1). The *proportions* of the four humors in the human body were thought to fluctuate with the four seasons, but also as

TABLE 1.1. Physical and Mental Characteristics Associated with Excesses of Individual Humors

	The four humors			
	Blood	Yellow bile	Black bile	Phlegm
Earth element	Air	Fire	Earth	Water
Season	Spring	Summer	Fall	Winter
Skin	Hot and moist	Hot and dry	Cold and dry	Cold and moist
Body type	Corpulent	Thin Fidgety	Thin	Sallow Corpulent
Temperament	Sanguine	Choleric	Melancholic	Phlegmatic
Traits	Cheerful Optimistic Sensuous	Enthusiastic Envious Argumentative	Reflective Artistic Depressed	Relaxed Sluggish Cowardly

Note. Based on Arikha (2007).

a function of physical and mental health. Thus, according to Hippocrates and his fellow physicians, both physical and mental illness were the result of imbalances among the four humors, and were evident from patients' body types and skin types.

In a treatise entitled *A Regimen of Health*, Hippocrates[1] outlined in detail various methods for bringing the four humors back into balance. Interestingly, some of the methods described by Hippocrates still make sense today, such as ingesting honey for its expectorant qualities to rid the body of excess phlegm. Others, such as bloodletting, are clearly less salubrious. Regardless of its effectiveness, or the lack thereof, this ancient tradition rapidly became the dominant medical theory in many cultures, making its mark on how medicine would be practiced around the world for over 2,000 years. So entrenched and beloved was this ancient theory that it has come to be known as the *doctrine* of the four humors, and, in fact, continues to be practiced to this day in parts of China, India, Pakistan, Bangladesh, and Sri Lanka (Bala, 2009). Even in the Western world, the doctrine of the four humors dictated how medicine was practiced until the 19th century, when it finally gave way to the more scientifically sound "germ theory" (Haller, 1986).

In the second century C.E., the theory of the four humors was further elaborated by the Greek physician Galen of Pergamon (ca. 130–ca. 200), who used the four humors as a framework for classifying human traits, personalities, and temperaments. He proposed that, for example, rosy cheeks and a chubby body were the reflection of high levels of blood, resulting in a "sanguine" (i.e., cheerful) personality (see Table 1.1). This psychological classification system proved to be even more resilient to change than its counterpart from physical medicine. Rather than being replaced by other theories, it was *incorporated* into newer conceptualizations of the human psyche. For example, William Sheldon (Sheldon & Stevens, 1942) and Hans Eysenck (Eysenck & Eysenck, 1958), as recently as half a century ago, relied on the nomenclature of the doctrine of the four humors in their classification systems of personality. In neuropsychology, the word "neuro*humors*" (Blair & Erlanger, 1936)—referring, of course, to neurotransmitters—was still in use as late as the mid-1980s (Goeders, Lane, & Smith, 1984) and can be seen in the writings of such prominent theoreticians as Karl Pribram (Pribram, 1967).

Interestingly, if one accepts the notion that the four humors represent a metaphor for hormones, neurotransmitters, vitamins, and other substances in the body that are crucial for normal functioning, it is easy to see how imbalances among such substances would be responsible not only for physical illness but for mental dysfunction as well. After all, neurotransmitter abnormalities, vitamin deficiencies, infections, and liver, kidney, or heart disease are only a few examples of the many "humoral" etiologies of cognitive and psychiatric dysfunctions that practicing neuropsychologists encounter in their clinics on a daily basis.

Defining the Soul and the Perfect Human: From Plato to Descartes

While the theory of the four humors focused on understanding the physical sources of personality and mental illness, other thinkers focused on trying to understand the *spiritual* underpinnings of emotions. Among these was Plato (427–347 B.C.E.) who, ironically, was not particularly interested in people's daily emotional strivings—in fact, he frowned upon dwelling on emotions. Instead, he was primarily interested in defining abstract ideal forms of the world, most notably, an ideal human society. In his famous tome *Republic*, he described three separate and necessary classes of citizens: the "ruling class," consisting of wise, rational philosophers; the "middle class," consisting of the determined, strong-willed military; and the "third class," consisting of workers, farmers, and businessmen who generated what was needed for the state's economic well-being. This *ideal state* would lend its structure to many of Plato's other writings, including those on human nature and the constitution of the human soul. Specifically, Plato proposed that the human psyche consisted of the "rational soul," corresponding to the ruling class of sage philosophers, the "spirited soul," corresponding to the strong-willed military, and the "appetitive soul," corresponding to the workers, farmers, and businessmen who provided sustenance for the state's citizens.

In the fifth century B.C.E., Plato's model of the three souls was further elaborated by his pupil Aristotle (384–322 B.C.E.), who was less interested in the abstract ideals and more interested in concrete ways in which any given person could strive toward achieving perfection. Aristotle believed, on the one hand, that emotions were undesirable or even evil, and, on the other, that emotions were an inextricable part of life. To reconcile these two views, he proposed the concept of *states*, or *predispositions to feel* emotions. This concept allowed him to propose that it was not the absence of emotions, but rather one's ability to regulate them, that defined the "perfect moral man" (Knuuttila, 2004; Schmitter, 2006).

Three aspects of these millenia-old reflections are rather striking. The first is the rather sophisticated distinction between emotions, on the one hand, and emotion regulation, on the other, proposed by Aristotle. As we will see in Chapters 7, 11, and 12, emotion regulation has been a hot topic of much recent research in behavioral medicine and affective neuroscience, representing a viable pathway toward truly holistic medicine.

The second interesting aspect of the ancient philosophies is that the same tripartite structure described by Plato and Aristotle likely served as a model for modern thinkers of the 20th century, most notably Freud and his psychosexual structure of personality (i.e., the concepts of the superego, the ego, and the id). Along the same lines, the notion of the three souls can also serve as a metaphor for key components of brain processing: crystallized intelligence (the sage philosophers), behavioral control (the military), and emotions or drives (the working class). If one accepts this metaphor, then the notion that the "appetitive soul" (i.e., emotions) is responsible for feeding and propagation may have inadvertently foreshadowed what would be articulated more than 2,000 years later by Charles Darwin: that emotions are the central force behind survival of both the individual and the entire species (Heinaman, 1997; Ryle, 1967). (See Table 1.2.)

Lastly, the ancient philosophies explicitly proclaim separateness between emotions and cognitions (i.e., the spirited and appetitive souls, on the one hand, and the rational soul, on the other). In fact, this same dichotomy between emotions and cognitions was revisited again in the 17th century by René Descartes, who, in his 1641 *Meditations*, described human behavior as being influenced by two separate entities: the *animal spirits* (i.e., emotions), and the *rational soul* (i.e., cognitions)[2] (Knuuttila, 2004). It is impossible to know today whether this presumed dichotomy between emotions and cognition is intuitively obvious to people, or whether it is a result of a doctrine that stems from the writings of Plato and Descartes, a doctrine that has become so entrenched in the human psyche that it is virtually impossible to break. One of the goals of this book is to challenge this doctrine and to demonstrate that the schism between emotions and cognition has been grossly overstated.

TABLE 1.2. Correspondence between Ancient Philosophy, Freud's Constructs, and the Structure of Cognition

Source	Overarching construct	Components		
Plato	Ideal state	Ruling class (philosophers)	Middle class (military)	Third class (workers)
Plato	Human soul	Rational	Spirited	Appetitive
Aristotle	Human soul	Rational	Sensitive	Vegetative
Freud	Personality	Superego	Ego	Id
Neuropsychology	Output of brain processing	Crystallized intelligence	Executive functioning	Emotions and drives

THE MIDDLE AGES

In medieval Europe, belonging to the Christian faith was a matter of survival. Non-Christian peoples (such as Jews) and religious heretics (such as scientists) were ostracized at best. At worst, they met with an untimely, and often painful, death. Love of Christ was the only emotion sanctioned by the Christian rule, and all other emotions were viewed as irrational or even subversive of religious faith (Knuuttila, 2004). It is against this politicoreligious backdrop that the medieval writings on emotions need to be considered.

Thomas Aquinas (1225–1274)

Thomas Aquinas is arguably the most prominent writer of the Middle Ages with respect to theories of emotions. Relying heavily on Aristotle, Aquinas accepted emotions as a necessary evil, viewing them as having a deleterious effect on people's lives. In general, according to his writing, prototypical emotions were all negatively valenced, such as despair or grief. In contrast, positive feelings, such as happiness, were not considered to be a part of the emotional phenomenology. Rather, Aquinas viewed happiness as a dispassionate, rational state, and he viewed God and the angels as rational, dispassionate, and therefore happy beings (Schmitter, 2006). Interestingly, by denying the existence of what would be viewed today as normal and necessary goals of appetitive drives, such as pleasure from food, drink, or sex, Aquinas essentially described a depressed society marked by anhedonia.

Niccolo Machiavelli (1469–1527)

Unlike Thomas Aquinas, who focused on the role of emotions in people's relationship with God, Machiavelli focused on how emotions could be exploited in the service of more secular masters. Machiavelli, of course, has *not* earned his prominence in history by writing scientific or philosophic treatises on emotions. Rather, he is known as the founder of political science and the author of *The Prince*, in which he expounds the virtues of taking all steps necessary, however evil or immoral, in the interest of preserving those in authority and power (Schmitter, 2006).

But in addition to these foundations for his fame (or infamy, whichever view the reader chooses to take), Machiavelli also made some rather astute observations about the role of emotions in motivating behavior. In a truly Machiavelian fashion, he recommended that some emotions, such as fear and envy, be exploited in military pursuits. In particular, he introduced the notion of publicly recognizing heroes, not as a deserved reward for heroic acts, but rather as an a priori manipulation of soldiers into desiring glory and thus desiring the opportunity to participate in combat (Schmitter, 2006).

In summary, emotions were judged in the Middle Ages as evil and immoral, an idea already introduced in Antiquity, and were considered to be appropriate only in the service of God or the politically powerful. Although the judgmental view of emotions still holds, to some extent, in people's daily lives even today, in academic writings, this view has given way to scientific pursuits about the purpose, source, and phenomenology of emotional processing. These are discussed next.

SCIENTIFIC APPROACHES OF THE 19TH AND 20TH CENTURIES

Starting in the 19th century, interest in emotions has become much more secular and scientific. Charles Darwin (1809–1882) was the first to *explicitly* point out the adaptive nature of emotions, which was in sharp contrast with the anhedonic society of Thomas Aquinas. Rather than pointing out how excesses of emotions can make one physically ill or morally weak (also see Introduction to Part I), he proposed that emotions not only help individuals communicate with one another, but also aid in their very survival. In *The Expression of the Emotions in Man and Animals*, Darwin detailed the virtues of experiencing emotions, as well as the parallels between emotions experienced by animals and those experienced by humans (Darwin, 1872/2009). By making the latter point, he opened the door for animal research, without which, as we shall see in Chapter 2, we would not have had the same understanding of the neuroanatomic underpinnings of emotional processing as we do today.

In the wake of Darwin's work, the importance of emotions as part of human experience came to be recognized and accepted. Emotions became an important topic of scientific interest, and researchers, spurred on by the empirical strides in physiology, anatomy, and neurology, were interested in linking emotions to what was known at the time about the workings of the human body. With positivism on the rise, psychology, the new kid on the scientific block, struggled to keep up with the advances in other fields, as it was thrust into the zeitgeist in which *only those phenomena that lent themselves to direct observation* were deemed worthy of study. In this positivistic milieu, psychologists focused on answering rather discrete, narrow questions about emotions. Among these was the chicken or the egg question, that is, the question of which comes first, emotions or reason.

The James–Lange Theory

William James (1842–1910), albeit a positivist at heart, took the revolutionary view that subjective feelings (as reported by people) were essentially raw data and as such *could* be studied. However, he also took the view that these data were actually *secondary* to some more basic, and perhaps *objectively* observable, processes. To explore these ideas further, he began collaborating with a physiologist named Carl Lange (1834–1900), with whom he shared the conviction that feelings and emotions were secondary to physiological phenomena. These collaborative efforts yielded what has come to be known as the James–Lange theory of emotional processing (Ellsworth, 1994).

In this theory, James proposed that perception of what he called an "exciting fact" (James, 1884, p. 449) led directly to a physiological response, and the cognitive interpretation of such a response *was* the phenomenon known as emotion (James, 1884, 1890). To account for different types of emotional experiences, James proposed that different emotions reflected our interpretations of *differentiated physiological states* (see Figure 1.1).[3]

Interestingly, the central tenet of the James–Lange theory—that different emotions are characterized by discernibly different physiological patterns—has proven to be more problematic than James could have predicted. Over the next 100 years, this tenet would be supported, refuted, or proclaimed untestable, depending on a given researcher's methodology, focus of interest, or perhaps even agenda. In fact, differences in agendas were at the very inception of the James–Lange theory itself: Whereas James aimed to gain an understanding of the *phenomenology* of conscious emotional experience (Lang, 1994), Lange aimed to trace the origins of physiological responses to specific loci within the brainstem, believing that emotional experience itself was a mere epiphenomenon[4] (Lange, 1922).

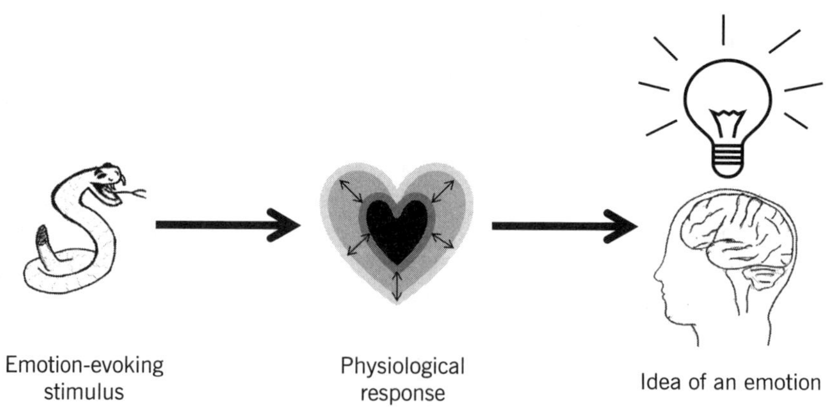

FIGURE 1.1. According to the James–Lange theory of emotion, an emotion-evoking stimulus triggers a physiological response, which is then interpreted as a particular emotion. According to the theory, this interpretation equals the experience of emotion.

The Cannon–Bard Theory

Walter B. Cannon (1871–1945) agreed with James and Lange that physiological responses played a crucial role in emotions. However, unlike James and Lange, he did *not* believe that physiological responses alone could explain subjective emotional experiences. For one thing, he argued, physiological responses were too slow and often imperceptible, and as such, could not possibly account for the relatively rapid and intense subjective awareness of emotion (Cannon, 1931). He also believed that the richness, variety, and temporal course of emotional experiences could *not* stem from physiological reactions that, in his view, reflected fairly *undifferentiated* fight or flight response (Cannon, 1927, 1929).[5]

But Cannon's criticism of the James–Lange theory did not stop there. His primary objection was that the James–Lange theory defied functional neuroanatomy, at least as functional neuroanatomy was understood at the time. In particular, based on research conducted by Cannon and his student Phillip Bard (1898–1977), *all* information, including sensory, motoric,

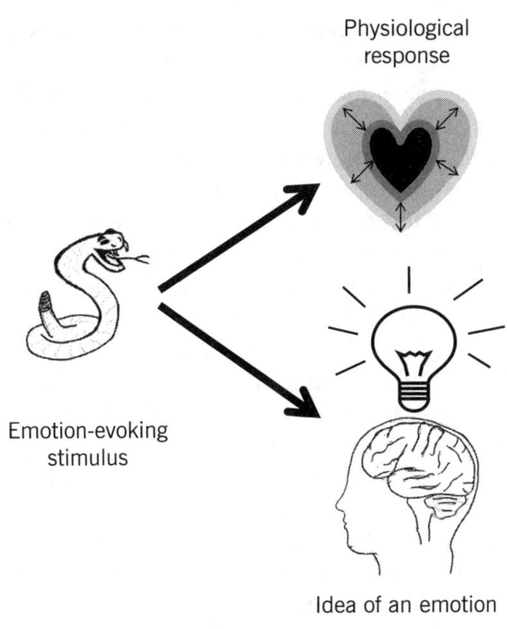

FIGURE 1.2. According to the Cannon–Bard theory of emotion, an emotion-evoking stimulus triggers simultaneously both a physiological response and a conscious experience of an emotion.

and physiological information, had to pass first through the diencephalon before being subjected to any further processing. Thus, Cannon argued, it was *not anatomically possible* for sensory events to trigger a physiological response *prior* to triggering conscious awareness (Cannon, 1929). In other words, emotional stimuli had to trigger both the physiological and the experiential aspect of emotion *simultaneously*. This interpretation came to be known as the Cannon–Bard theory of emotion (see Figure 1.2).

The Two-Factor Theory

Stanley Schachter (1922–1997), unlike William James, had the benefit of a half century's worth of research pointing to the nonspecificity of physiological reactions. He also had the benefit of research conducted in 1924 (i.e., *after* James's death) by Spanish physician Gregorio Maranon. Interested in testing the James–Lange theory, Maranon injected some 200 hospital patients with epinephrine and subsequently asked them how they felt. Interestingly, although some patients described what appeared to be genuine emotional experiences, the vast majority of them responded with "as if" statements: "I feel as if I'm afraid, but I'm not" (described in Schachter & Singer, 1962). In other words, in the absence of an emotion-evoking stimulus, most patients were *un*able to interpret their physiological arousal as genuine subjectively experienced emotions.

Nevertheless, like others before him, Schachter felt that physiology did play an important role in the generation of emotions. He suggested that physiological reactions contributed to emotional experience by facilitating a focused cognitive appraisal of a given physiologically arousing event, and that this appraisal was what defined the subjective emotional experience. In other words, emotions were a result of a two-step process: first, physiological arousal in response to a stimulus, and second, cognitive elaboration of the context in which the stimulus occurred.

To test his theory, Schachter, along with his student Jerome Singer, conducted a study that, to this day, represents possibly one of the most recognizable experiments in all of psychology (Schachter & Singer, 1962). As part of this well-known experiment, Schachter and Singer invited undergraduate volunteers to participate in a study that presumably examined the effects of vitamins on visual acuity. Under the guise of being given a vitamin shot, the participants were injected with either epinephrine or a placebo. Following the injections, while waiting for the presumed vision test to take place, the participants were asked to fill out some questionnaires. A confederate of the experimenters, masquerading as another subject, joined the other participants and proceeded to act either as though he was enraged, or as though he was amused, by the questionnaire items. The naïve participants unwittingly joined in, alternately laughing or cussing at the questionnaire. They were unaware, of course, that their reactions to the confederate were the *actual* focus of the study.

In support of Schachter and Singer's (1962) hypothesis, the results of the study showed that those participants who had been injected with epinephrine (and were thus more physiologically aroused) reported experiencing higher levels of anger or happiness in response to the angry or happy confederate. In other words, undifferentiated arousal, combined with a particular context, resulted in context-specific emotional experiences. To highlight the notion that emotional experience is a function of two independent processes (i.e., physiological arousal and context), the theory proposed by Schachter and Singer came to be called the "two-factor theory of emotion."

Subsequent research demonstrated that the two-factor theory held even when levels of adrenaline were manipulated naturalistically. In a series of experiments conducted by Dutton and Aron (1974), male college students were interviewed by an attractive young female. The interviews took place either in a safe, comfortable place, or in settings that were anxiety-producing, such as on a high, narrow bridge. As predicted by the two-factor theory, those participants whose interviews took place under anxiety-producing conditions reported greater levels of sexual attraction to the interviewer than those who were interviewed in a safe, comfortable place (Dutton & Aron, 1974). In other words, physiological arousal, albeit unrelated to sexual arousal, was interpreted by the participants as stemming from a greater attraction to the experimenter.

Interestingly, James and Lange, Cannon and Bard, and Schachter and Singer all made assumptions about the specificity, or the nonspecificity, of physiological arousal in relation to different types of emotions—a question that has yet to be answered. This question was revisited again in the 1980s and 1990s, with inconsistent findings. Robert Levenson, a prominent researchers in this area, wrote: "It is my belief that despite more than 50 years of empirical work, we still do not have a definitive answer as to the extent of autonomic specificity in emotion [because] there still does not exist a body of well-replicated, well-designed research that would settle this issue" (2003, p. 220). Thus, although physiological arousal represents one of the longest studied aspects of emotion, it arguably continues to be one of the least understood.

Richard Lazarus and Cognitive Appraisal

Richard Lazarus (1922–2002), one of the most influential figures of American psychology in the second half of the 20th century, was less interested in the relationship between emotional experience and physiology. Rather, he sought to understand the distinction between emotions and cognition, and the primacy of one over the other. Lazarus argued that emotions were a result of cognitive assessments, and that the role of these assessments was to calculate the degree to which any given situation was favorable or unfavorable in relation to one's short-term or long-term goals. Lazarus demonstrated that such appraisals took place by conducting a series of studies in which he manipulated participants' cognitive sets prior to presenting them with films designed to evoke emotions. The results showed that identical films resulted in different subjective emotional experiences and even different physiological states, depending on a given participant's assumed cognitive set (Lazarus, 1982). Lazarus's work demonstrated not only the primacy of cognitions over emotions, but also the power of cognitions in evoking or dampening emotional experiences, thereby forming the theoretical foundation for cognitive-behavioral therapy. But Lazarus's suggestion that cognitions essentially preceded subjective emotions came under attack from another researcher, Robert Zajonc, whose own research pointed to a very different interpretation.

Robert Zajonc and the Mere Exposure Effect

In a series of studies, Robert Zajonc (1923–2008) demonstrated what came to be known as the *mere exposure effect.* This effect refers to people's preference for stimuli that are familiar, or to which they have been exposed more than once, even if they have no explicit memory of such prior exposure. In a classic experiment, Zajonc presented participants with a series of nonsense words and Chinese characters. Each word and character was presented a varied numbers of times. Subsequently, Zajonc asked participants to rate their liking of both the words and the characters. The results showed that the number of times participants were exposed to the stimuli correlated positively with their liking of those stimuli (Zajonc, 1968).

Aside from being interesting, Zajonc's work was in direct contrast to Lazarus's theory of the primacy of cognition, demonstrating, at least by Zajonc's standards, that emotions, not cognitions, came first. After all, Zajonc's participants experienced emotional preferences for certain stimuli *without* any conscious awareness of having processed those stimuli previously; consequently, they could not possibly exert cognitive control over how they felt. A heated intellectual debate between the two researchers ensued, lasting for more than a decade and capturing the imagination of the scientific community. Many thoughtful commentaries have been written on the two competing theories, attempting to disentangle the differences and similarities between the positions held by Zajonc and Lazarus (Ellis, 1985; Kappas, 2006; Kleinginna & Kleinginna, 1985; Plutchik, 1985; Scheff, 1985). The ultimate resolution of the debate, which has generally been accepted by the field, was rather prosaic: The two researchers agreed that their whole debate hinged on semantics. On the one hand, according to Zajonc, cognition was a *deliberate process* that manipulated, in some manner, initial perceptions. Such a deliberate process clearly could *not* take place in his experiments, as the participants were not even aware that they had perceived some of the stimuli a greater number of times than others. On the other hand, according to Lazarus, the simple *act of perceiving* constituted cognition. By these standards, of course, cognition *was* a part of Zajonc's experiment, as the act of perceiving was, necessarily, taking place. And so, in the end, the two researchers simply agreed that for emotions to take place, processing of sensory information was required. In other words—back to what William James, Cannon and Bard, and Schachter and Singer said all along—emotions required perception of an emotion-evoking stimulus. This notion is the focus of Chapter 3 of this book.

Of course, the fact that stimuli can be perceived and emotions evoked *unconsciously* should not be a surprise to a neuropsychologist. Emotional reactions without conscious awareness of the emotion-eliciting stimulus have been described in split-brain patients (Ladavas, Cimatti, del Pesce, & Tuozzi, 1993) and in patients with cortical blindness (Morris, de Gelder, Weiskrantz, & Dolan, 2001; Tamietto & de Gelder, 2008). This does not mean that the Zajonc–Lazarus debate is irrelevant to neuropsychology. Rather, it demonstrates the contributions that neuropsychology can make to the theory and research of emotional processing.

On a final note, in recent decades Richard Lazarus has altered his views, proposing that emotions are an *inextricable* part of our cognitive system (Lazarus & Lazarus, 1994). Thus, Lazarus has ultimately defied the traditional notion about the dichotomy between emotions and cognitions—the notion that began with ancient philosophers and represented the mainstream view in literature, arts, and sciences throughout the 20th century.

NOTES

1. Hippocrates' name has been associated with over 60 medical treaties (known today as the Hippocratic Code). However, in reality these writings spanned a period of nearly 200 years, suggesting that they were a product of multiple writers.
2. In this same vein, Descartes also viewed cognition as being superior to emotions, proclaiming famously, "I think, therefore I am."
3. James was criticized for not giving credit to Renaissance philosophers such as René Descartes when proposing his theory, as the notion that emotions are derived from bodily sensations can be found in Descartes' writings as well (Titchener, 1914).

4. Regardless of their differences, and despite their positivistic leanings, neither James nor Lange actually ever tested their theory empirically, although Lange did conduct research on neural pathways of "emotional" physiological reactivity, tangentially related to their theory (Lang, 1994).
5. Cannon's opinions about the richness of the phenomenology of *human* emotions were based on introspection and anecdotal evidence, rather than empirical research, as *all* of his work was done with laboratory animals.

CHAPTER 2

Early Neuroatomic Models of Emotional Processing

In the previous chapter, we reviewed early philosophic and psychological models of emotions. In this chapter, we review when and how the *central nervous system* began to play a role in theories and hypotheses about emotional substrates—from the initial acknowledgments of the brain as the center of emotional processes, to the "centers within the center," to the complex neuroanatomic networks emerging early in the 20th century. The reader will notice that the path linking structure and function was not always straightforward. Often, accidents of nature, incidental observations, or happenstance discoveries served as the springboard for future, more goal-directed research. From the musings of the ancient philosophers to the cold, brutally scientific methods of animal, as well as human, ablations, the brain replaced the heart as the presumed seat of the emotional soul.

THE BRAIN AS THE CENTER OF EMOTIONS

Philosophy and Pseudoscience

The first to suggest the potential role of the brain in emotional processing was Hippocrates, the same Hippocrates who was the central figure in the doctrine of the four humors (see Chapter 1). Hippocrates' introduction of the brain as the seat of emotional experience was actually inspired by yet earlier writings (around 500 B.C.E.) of a fellow philosopher, Heraclitus. Heraclitus, as if anticipating the empiricism of the 19th century and the psychophysiological methods of the 20th century (e.g., detection of perspiration via measurement of the Galvanic skin response), attempted to define emotions by imposing clear, *measurable* parameters. He proposed that the amount of emotion one was experiencing could be directly assessed by measuring the temperature of the body and the amount of perspiration one produced. More specifically, Heraclitus believed that the absence of emotion was characterized by dry, cool skin, whereas high levels of emotional excitation were characterized by skin that was moist and radiating heat (Arikha, 2007).

Around 460 B.C.E., Hippocrates elaborated on this model in two ways (Arikha, 2007). First and foremost, *he added the brain into the equation*. In particular, according to him, the quality of the skin was just a reflection of the state of the brain, a notion that foreshadowed what we know today about the thermoregulatory functions of the hypothalamus. Second, he matched specific permutations of Heraclitus's variables with discrete types of emotions, such that, for example, fear was thought to be the result of the brain being overheated, whereas grief and anxiety were the result of the brain cooling down. Thus, in addition to foreshadowing hormones and neurotransmitters (with the theory of the four humors), Hippocrates also foreshadowed the debate that is generally thought to originate with William James, that is, the debate about whether specific autonomic responses (e.g., vasodilation and perspiration) correspond to specific emotions (see Chapter 1).

Although only 100 years later Aristotle disagreed with Hippocrates and argued that the *heart*, not the brain, was the seat of all mental processes (Arikha, 2007), only 50 years after that the brain was back in the picture, and this time, it came with a localizationist twist: The seat of the soul (and the source of emotions) was, in turn, assigned to the fourth ventricle (Horophilus, ca. 300 B.C.E.), the frontal lobes (Galen of Pergamon, ca. 150 C.E.), and the pineal gland (René Descartes, 17th century) (Harkins & Riese, 1963; Hankinson & Everson, 1991; Jefferson, 1949).

Early Scientific Attempts

In the early 19th century, Franz Joseph Gall (1758–1828), the father of phrenology, offered detailed maps that presumably localized discrete emotions, temperaments, and traits within discrete loci of the brain (Knott, 1911). After that, it was only a matter of time before the pseudoscientific claims of phrenology would spur empirical scientific investigations. Among the first such investigations, undoubtedly inspired not only by both Franz Joseph Gall but also by Hippocrates, was the science of *cerebral thermometry*. Practiced at the end of the 19th century in Western Europe and in the United States, this crude precursor to psychophysiology involved measurements of temperature fluctuations on different parts of the skull, with the assumption that such fluctuations reflected brain temperature changes during mental and emotional activity. This method, not surprisingly, did not yield particularly notable findings, at least not until it was adopted by the Italian physiologist Angelo Mosso (1846–1910). Mosso, who would later be hailed as one of the forefathers of modern functional neuroimaging (Nicholson, 2006), proceeded to measure the temperature of the brain *directly*, that is, *not* through the skull. Although his first experiments were conducted with animals, his fame stems from his later work with humans. In the late 19th century, Mosso convinced a 12-year-old girl named Delfina Parodi to become a research participant. To his defense, Mosso did not drill a hole into Delfina's skull, as Delfina had been born with a skull defect that already provided an opening into the brain. While prodding inside her cranium with a thermometer, Mosso attempted to systematically elicit emotional responses from the girl. Although the details about Delfina's own point of view do not appear to be part of the written history, the results of Mosso's experiments are: In a scientific publication in 1894, Mosso reported a brain temperature increase of .09 degrees Celsius, brought about by emotional arousal (Dror, 2001).

But Delfina Parodi was not the first human participant whose brain was under Angelo Mosso's direct scrutiny. Earlier, in the 1870s, Mosso treated a 37-year-old man named Michele Bertino, who, following an accident, was left with only a thin layer of skin covering an inch-long gap in his skull. As luck would have it, Mosso was Bertino's physician. During a follow-up office visit, Mosso noticed that the gap on Bertino's head noticeably swelled with pulsating blood when the bells on the church across the street rang. Mosso inquired whether the bells made Bertino think of prayer, and he answered yes. Mosso then asked Bertino to multiply 8 by 12 and, as Bertino responded "96," the gap in his skull again swelled with blood. Mosso deduced that mental activity and emotional excitation were accompanied with increased blood circulation in the brain (Nicholson, 2006). To test this hypothesis, Mosso developed an apparatus that could be placed over the gap on Bertino's head while recording changes in pressure, reflecting the underlying pulsation of the blood. Once attached to the apparatus, Bertino would be seated facing the wall so as to avoid distraction by irrelevant stimuli. While changes in blood pulsation were recorded, Mosso systematically chided or startled Bertino from time to time, so as to evoke emotional responses. Using this method, Mosso did demonstrate that there, in fact, was a relationship between blood circulation and emotional upset, and, in

1881, published his findings in a scientific treatise entitled *Blood Circulation in the Human Brain* (Dror, 2001).

Mosso was hailed by his contemporaries as "one of the best known living physiologists [to whom] the world owes some of the choicest methods and apparatus invented" (Nichols, 1896, p. 445). During his time, however, his methodology did not gain much following, undoubtedly due to the difficulty of finding appropriate human subjects. But then, following Darwin's publication of *The Expression of the Emotions in Man and Animals* in 1872, research on emotion did not need to be limited to the examination of human subjects. As discussed in the next section, animal research came to play a central role in the quest for finding the seat of emotions.

THE CENTERS WITHIN THE CENTER

The Diencephalon

The first scientific demonstration of the localization of emotions within a specific area of the brain, namely the diencephalon, came from a Russian physiologist, Vladimir Bekhterev (1857–1927), less than a decade after Mosso's blood circulation experiments. In 1887, Bekhterev conducted ablations on live animal brains, demonstrating that apparently normal emotional responses took place even after the brain was "truncated" above the thalamus. Based on these findings, Bekhterev reasoned that the thalamus must be the center of emotional expression (Sirotkina, 2007). Bekhterev's work, however, went virtually unnoticed by the then-small scientific community, and although a number of other researchers would report similar results shortly after him, it would be another 30 years before anyone else would conduct this line of research with the explicit goal of localizing emotions within the brain. Meanwhile, researchers with altogether different scientific agendas would replicate Bekhterev's findings incidentally, and still without much notice by the scientific community.

The first such incidental replication took place in 1892, less than a decade after Bekhterev's experiments, when Friedrich Goltz followed up on earlier research on localization of motor functions within the neocortex (Fritsch & Hitzig, 1870). To examine the extent to which cortical functioning was necessary for motor output, Goltz conducted ablations of some, or all, of dogs' cerebral cortices (Goltz, 1892). He found that the decorticated animals maintained many normal functions, such as a nearly normal sleep–wake cycle, normal responses to changes in temperature (e.g., panting or shivering), normal spinal reflexes, virtually normal ability to respond to certain sensory stimulation, and functional, albeit not normal, locomotion. What he also found, quite incidentally, was that these animals exhibited *emotional reactions* in response to pain.

Twelve years later, Goltz's and Behkterev's observations of emotional displays in decorticated animals were replicated again, still not as an inquiry into the seat of emotions, but rather as a *method*. Specifically, in the late 1800s, many scientific inquiries into the workings of the human body relied on animal vivisection, a method that did not go over well with animal activists even then (Dror, 2001). Thus, when R. C. Woodworth and Charles Scott Sherrington (Woodworth & Sherrington, 1904) set out to study the pathways of pain-related reflexes within the central nervous system, the use of decorticated, as opposed to intact, animals seemed a politically perfect solution: On the one hand, according to the James–Lange theory of emotion (see Chapter 1), such animals were *in*capable of *experiencing* pain; on the other hand, according to Goltz's work, decorticated animals were capable of *expressing* pain reflexes. Perhaps to further drive home the point that the animals' responses to pain stimulation were not reflecting a true emotional experience, Woodworth and Sherrington termed these responses *pseud-affective*[1] *reflexes*. After completing this series of studies, which involved transecting various columns in the spinal cord with the goal of abolishing the pseud-affective response, 10 years went by before another handful of researchers produced additional replications. Once again, however, pseud-affective reflexes were described only incidentally, in the course of studying sensory functions (Dusser de Barenne, 1915), temperature regulation (Isenschmid & Krehl, 1912), and pain pathways (Bazett & Penfield, 1922).

Meanwhile, those researchers who *were* actually interested in the study of *emotions* focused on physiological responses and blood chemistry changes, often elicited by the then popular cat–dog paradigm (Dror, 2001). This paradigm involved placing a cat in a cage and a dog outside the cage. The dog was allowed to approach the cage, becoming frustrated and enraged by the inability to reach the cat; the cat, meanwhile, was experiencing intense fear, caused by the close proximity of a snarling, growling, salivating dog. And all the while, the potential for identifying neuroanatomic underpinnings of emotions, suggested by the work with decorticated animals, went unnoticed. That is, until Walter B. Cannon stepped on the scene.

While Cannon (1871–1945) was keenly interested in the study of emotions, he found the cat–dog paradigm unsatisfactory (Cannon, 1915, 1929). His primary objection was that emotionally excited animals did not lend themselves to collections of blood samples and measurements of blood pressure—the very indices that were of interest to Cannon at the time. Unfortunately, these same indices were also very unstable because physiological responses tended to dissipate quickly once emotionally aroused animals have calmed down and were thus ready for data collection. In search of a better method, Cannon discovered the research that described pseud-affective reflexes in decorticated animals, and determined that such animals represented a much more controllable and therefore more viable paradigm. As he embarked on this new path, Cannon separated himself from the incidental findings of prior investigators, not only by focusing his research specifically on the emotional reactions, but also by coining the term "sham rage" as a replacement for the older term "pseud-affective reflexes" (Cannon & Britton, 1925). The term "sham rage," of course, has been with us to this day.

Soon thereafter, Cannon's student Phillip Bard (1898–1977), who shared Cannon's interest in the study of emotions, came to realize that although the phenomenon of sham rage was described by several earlier researchers, its exact neuroanatomic underpinnings had never been studied systematically. He set forth to examine the subject more closely. After conducting literally hundreds of brain surgeries on cats and dogs, with the ablations ranging from unilateral portions of the neocortex to nearly complete removal of the thalamus (Bard, 1928, 1929, 1934), Bard concluded that the apparent emotional reactions, most notably *sham rage* and fear, represented "motor activity" dependent on the caudal hypothalamus, and that such motor activity was differentially associated with different types of emotions (Bard, 1928, 1929, 1934).[2] In drawing these conclusions, Bard also noted that no stimuli elicited motor signs of pleasure, such as purring in cats or tail wagging in dogs, suggesting that such emotions required processing by brain regions above the diencephalon, consistent with the outcomes of frontal lobotomies discussed later in this chapter.

The notion that the diencephalon was the center of emotional processing remained popular for several decades and was later corroborated via electrical stimulation of the hypothalamus (Hess & Akert, 1955; Levison & Flynn, 1965; Macdonnell & Flynn, 1964). With the increased popularity of this structure as an emotional center, a variety of emotional and psychiatric problems, including mood disorders (Abely, 1951; Spiegel, Wycis, Freed, & Orchinik, 1951) and psychosis (Garcia, 1951), came to be blamed on diencephalic abnormalities. However, with time, the focus of hypothalamus research began to shift from emotions to vegetative functions, as the hypothalamus came to be known in turn as the sleep center, the wake center, the hunger center, and the temperature center of the brain (Chatfield & Lyman, 1950; Lafora, 1940; Nauta, 1946; Serota, 1939; Teitelbaum, 1964). And, gradually, at least with respect to emotional processing, the hypothalamus gave way to the new kid on the block, the amygdala.

The Amygdala

The first evidence that the amygdala may play a role in emotions came from the seminal research conducted by Heindrich Klüver (1897–1979) and Paul Bucy (1904–1992), who described rhesus monkeys' behavioral alternations following bilateral anterior temporal lobectomies. These monkeys, in addition to experiencing visual agnosia and indiscriminate eating, also exhibited unusual emotional and social behaviors, such as tameness and loss of fear, hypersexuality, aberrant maternal behavior, blunted affect, social disinterest, rejection from their social group, and a decline in social status (Klüver & Bucy, 1937, 1938, 1939). These experimental findings were further buttressed by later reports of patients with bilateral anterior temporal damage, who evidenced a syndrome that was similar to that reported by Klüver and Bucy (Hierons, Janota, & Corsellis, 1978; Lilly, Cummings, Benson, & Frankel, 1983).[3] However, Klüver and Bucy did not specifically isolate the amygdala in their surgeries, and the extent to which the amygdala, versus other adjacent brain structures, contributed to different components of the syndrome described by Klüver and Bucy was not clear.[4]

The first inklings that tameness and loss of fear were caused specifically by ablations of the amygdala came from the work of José Delgado, whose research utilized electrical stimulation of various subcortical structures. He found that electrical stimulation of the amygdala, particularly the medial nucleus, resulted in fear responses in the studied animals (Delgado, 1955). Additionally, as a purely incidental finding, he noticed that the animals acted in a fearful manner not only when their amygdala was being stimulated, but also when they were exposed to the cage or the apparatus that was used for the stimulation experiments. This observation was the first to suggest that the amygdala played a role in fear conditioning (Delgado, Rosvold, & Looney, 1956). Around the same time, independent of Delgado's work, Lawrence Weiskrantz set out to investigate the substrates of the emotional aspects of the Klüver–Bucy syndrome and also found that tameness and loss of fear were specifically linked to ablations of the amygdala (Weiskrantz, 1956).

These clinical and experimental findings together served as a springboard for research of the role of the amygdala in emotional processing. This research question became particularly popular in the 1970s and 1980s, making the amygdala arguably the most studied brain structure in the history of neuroscience (Phelps, Fiske, Kazdin, & Schacter, 2006). Given the complex circuitry within this relatively small brain area, it should not be surprising that research on the amygdala quickly became quite specialized, with different laboratories focusing on the role of the amygdala in different discrete aspects of emotional processing, such as emotional memory and learning (Phelps et al., 2006), aggression and fear (Panzer, Viljoen, & Roos, 2007), and social and facial processing (Olson, Plotzker, & Ezzyat, 2007). Although the early research relied almost entirely on animal models, generalization of such models to human emotions became possible with the advent of noninvasive functional imaging (i.e., functional magnetic resonance imaging [fMRI]) in the 1990s.

Given the role of the amygdala in clinically relevant aspects of emotional processing, including social functioning and the experience of fear or anger, it was only a matter of time before linkages between this structure and psychiatric disorders would be drawn. Specifically, the amygdala and related circuitry have now been linked to abnormalities in autism (Stanfield et al., 2008), psychopathy (Kiehl, Bates, Laurens, Hare, & Liddle, 2006), and anxiety disorders (Grillon, 2008), to name a few.

Interestingly, social and emotional deficits associated with the ablation of the amygdala, with the exception of hypersexuality, have also been shown to be present even with partial lesions of the anterior temporal lobe (excluding the amygdala) or prefrontal (particularly orbitofrontal) cortex. Such findings illustrate the fallacy of earlier quests to identify a *single center* of emotional processing, demonstrating that appropriate emotional and social conduct must be subserved by much more extensive circuitry (Olson et al., 2007).

THE EMOTIONAL CIRCUITRY

The Papez Circuit

In 1937, the same year the first descriptions of what would come to be known as the Klüver–Bucy syndrome hit the press, and only a few years after the systematic description of sham rage by Philip Bard, an alternative, and arguably more sophisticated, notion was being introduced, one of an entire emotional *system.* This notion was proposed by an American neuroanatomist, James Papez (1883–1958). In his seminal 1937 paper, Papez stated that the structures that constituted what would later come to be known as the Papez circuit "constitute a harmonious mechanism which may elaborate the functions of central emotion, as well as participate in emotional expression" (p. 743). Papez developed his model, the precursor of today's limbic system, by tracing connections between the hippocampus and other brain structures[5] (see Figure 2.1).

In building his circuit, Papez relied heavily on Bard's work with decorticated animals, particularly the notion that motoric and physiological responses (i.e., sham rage) were separate from the *experience* of emotion (i.e., "real" rage). He also built upon other new developments in neuroanatomy, which described (1) the medial aspects of the brain (e.g., the medial temporal lobe) as being closely linked to the hypothalamus and its role in controlling visceral functions, and (2) the lateral aspects of the brain (i.e., the dorsolateral aspects of the neocortex) as closely linked to the thalamus and its role in experiential, or sensorimotor, functions. Consequently, Papez integrated this knowledge into a theory that required an interface between

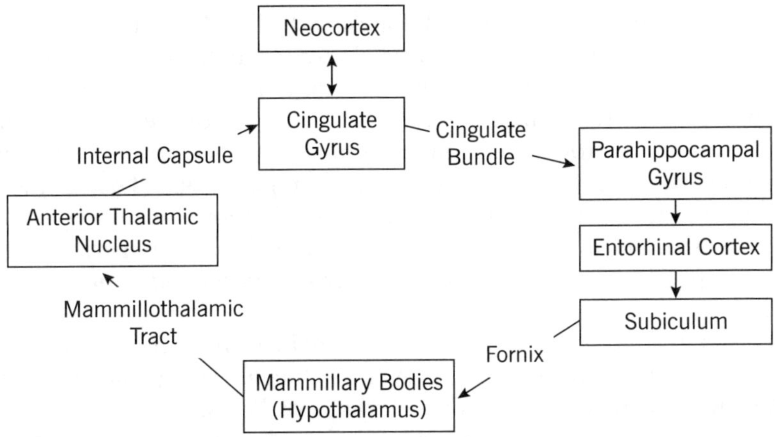

FIGURE 2.1. The Papez circuit.

the visceral and the experiential systems, proposing that such an interface resided in the cingulate gyrus (Lautin, 2001). Papez's decision to designate the cingulate gyrus as a candidate for the visceral–experiential interface was based in part on its neuroanatomic location between the limbic structures and the neocortex, and in part on clinical findings of emotional disturbance among patients who had lesions along the cingulate–hippocampal stream. Later research, primarily by Paul MacLean, supported much of the connections proposed by Papez, but further extended the circuitry to include the prefrontal cortex and the septum, as well as the amygdala.

The Limbic System

In 1947, 10 years after Papez first introduced his circuit, Paul MacLean (1943–2007) came across Papez's 1937 paper. There were good reasons for MacLean to take a full ten years to discover Papez's work, the very work that would become the springboard for the most prominent theoretical contribution of MacLean's entire career. For one thing, MacLean had not been interested in the study of emotions. Until 1946, his research interests were far from the human psyche, focusing on the study of the diphtheria virus and its role in tropical ulcers. Furthermore, he had enough to worry about during the intervening decade. In the 1930s, he was busy completing his undergraduate English degree at Yale University, his premedical studies in Edinburg, Scotland, and his medical studies back at Yale; and, in the first half of the 1940s, during World War II, MacLean traveled the world as a medical officer in the U.S. Army (Lambert, 2003).

After his return to the United States, in 1947, MacLean became a fellow at the Brain Wave Laboratory at Harvard Medical School, where he worked on the development of an electrode that would facilitate electroencephalographic recordings from the basal regions of the brain. With the use of his new electrode, MacLean and his colleagues were able to collect recordings from the medial portions of the temporal lobe. They found that the greatest "bioelectrical disturbances" in this region were exhibited by patients with epilepsy who, as part of their epilepsy aura, experienced vivid sensory experiences accompanied by *strong emotional reactions* (described in MacLean, 1990).

It was around that same time that MacLean happened upon Papez's 1937 paper, which he later described as "neglected" (MacLean, 1990, p. 265). MacLean recognized the relevance of Papez's work for the emotional symptoms of patients with epilepsy, but also for its failure to propose any connections with the sensory areas. Based on his subsequent discussions with Papez, as well as the research efforts of the intervening decade, MacLean developed his own elaboration on Papez's circuitry. He presented his model soon thereafter at his departmental seminar under the title, "Psychosomatic Disease and the 'Visceral Brain': Recent Developments Bearing on the Papez Theory of Emotion" (MacLean, 1949, 1990). In it, he proposed a mechanism whereby the phylogenetically older "visceral" cortical areas (i.e., what is known today as the limbic areas) receive sensory information from the phylogenetically newer neocortex.[6]

The term *visceral*, in MacLean's view, nicely captured the role of these brain areas in both the "feelings" of emotion and the accompanying physiological reactions. After all, it was not lost on MacLean that the auras experienced by patients with medial temporal lobe epilepsy were characterized not only by subjective emotional experiences, but also by epigastric phenomena. However, the term, as used by MacLean, was widely misunderstood at the time by the scientific community, which associated *visceral* with glands and hollow organs. Additionally, Karl Pribram, a close collaborator of MacLean during that period, criticized the notion that any part of the brain would be uniquely and distinctly involved in visceral functions. And thus, by 1952, MacLean abandoned the term *visceral* and replaced it with one that would enter and find a permanent place in the parlance of neuropsychology: the "limbic system" (MacLean, 1952).

In his 1952 paper, MacLean simultaneously coined the term *limbic system* and brought the Papez circuit into prominence (Lautin, 2001). In his work, he referred to the Papez circuit, not the limbic system, when proposing that additional structures (the posterior orbitofrontal cortex, the amygdala, the anterior insula, and frontotemporal and pyriform cortices) were integral parts of the limbic circuitry. His elaboration of the Papez circuit was based on (1) his own work (some of it in collaboration with Pribram) using strychnine for identification of connections between the Papez circuit and other brain structures, as well as on (2) impressive integration of clinical case studies and electroencephalographic (EEG) findings in patients with epilepsy (Lautin, 2001). The case studies described by MacLean are of particular significance for the study of emotion because they describe patients who, during their epigastric epileptic auras, experienced what MacLean (1952, p. 412) described as "raw, poorly differentiated, and impersonalized feelings" of sadness, fear, or desire—feelings that occurred in the absence of a clear target or source. In other words, these patients appeared to experience something that was quite akin to the "as if" emotions described by Maranon's patients following epinephrine injections (Schachter & Singer, 1962; see Chapter 1). These observations drive home the point that human emotions require higher-level, more elaborate processing, beyond what can be afforded by the limbic structures that are capable of generating only pseud-affective reflexes and "as-if" emotions.

THE CEREBRAL CORTEX

Hemispheric Asymmetry

The precursors of the notion that the two hemispheres differ in how they process emotional information date back to the 19th century. In 1885, Russian-Swiss neuropathologist Constantin von Monakow (1853–1930) described a patient who exhibited a denial, or a lack of awareness, of hemiplegia. Within the next three decades, other similar cases characterized by a lack of awareness, or *anosognosia*, were reported by Austrian neurologist and psychiatrist Gabriel Anton, Czech neurologist Arnold Pick, and French neurologist Josef Francois Babinski (1857–1932) (Papagno & Vallar, 2001). Together, these cases began to provide the first inklings about the key role the right hemisphere plays in an important aspect of emotional processing, self-awareness. But perhaps even more central to the present discussion, in 1885, von Monakow described patients with hemiplegia who, in the absence of anosognosia, exhibited an unusual emotional state characterized by the *lack of concern* about their paralysis (Koehler & Jagella, 2002). In 1914, Babinski presented similar cases, calling this condition "anosodiaphoria" (Papagno & Vallar, 2001), a term that is still with us today.

The observations of a lack of awareness and a lack of concern among patients with right-hemisphere damage were followed in 1939 by observations offered by German neurologist and psychiatrist Kurt Goldstein, who noted that patients who had suffered a stroke in the left hemisphere often exhibited what he described as a "catastrophic reaction." These patients were the diametric opposite of patients who showed no concern, reacting to even minor instances of cognitive or physical difficulties by uncontrollable crying, as well as an apparent inability to appreciate praise, signs of improvements, or clear signs of cognitive or physical strengths.

However, despite the ample evidence that patients with right-hemisphere damage were characterized by considerable lack of concern about their deficits, whereas patients with left-hemisphere damage were characterized by excessive catastrophizing, these hemispheric differences went virtually unnoticed by the larger neuropsychological community until the 1960s. At that time, a number of researchers began to report that patients undergoing intracarotid amytal injections exhibited different emotional reactions depending on which hemisphere was pharmacologically immobilized (Gainotti, 2001). That is, left-hemisphere injections led to depressive reactions, whereas right-hemisphere injections led to euphoric or manic reactions. After that, it would be another 10 years before the first serious theoretical attempts at explaining the hemispheric differences in emotional processing would begin to emerge (Gainotti, 1972). These differences are addressed throughout the remainder of this book.

The Frontal Lobes

As seen from the previous sections, it was often decades before key scientific discoveries began to be noticed by the broader scientific community. But this slow progress pales in comparison to the more than 100 years and the more than 100,000 human ablation patients that would come and go before the indispensibility of the frontal lobes for healthy emotional functioning would come to be fully recognized.

Phineas Gage

The first well-publicized case of emotional disturbance following a lesion in the frontal lobes was that of a 25-year-old railroad gang foreman named Phineas P. Gage. On September 13, 1848, at 4:30 P.M., Mr. Gage sustained an explosion injury in which a tamping iron, 3 feet and 7 inches long and 1.25 inches in diameter, penetrated the left side of his face and exited on the dorsal part of his skull, landing some 25 yards behind him. The nature of the injury, as well as the initial recovery, were described 2½ months later by Mr. Gage's physician, Dr. John Martyn Harlow, in a letter to the editor of the *Boston Medical and Surgical Journal* (Harlow, 1868). Contrary to popular belief, Mr. Gage's personality is barely addressed in this fairly extensive letter.

Dr. Harlow began his letter by describing the events prior to his arrival to Mr. Gage's aid. As Dr. Harlow gathered from the report of those at the scene, the explosion apparently threw Mr. Gage onto his back, but he remained conscious, or, at most, had lost consciousness only momentarily.

He was picked up and carried by his men and placed onto an ox cart, in which he rode, sitting upright, to a nearby village. Once there, he apparently got up and walked, with minimal assistance, up a long flight of stairs into the hallway of a local hotel. There, he was cleaned up, changed, and cared for while waiting for his physician, Dr. Harlow, to arrive. Mr. Gage was weakened from profuse bleeding, both externally and into his stomach via the wound at the base of his skull, causing him to vomit blood periodically. Nevertheless, he apparently recognized his physician immediately and conversed with him about the accident and its aftermath.

According to Dr. Harlow's account, in the days following the accident, the bleeding gradually subsided, as did vomiting of blood. Mental status, however, fluctuated from lucid to delirious to comatose for the next 3 weeks, during which time the wound appeared infected, then drained through the openings at either end and eventually began to heal. On October 11, when asked if he knew how long it had been since his accident, Mr. Gage correctly responded, "Four weeks this afternoon, at half past four o'clock." By early November, Mr. Gage was able to walk unassisted, and, following a brief temporary setback caused by his noncompliance with Dr. Harlow's orders, he eventually fully recovered physically.

At that point of Mr. Gage's recovery, Dr. Harlow's letter ended. Throughout his detailed case study, Dr. Harlow made only three mentions of Mr. Gage's demeanor. The first occurred early in the case description. Dr. Harlow, who had known Mr. Gage prior to the accident, described him as a man of "vigorous physical organization, temperate habits, and ... considerable energy of character," who bore "his sufferings with most heroic firmness" and had retained "full possession of his reason" (Harlow, 1848, p. 390). The second mention of Mr. Gage's personality can be found in the portions of the letter reporting on progress at about 2 months following the accident, when, rather matter-of-factly, Dr. Harlow described Mr. Gage's behavior as "childish." And finally, at the close of his letter, Dr. Harlow promised that he would speak to the patient's "mental manifestations" in future letters.

According to others who came into contact with him over the next decade, Mr. Gage was unable to regain employment with the railroad and spent the following years holding a variety of jobs, including as an "attraction" at the Barnum's American Museum in New York and a medical exhibit at lectures in a number of major U.S. cities. He also helped out on his parents' farm and was occasionally examined by interested physicians, most notably Dr. Henry Jacob Bigelow, who is the author of additional descriptions of Mr. Gage's injuries. Similar to Dr. Harlow, Dr. Bigelow seemed more focused on Mr. Gage's physical recovery, noting only briefly that Mr. Gage seemed "quite recovered in faculties of body and mind" (Bigelow, 1850, p. 14). In February 1860, 11½ years after his accident, Mr.

Gage began to suffer from epileptic seizures and on May 21 of that year, passed away (Macmillan, 2008).

Although Dr. Harlow promised in his initial publication to provide more information about Mr. Gage's mental status, it was not until 1868, 8 years after Mr. Gage's death, that this came to bear. In a brief (less than 200-word) summary, Dr. Harlow enumerated the ways in which it was apparent that Mr. Gage had lost "the balance between his intellectual faculties and animal propensities" (Harlow, 1868, p. 13). He described, almost telegraphically, what has come to be a well-known and unduly elaborate story that can be found in textbooks as well as popular media. In this short piece, Dr. Harlow simply described Mr. Gage as previously being a man of iron will, temperate, efficient, capable, well balanced, and a favorite with others. Equally simply, he stated that following the accident, Mr. Gage's demeanor became fitful, irreverent, profane, impatient, and capricious, "a child intellectually with the animal passions of a strong man" (Harlow, 1868, p. 14).

Interestingly, the case of Phineas Gage and the brief account of his personality change may have fallen into obscurity, if it weren't for David Ferrier, an early localizationist, who was conducting ablations on the frontal lobes of monkeys. In 1878, he happened across the brief, obscure write-up by Dr. Harlow and used the case to point out that the personality changes he had seen in monkeys following frontal lobe ablations may have a human counterpart (Ferrier, 1878). And so, ultimately, it was Ferrier who brought Dr. Harlow's accounts of Phineas Gage's injuries into both the scientific and the popular limelight, making Dr. Harlow's letters among the most cited scientific contributions of the 19th century (Macmillan, 2008).

Psychosurgery

Psychosurgery, or, more specifically, frontal lobotomies, contributed what seems like countless case studies to our understanding of the role of the frontal lobes in emotional processing. During its heyday, more than 100,000 psychosurgeries were conducted, leaving in their wake volumes of data, but also scores of vacant shells instead of human beings. The outcomes of frontal lobotomies ranged from down-right tragic to, well, not so good. Some patients died in surgery; some suffered severe declines in cognitive functions; some (typically patients with schizophrenia who had prominent negative symptoms) remained virtually unchanged; and some "improved" by becoming less concerned, less anxious, and less agitated. The latter group, however, had also clearly lost the ability to experience *positive* emotions, becoming lethargic, apathetic, and directionless (Hoffman, 1949). This loss of positive emotions should, of course, have been expected: After all, only a few decades earlier Phillip Bard had taken note of the fact that decorticated cats did not purr, and decorticated dogs did not wag their tails (Bard, 1934).

Although the initiation and propagation of psychosurgeries were spearheaded by a few strong individuals, it was likely inevitable that psychosurgeries would come to be practiced at some point in human history. The earliest well-documented example of psychosurgery is the work of a Swiss psychiatrist and surgeon, Gottlieb Burckhardt (1842–1928) (Whitaker et al., 1996). In 1890, Burckhardt performed partial cortical ablations on six "highly excitable" patients with schizophrenia, with the goal of ameliorating some of their psychiatric symptoms. The procedure not only failed to produce much relief from "excitability," but also led to seizures and two deaths. These outcomes led to a widespread opposition among the European medical community, and Burckhardt's psychosurgical practice ended before it had a chance to take off. But 45 years later, Portuguese physician Antonio Egas Moniz (1874–1955) reintroduced the once-condemned procedure under the term *psychosurgery*, marking the beginning of the 50-year era of the most devastating medical practices in modern history.

Prior to becoming famous for spearheading psychosurgery, Moniz had already lived what some might consider more than one lifetime's worth. He had worked as a physician and a professor of internal medicine and neurology, had achieved some fame with his scandalous book on sexology, and had launched a distinguished 15-year career as a politician. After leaving politics in 1918, Moniz went back to practicing medicine, and, by the 1920s, began a prolific research career. The focus of his early investigations, however, was neither psychosurgery nor the plight of the mentally ill, but rather the quest for developing better methods for brain imaging.

Neuroimaging during Moniz's time was limited to pneumoencephalography, an invasive, painful, and minimally effective practice that consisted of draining the cerebral-spinal fluid and replacing it with gas. Moniz experimented with different methods of depositing bromide (radio-opaque material) into the brain parenchyma, and finally, in 1927, arrived at a formula that allowed him to visualize portions of the internal carotid artery along the Sylvian fissure. During the next 4 years, Moniz perfected the technique, expanding it to pulmonary angiography and generating 61 scientific papers and numerous conference presentations during that brief period of time. This effort earned Moniz a nomination for the Nobel prize in 1928, but the prize itself ended up going to someone else (Doby, 1992).

Moniz's frustration over not winning the Nobel prize for his work in radiology can arguably be credited with propelling him from angiography to psychosurgery. In 1935, while attending the Second International Neurological Congress in London, Moniz was in the audience when two Yale physicians, John Fulton and Carlyle Jacobsen, presented the results of their work with chimpanzees. Among other things, they reported an incidental observation that two of their somewhat neurotic chimps, Becky and Lucy, became much calmer following frontal lobe ablations. This presentation translated into a moment of epiphany for Moniz, and immediately upon returning home he began conducting experimental frontal lobotomies directly on the brains of mentally ill patients. True to his propensity for getting a lot done in a short period of time, he worked tirelessly on his project, and by 1936, only 1 year after his initial epiphany, Moniz had acquired lobotomy data from 20 psychiatric patients (Berrios, 1997; Mashour, Walker, & Martuza, 2005).

In his lobotomy publications, Moniz detailed what he considered an improvement in the patients' condition, such as decreases in agitation, worry, and paranoia. Although Moniz (1937) also admitted that in most cases the outcome included apathy and disorientation, he nevertheless described his patients as "cured." In 1942, 14 years after having been snubbed by the Nobel Assembly, Antonio Egas Moniz was awarded the Nobel prize in physiology and medicine for his "discovery of the therapeutic value of leucotomy in certain psychoses" (*Nobel Lectures, Physiology or Medicine 1942–1962*, 1964). Ironically, within only a decade after Moniz was awarded the prize, psychosurgery began falling out of favor (and was actually banned in the Soviet Union as early as 1943), while Moniz's first real contribution to medicine, angiography, continues to be an invaluable diagnostic tool to this day.

Meanwhile, in the United States, Moniz's work was adopted by the physician Walter J. Freeman and neurosurgeon James W. Watts, and, despite its declining reputation in Europe, was heavily promoted in their 1942 book *Psychosurgery*. Based on their observations, Freeman and Watts advanced a new theory for why lobotomies worked—that is, due to the disconnection of the frontal lobes from the diencephalon, the presumed seat of human emotions (see "The Diencephalon" section earlier in this chapter). Additionally, Freeman developed a new method, known as transorbital lobotomy, which did not require surgical staff or general anesthesia[10] (Freeman & Watts, 1948), leading to an exponential growth in the numbers of neurosurgeries performed in the years to follow (Berrios, 1997; Mashour et al., 2005).

The initial reports on the successes of lobotomy, published primarily by Freeman and Watts, described the patients' psychiatric status as improved (Freeman & Watts, 1942a, 1942b). However, starting in the late 1940s, evidence of cognitive problems (Rylander, Fulton, Aring, & Wortis, 1949), high rates of mortality and seizures (Barahal, 1958), and poor psychiatric outcomes (Robin, 1958, 1959) began to mount. Although these reports were followed by a precipitous decrease in the number of psychosurgeries, lobotomies nevertheless continued to be practiced on a small-scale basis in the United States and in many European countries until as late as the mid-1980s (Berrios, 1997; Mashour et al., 2005).

In the final analysis, what have the thousands of frontal lobotomies taught us about the neuroanatomic substrates of emotions? For one thing, we have come to appreciate that the connections between the frontal lobes and the rest of the brain are crucial for the ability to exhibit, and experience, normal emotions. Second, we learned that animal models are not always adequate when it comes to examining the phenomenology of the human experience of emotions. Specifically, the few animal studies that examined whether anxiety and neurotic responses could be abolished by severing the connections between the frontal lobes and the diencephalon have shown positive results (Lichtenstein, 1950; Streb & Smith, 1955). Lastly, in spite of the encouraging findings of animal research, the necessity of emotions for healthy *human* functioning has become abundantly apparent, even if, for some decades, conveniently ignored. Freeman and Watts (1939) put it well when they described the human frontal lobes *not* as the *center* of emotion, but rather as being "equipped with appropriate affective tone," which allows the frontal lobes to "project the individual into the future, direct him toward his goals—and criticize his shortcomings" (p. 527). This last point became further buttressed when the frontal lobes of people who were *not* deemed mentally ill were increasingly placed at peril on the autobahns and highways of the modern Western world.

The Frontal Lobes and the Automobile

There are no mad, overzealous, or deluded scientists to blame for the next natural experiment with the human frontal lobes—only the desire to move through space at speeds that exceed the cushioning capabilities of cerebrospinal fluid. In the second half of the 20th century, as the automobile industry produced cheaper and faster cars and the department of transportation produced better and smoother highways, so did the brain injuries from car accidents increase. In most Western settings, between 30 and 50% of all traumatic brain injuries are caused by motor vehicle accidents (Andersson, Bjorklund, Emanuselson, & Stalhammar, 2003; Appleton & Baldwin, 2006; Burns & Hauser, 2003; Koskinen & Alaranta, 2008). As we well understand today, because of the mechanics and structure of the skull and the brain, traumatic brain injuries frequently lead to injuries of the frontal lobes, particular the orbitofrontal cortex (Eslinger, Grattan, & Geder, 1996), as well as damage to the white matter tracts that connect the frontal lobes with subcortical structures (Bigler, 2004; Wilde et al., 2006). It is these types of injuries, affecting individuals who are not hospitalized for mental illness, that provide the final piece of evidence that personality change and psychiatric symptoms are a likely outcome of damage to the prefrontal cortex and related circuitry (Handel, Ovitt, Spiro, & Rao, 2007; Max, Robertson, & Lansing, 2001; Persinger, 1993; Tate, 2003).

SUMMARY AND CONCLUSIONS

As alluded to in the introduction to this chapter, our initial understanding of the brain as the substrate for emotional experience was based on random accidents, happenstance discoveries, and the incidental crossing of paths of scientists with diverse sets of interests, skills, and experiences. After ancient philosophies and the pseudoscience of the 19th century gave way to true scientific inquiry, it took more than 100 years to come to the conclusion that virtually all of the brain is, in one way or another, involved in emotional processing. Such an undifferentiated notion harks back to Hippocrates, who was the first to propose that the brain *as a whole* was the principal substrate of emotions. In the next section of this book, we examine the more focused, goal-directed inquiries into how discrete aspects of emotions relate to discrete circuitries.

NOTES

1. Woodworth and Sherrington did, in fact, use the term *pseud-affective*, rather than *pseudo-affective*, which would be more common usage today.
2. In his 1934 publication, Bard described, in excruciating detail, the condition, personality, behavior, and daily life of four cats and three dogs, whose survival, following extensive cerebral ablations, ranged from 6 weeks to 26 months. Bard found that painful stimuli elicited normal rage and fear responses in all such animals.
3. In recent years, even more direct clinical evidence has become available, as reports of personality changes and social and emotional deficits among patients with bilateral or right-sided amygdalar lesions have begun to emerge (Olson et al., 2007). In fact, such patients not only exhibited flat affect and social withdrawal, but also inappropriate sexual behavior, such as excessive sexual advances toward hospital staff, or sudden onset paraphilic and pedophilic behaviors (Kawashima et al., 1999; Mendez, Chow, Ringman, Twitchell, & Hinkin, 2000).
4. By the 1950s it was becoming clear that brain regions outside of the amygdala played a role in at least some components of the syndrome described by Klüver and Bucy. For example, it became clear that visual agnosia could be elicited by lesions in the ventrolateral aspects of the temporal lobe (Chow, 1952), and tameness and indiscriminate eating could be elicited by anteromedial temporal lesions (Pribram & Bagshaw, 1953).
5. Interestingly, the Papez circuit conformed quite closely to what Paul Broca, some 60 years earlier, described as the "great limbic lobe." In fact, not only did Broca describe the same structures as forming a unified circuit, he even foreshadowed their role in emotion, describing them as "animalistic" and "motivational" (Lautin, 2001, p. 57). Papez's work was not based on the limbic lobe

described by Broca, however, but rather on the empirical findings of researchers who were his contemporaries.

6. This lecture lay the basis for what would later become the theory of the *triune brain* (MacLean, 1990), which represented an attempt to place the limbic system into an evolutionary context. In it, MacLean introduced the notion of three phylogenetically distinct "brains": (1) the protoreptilian formation (or the R-complex), present in reptiles, birds, and mammals, which consisted primarily of the diencephalon, but also the basal ganglia and the nucleus accumbens; (2) the protomammalian formation (or the limbic system), present in early mammals; and (3) the neomammalian formation (or the neocortex), present in higher mammals.
7. Von Monakow also coined the term *diaschisis* (i.e., loss of function in an area of the brain that is distant from the lesion), and was the first to describe the thalamus as the relay between the retina and the primary visual cortex.
8. During that same time, Anton also described patients who were unaware of their cortical blindness (a phenomenon known today as Anton's syndrome).
9. Arnold Pick is primarily known for his description of the Pick's bodies that define Pick's disease.
10. Electroconvulsive therapy (ECT) was used during these surgeries to render the patient unconscious (Freeman & Watts, 1948).

PART II

Anatomy of an Emotional Event

From Emotional Trigger to Emotion Regulation

INTRODUCTION TO PART II

The purpose of Part II of this book is to propose five domains that make up an emotional response, domains that are relevant for us as clinical neuropsychologists when evaluating patients: (1) emotional trigger mechanism, (2) reflexive emotional response, (3) conscious awareness of emotional response, (4) emotional communication, and (5) emotion regulation. Although these five domains clearly interact with one another, with none of them really ever expressed in isolation, they are nevertheless considered separately here, much like cognitive domains are typically considered separately, toward conceptual, theoretical, and clinical ends.

An overview of relevant *theoretical background* is provided for each domain, including a conceptual analysis of the constructs that make up the domain, the interface of the domain with cognition, as well as the underlying neuroanatomy. Please note that each domain could be reduced to many additional minute processes, just as, for example, visual perception could be reduced to the firing in the cones and rods in the retina of the eye, the "blob" columns in the primary visual cortex, or each neuron's exqui-

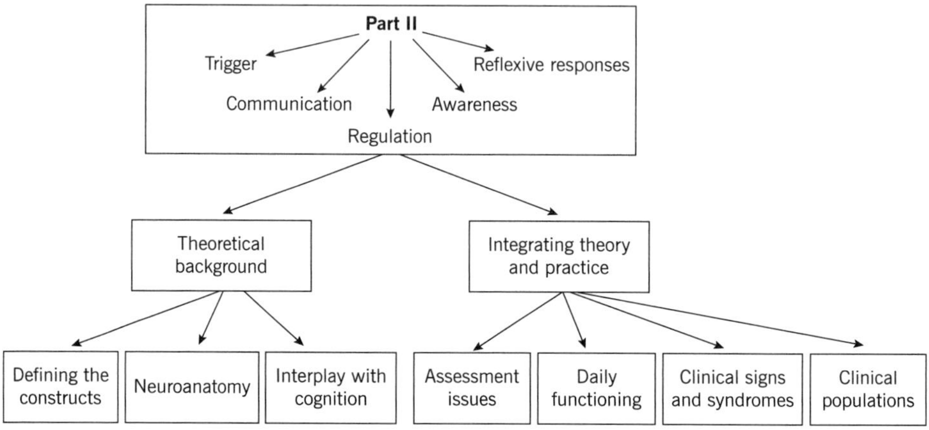

FIGURE II.1. A graphical overview of the organization of Part II of this book, as well as a general organization of each of the next five chapters.

sitely fine-tuned receptive fields. While such a molecular level of analysis is important for our understanding of how the brain works, this is *not* the level of analysis that is helpful in the everyday practice of clinical neuropsychology. Rather, as clinicians, we focus on domains that are measureable or observable within a clinical context, diagnostically informative, and relevant for daily functioning.

Lastly, a section on *integrating theory and practice* is provided for each domain, examining how understanding of a given domain informs *clinical practice*, including ways in which emotional deficits affect cognition and test performance, descriptions of syndromes associated with each domain, an overview of typical clinical populations that are deficient in a given domain, and, if relevant, methods for assessing a given domain or its subcomponents. See Figure II.1.

CHAPTER 3

The Trigger Mechanism and the Detection of Emotionally Salient Stimuli

From the first glimmer of consciousness as we wake up in the morning, until the last faint awareness of drifting off into sleep at night, our senses are bombarded with information: the somewhat disorienting beep of the alarm clock; the first glimpse of the morning sky; the comforting scent of coffee beginning to brew. All day, sounds, sights, scents, and touches provide us with information about the world. How are we to make sense of it all? How are we to know what matters?

Some information seems hard-wired, and we deal with it reflexively, the same as a moth flying toward the lightbulb or a newborn baby turtle marching toward the sea. Some information has an entrenched and clearly delineated role in our plans and goals for the day, like the landmarks on our daily route to work. Other information screams to us for attention, like a tripped up smoke detector screeching overhead.

But what about the rest of it—the less reflexive, less routinized, less demanding, less goal-related objects, sensations, and events? Consider the following scenario.

You are at a summer picnic. You feel relaxed, not a care, not a worry in the world. A multitude of sounds and sights surrounds you: the twang of Janis Joplin's *Summertime*; the red and white impatiens blossoms, spilling over the edges of a terra cotta flower pot; the cool, gentle breeze on your nape; the tart, biting flavor of red wine on your tongue; the delicious scent of scorching meat. ... Then, with the suddenness of a thunderbolt out of a blue sky, the twang of Janis Joplin, the impatiens, the scent of scorching meat—it all disappears from your attentional radar, and you, heart pounding and muscles stiffened, focus all of your attention on a single tiny stimulus: a yellow-jacket that has entered your personal space and is now flying in jagged lines about your face.

How is it that you responded so extremely to its presence?

It wasn't its movement or its buzzing, because, after all, other insects have flown in and out of your immediate surroundings, unnoticed, or at most shooed away by a half-hearted swipe of your hand. It wasn't its appearance, because, after all, the napkin you are holding is adorned with cartoons of bumblebees and yellow-jackets. Now, you do have a clear memory of your last encounter with a yellow-jacket only a few days earlier, during which you had been stung and you most definitely did not like it. But still: How could such a miniscule creature amid so many other engaging stimuli so completely monopolize your attentional resources? The mechanism behind the ability to detect, and respond to, emotionally significant stimuli—what we will call the *emotional trigger*—is the topic of this chapter.

THEORETICAL BACKGROUND

Defining the Constructs

In this chapter, and for the remainder of this book, the term *trigger* does *not* refer to the emotion-evoking *stimulus*, but rather to the *brain mechanisms* that detect emotionally relevant stimuli. In other words, the emotional trigger, like a trigger of a gun, initiates a reaction, while the emotionally relevant stimulus, like the index finger, "trips" the trigger into firing. The notion that the trigger is *not* inherent in the stimulus, but rather is contained within the organism itself, can be gleaned from the fact that the same stimuli have different impacts on different species, or even on different individuals within the same species. For example, the sound of a baby's cries evokes an emotional response that is in proportion to the levels of hormones in one's bloodstream, which itself is partly dependent on one's past experiences with babies (Delahunty, McKay, Noseworthy, & Storey, 2007; Giardino, Gonzalez, Steiner, & Fleming, 2008).[1]

Properties of an Emotional Trigger

For a brain mechanism to be able to function as an effective emotional trigger, it must possess several important properties. First, it must be able to detect emotionally relevant stimuli rapidly, perhaps even preconsciously, so as to facilitate a rapid, adaptive response. Second, it must be able to initiate the complex cascade of cognitive, behavioral, and physiological events we call emotion. And third, it must be able to learn about emotionally relevant properties of stimuli that may have previously been emotionally neutral. As such, a trigger mechanism must have a ready and immediate access to the information from the outside world, as well as to neural circuits that employ various components of an emotional response.

Properties of Emotionally Relevant Stimuli

Stimuli that are emotionally relevant, or emotionally *loaded*, carry information that is important for the survival of a given organism. Emotionally relevant stimuli can be classified along several dimensions.

First, the affective loading of some stimuli, such as spiders or snakes, is *inherent* (Ohman & Mineka, 2001), whereas the affective loading of others, such as guns, electricity outlets, or oncoming traffic, must be *learned*. Stimuli from the latter category can trip the emotional trigger only if an organism has the capacity to learn the associations between them and the emotionally relevant outcomes. Note that the affective loading of certain species-specific responses, such as affective facial expressions, vocalizations, or postures, is always inherent for all normally developed members of the same species. Thus, out of convenience, facial expressions are commonly used in research to elicit activation of the emotional trigger.

Second, emotionally loaded stimuli can be classified based on their *valence* (i.e., whether the stimulus signals "good" or "bad" outcomes). As discussed later in this chapter, the question of whether the same trigger mechanism can respond to both positive and negative emotional stimuli continues to be a source of controversy. Also note that the valence of a stimulus does not necessarily determine the direction of a behavioral outcome. For example, stimuli that evoke anger and stimuli that evoke happiness can both elicit approach behaviors, despite their differences in valence. In contrast, stimuli that evoke anger and those that evoke fear, although both being negatively valenced, may lead to opposite behavioral responses.

Third, stimuli can be classified based on the *intensity* of the emotional arousal they typically elicit. Although threatening stimuli, in general, tend to be higher in intensity than positive or pleasant stimuli, valence and intensity should nevertheless be viewed as mutually orthogonal, and it is important to avoid confounding the two when interpreting research findings. In fact, confounding of valence and intensity is likely responsible for some considerable controversies in research, reviewed later in this chapter.

Neuroanatomic Substrates

It seems that a single trigger mechanism could not possibly account for the multitude of emotional reactions an organism can experience. And, in fact, a network of at least two related brain circuits plays a role in triggering emotions. These circuits are (1) the amygdala, which triggers emotions in response to external stimuli or cognitive states, and (2) the hypothalamus, which triggers emotions in response to threats to internal homeostasis. The present chapter focuses on responses to external events.

The Amygdala[2]

The role of the amygdala as the emotional trigger mechanism can be surmised from its efferent and afferent connections with other structures in the brain. First, the amygdala (specifically the basolateral amygdala) receives afferents from virtually every step along the routes of sensory processing, including the thalamus, the primary and secondary sensory areas, the association cortices, as well as the hippocampus (Davis & Whalen, 2001). This wide receptivity range allows the amygdala to receive information at any level of processing. In addition to the relevant afferents from the senses, there are rich projections (originating in the central nucleus of the amygdala) to the hypothalamus, which controls initiation of hormonal releases, and to a number of brainstem nuclei, which control species-specific motor (e.g., aggressive posturing, defensive freezing) and visceromotor responses (e.g., heart rate and blood pressure changes) (Davis, 1997).[3]

This input–output circuit is what makes very rapid, "preconscious" responses to even crudely processed stimuli possible. A well-known illustration of this concept is an encounter with a snake, described by the prominent affective neuroscientist Joseph LeDoux (1996). The story goes like this: Imagine that you are walking through the woods. Suddenly, you hear a crackling sound, just as you catch a glimpse of a slender curved object on the path in front of you. Before you have a chance to give this object any thought or any further examination, your next step is aborted as the muscles in your legs, arms, torso, and neck stiffen into a frozen stance.

Meanwhile, as you stand frozen on the path in the woods, the neural code of the crude visual image of the elongated object travels via the neural superhighway of the optic radiation, taking a mere few milliseconds to complete its journey to the primary visual cortex. Once there, the code is broken down into its smallest components, lines, angles, colors, and movement, taking a few more milliseconds for this analytical process to be complete. Next, the broken down visual information is subjected to the comparatively snail-paced cortical conduction while it travels to the secondary visual cortex, where it is synthesized into a unified form, though still lacking a clear meaning. Then, several dozen painstaking milliseconds later, the code reaches the tertiary association areas, where the image *becomes a snake*, with the word *snake* attached to it, along with all your past memories and knowledge of what snakes represent (Nowak & Bullier, 1997). In all, it will be about 100–200 milliseconds (Thorpe, Fize, & Marlot, 1996) from your initial reaction to the time you fully process the image and figure out whether what you saw was indeed a snake or, as is the case in Joseph LeDoux's scenario, just a stick in the middle of the path. It will be longer yet before you react behaviorally to what just happened—in other words, before you loosen your frozen stance and proceed with a more reasoned response.

The question is, how is it that your muscles reacted long before all that processing had a chance to take place? As described in the Figure 3.1,

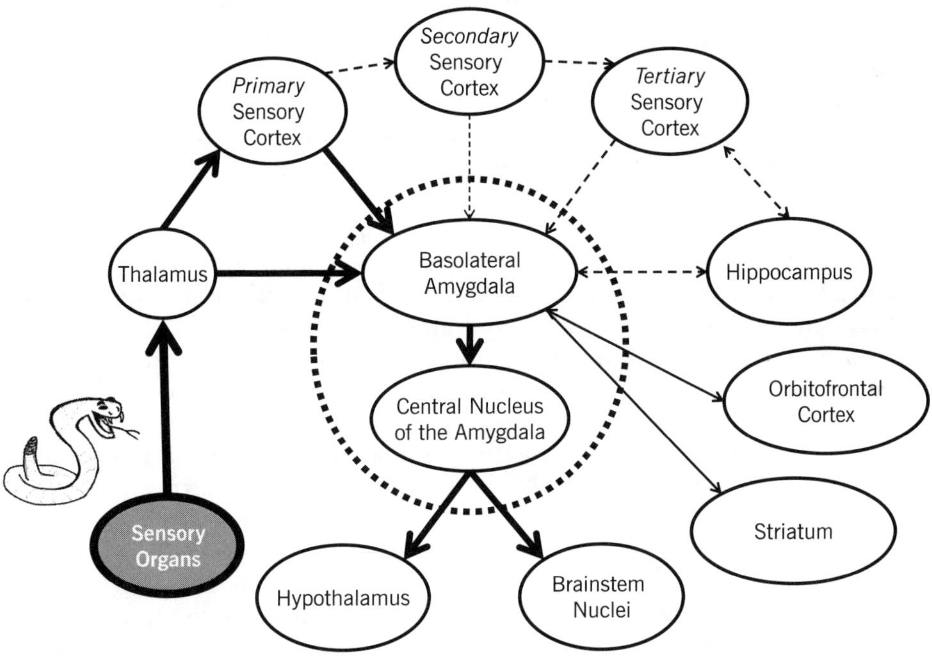

FIGURE 3.1. The so-called "slow route" of information processing (indicated by arrows with broken lines) and the so called "fast route" of information processing (indicated by solid bold arrows) leading from the sensory organ to the amygdala. Specifically, the thalamus and the primary visual cortex provide information about the basic crude sensory characteristics of a stimulus; unimodal association cortices provide information about the object that is perceived; supramodal association cortices provide information about the meaning of the stimulus; and the hippocampus provides information about the context in which the stimulus is encountered. The output from the amygdala to the hypothalamus and the brainstem nuclei accounts for behavioral and physiological responses, covered in detail in Chapter 4. The connections with the orbitofrontal cortex and striatum reflect aspects of emotional learning circuitry, covered in more detail in Chapter 9.

this rapid processing is possible because of the so-called "fast route," or "low road," of visual information transfer that bypasses the primary visual cortex and leads directly from the thalamus to the amygdala (LeDoux, 1996). The existence of this fast route is suggested not only by the snake-in-the-woods scenario described above, but also by a clinical phenomenon known as affective blind sight. In this condition, individuals who are cortically blind can nevertheless detect the emotional valence of stimuli that they, for all intents and purposes, cannot see (de Gelder, Vroomen, Pourtois, & Weiskrantz, 1999, 2000; Morris et al., 2001). As an analogue to the research with cortically blind patients, studies with normally sighted individuals have demonstrated that emotionally significant stimuli can be detected and classified according to their valence even if presented subliminally (Naccache et al., 2005; Ohman, 2002, 2005). The evolutionary advantage of this alternate fast route for information transfer is quite clear. As Joseph LeDoux has put it, "The cost of treating a stick as a snake is less, in the long run, than the cost of treating a snake as a stick" (1996, p. 165).[4]

But the evidence for the fast route alone does not represent proof that the amygdala is what actually detects emotional stimuli, or that the amygdala is responsible for rapid communication with other brain areas that control hormonal cascades and archetypal motor programs such as freezing or flight. To prove that, research needs to demonstrate that the amygdala is (1) necessary and sufficient for *detection* of affective aspects of stimuli, (2) necessary for *triggering* affective physiological and motor responses, and (3) capable of *learning* the associations between affective outcomes and neutral stimuli. We examine such evidence next.

DETECTION OF AFFECTIVE STIMULI

Evidence supporting the key role of the amygdala in detection of emotionally loaded stimuli comes from both functional imaging and lesion research. Functional imaging has shown that the amygdala becomes reliably activated in response to stimuli that are inherently emotionally loaded, such as spiders (Ohman, 2005), facial expressions (Derntl et al., 2009; S.-E. Kim et al., 2007; LaBar, Crupain, Voyvodic, & McCarthy, 2003), or affectively expressive body movements (Hadjikhani & de Gelder, 2003), as well as stimuli that have become affectively loaded via fear conditioning (Herry et al., 2007; Moses et al., 2007; Tabbert, Stark, Kirsch, & Vaitl, 2005). Such activation occurs even when the stimuli are presented subliminally, without the participants' conscious awareness (Diaz & McCarthy, 2007; Naccache et al., 2005; Ohman, 2002, 2005). Furthermore, damage to the amygdala has been shown to interfere with the detection, or understanding, of the emotional aspects of stimuli. For example, individuals with bilateral amygdalar damage show impaired processing of the emotional aspects of facial and verbal expressions (Adolphs, Baron-Cohen, & Tranel, 2002; Adolphs, Russell, & Tranel, 1999; Adolphs & Tranel, 2003, 2004; Adolphs, Tranel, et al., 1999; Anderson & Phelps, 2000; Graham, Devinsky, & LaBar, 2007; Sato et al., 2002; Siebert, Markowitsch, & Bartel, 2003), as well as the emotional aspects of music (Gosselin, Peretz, Johnsen, & Adolphs, 2007). Together, these findings show that the amygdala is (1) necessary for detection of the emotional content of stimuli, and (2) sufficient for detection of emotional stimuli, given that it becomes active even when stimuli are presented subliminally.

TRIGGERING OF MOTOR AND PHYSIOLOGICAL RESPONSES

Although sensitivity to, or metabolic activation in response to, emotional stimuli demonstrates that the amygdala plays a role in detection of emotional content, it does not, in and of itself, prove that the amygdala is what actually *triggers* an emotional response. For that, as mentioned above, abolishment of such a response by disrupting the functioning of the amygdala needs to be demonstrated. This, in fact, has been shown. For example, subsequent to amygdalar lesions, rats fail to exhibit normal avoidance, escape, and freezing when exposed to cats (Blanchard & Blanchard, 1972; de Oca & Fanselow, 2004), and monkeys fail to exhibit the normal behavioral and physiological responses when exposed to snakes (Izquierdo & Murray, 2004; Izquierdo, Suda, & Murray, 2005; Kalin, Shelton, & Davidson, 2004). Similarly, humans with bilateral amygdalar damage fail to exhibit normal physiological and/or cognitive responses when exposed to emotional pictorial stimuli (Adolphs, Tranel, Damasio, & Damasio, 1995; Adolphs, Tranel, et al., 1999; Berntson, Bechara, Damasio, Tranel, & Cacioppo, 2007; Young, Hellawell, Van De Wal, & Johnson, 1996), emotional words and sentences (Adolphs, Russell, et al., 1999), and scary or sad music (Gosselin et al., 2007; Khalfa et al., 2008). Together, this research shows that the amygdala is necessary[5] for the triggering of physiological and behavioral cascades, known as emotions, in response to emotionally loaded stimuli.

LEARNING THE ASSOCIATIONS BETWEEN AFFECTIVE AND NEUTRAL STIMULI

Lastly, as mentioned before, the trigger mechanism needs to accomplish more than just a rapid detection of emotionally significant stimuli. It also needs to *learn* about the emotional significance of stimuli that may appear neutral but are associated with emotionally significant outcomes. The most commonly used paradigm for demonstration of such learning is fear conditioning. In the fear-conditioning paradigm, human or animal subjects are exposed to a neutral stimulus, such as a particular tone or object, which is paired with a noxious stimulus, such as a mild electric shock. Fairly quickly, often in a single trial, such paradigms cause the subjects to experience fear even when exposed to the neutral stimulus alone. Importantly, amygdalar lesions prevent such associations, or conditioning, from taking place both in animals (Davis & Whalen, 2001; Ito, Robbins, McNaughton, & Everitt, 2006; Maren & Hobin, 2007; Zimmerman, Rabinak, McLachlan, & Maren, 2007) and in human patients (Adolphs et al., 2005).[6]

Of note, the role of the amygdala in fear conditioning is *not* limited to personal experiences with the emotionally significant stimuli; rather, it also includes social learning or learning by example. In other words, the amygdala responds to conditioning experiments conducted on others, as well as to verbal explanations of relationships between apparently emotionally neutral stimuli and potential dangers (Phelps et al., 2006). It is this vicarious learning that allows us to have the appropriate emotional response to, say, a pointed gun, without the need for the past experience of actually having been shot.

Importantly, however, the amygdala alone is not responsible for *all* affective learning. As can be seen in Figure 3.1, the amygdala has mutually reciprocal connections with the hippocampus, suggesting mutual modulation of function. Specifically, whereas the amygdala is sensitive to *discrete* emotionally significant stimuli, the hippocampus is sensitive to emotionally significant *contexts* (Ito et al., 2006; Maren & Hobin, 2007; Phelps, 2004). Thus, for example, animals with amygdalar lesions fail to develop normal fear conditioning to a discrete stimulus such as the sound of a buzzer, but do develop a normal conditioned response to the cage or even the room in which the experiments have taken place (see Table 3.1). The opposite pattern is seen in animals with hippocampal lesions—in other words, the animals condition normally to the discrete warning sound, but are unaffected by the greater context, such as the cage or the room. Thus, in a healthy brain, the two structures work in concert. The hippocampus primes the amygdala to contexts that are more likely to contain emotionally relevant stimuli (prompting the organism to be vigilant or anxious and to startle more easily), while the amygdala modulates explicit episodic memories

TABLE 3.1. Fear Conditioning to a Buzzer versus a Context as a Function of Lesion Location

	Response to context conditioning (cage, room)	
Response to buzzer conditioning	Normal	Impaired
Normal	No lesion	Hippocampal lesion
Impaired	Amygdalar lesion	Amygdalar and hippocampal lesions

laid down by the hippocampus so as to enhance recall of events that have emotional significance. Along these same lines, it has been argued that the amygdala mediates phobic reactions to specific stimuli, whereas the hippocampus mediates the anticipatory and contextually driven generalized anxiety (Etkin & Wager, 2007; Hasler et al., 2007; Straube, Mentzel, & Miltner, 2006).

Lastly, the orbitofrontal cortex also appears to contribute to emotional learning. In fact, affective conditioning is impaired in populations characterized by orbitofrontal damage (Hoefer et al., 2008; Mitchell et al., 2006), and both the amygdala and the orbitofrontal cortex are metabolically activated by presentation of conditioned stimuli (Gottfried, O'Doherty, & Dolan, 2003; Tabbert et al., 2005). However, the role of the orbitofrontal cortex in affective learning is different from that of the amygdala. Specifically, the orbitofrontal cortex has been implicated in *updating* the current reinforcement value of a given stimulus (Cox, Andrade, & Johnsrude, 2005; Gottfried & Dolan, 2004; Salzman et al., 2007), as well as *allocating* attentional resources to the stimulus based on its current reinforcement value (Grossberg, Bullock, & Dranias, 2008). Thus, when fMRI signals are collected during the acquisition (or learning) phase of fear conditioning, the orbitofrontal cortex actually responds to the conditioned stimulus earlier than the amygdala (Tabbert et al., 2005).[7]

CONTROVERSIES IN AMYGDALA RESEARCH

Although the three components of the trigger mechanism discussed above have all been extensively studied by research on the functioning of the amygdala, many inconsistencies, or even controversies, in findings remain. A thorough treatment of these is beyond the scope of this chapter, but we will briefly touch on two perennial, and as yet to be definitively answered, questions. These have to do with (1) the emotional valence of stimuli to which the amygdala responds, and (2) the hemispheric asymmetry in amygdalar processing.

Valence of Stimuli. Traditionally, it has been thought that the amygdala plays a role *only* in triggering *negative* emotions (Adolphs, Russell, et al., 1999; Adolphs, Tranel, et al., 1999), and, even more concretely, fear (Murphy, Nimmo-Smith, & Lawrence, 2003). This interpretation is based in part on research showing that individuals with amygdalar dysfunction tend to demonstrate greater difficulties with recognizing negative, as opposed to positive, emotional facial expressions, and are generally *un*impaired in the ability to discriminate the valence of positive versus negative emotional faces (Adolphs, Russell, et al., 1999). These findings, however, can be explained in ways other than the amygdala's specificity to negative emotions.

The first alternative explanation relies on the manner in which people process facial information. In particular, when discriminating among various facial expressions, most healthy individuals tend to focus on the expressive changes reflected in the eye region of the face (Hernandez et al., 2009); in contrast, individuals with amygdalar abnormalities tend to focus their attention on the mouth. Interestingly, this abnormal pattern of processing seems to be true both for individuals with congenital (Dadds, El Masry, Wimalaweera, & Guastella, 2008) and acquired (Adolphs et al., 2005) amygdalar dysfunction. Consequently, this style of facial processing does not appear to reflect a neurodevelopmental anomaly, but rather a compensatory mechanism. As can be readily seen in Figure 3.2, examination of the mouth region easily accomplishes simple discrimination of valence. In fact, if a person were asked to identify the face in which mouth corners point up, the smiling face would likely be selected regardless of whether the examinee understood the meaning of a smile. In other words, the hallmarks of a smile can be encoded semantically.

However, as can be seen in the figure, such semantically coded distinctions cannot be easily accomplished among the negative emotions. In fact, fine-graded distinction among the negative emotions can only be gleaned

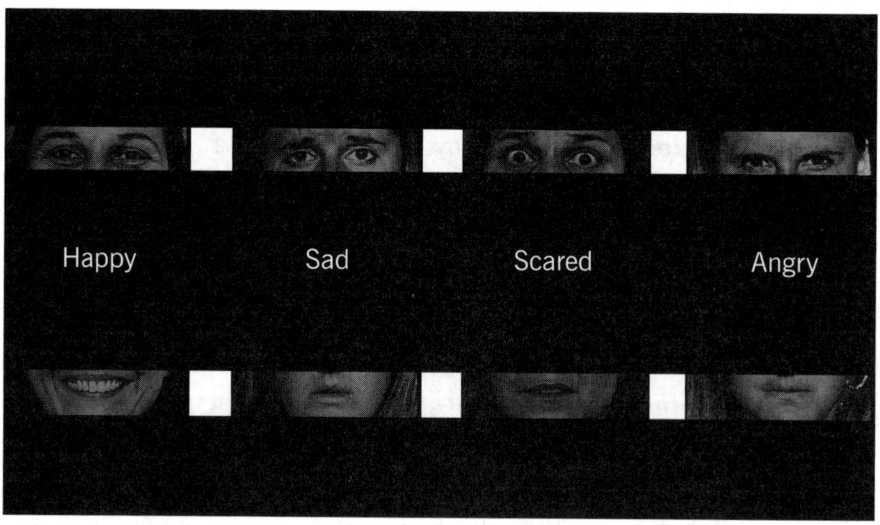

FIGURE 3.2. Illustration of the difficulty of differentiating among negative emotions when relying on the mouth region of the face. In contrast, a smile is easier to recognize from the mouth region alone. Faces reprinted with permission from Paul Ekman Group, LLC.

from the eyes. Consequently, it has been suggested that the inability to recognize fear (i.e., the most common finding in this line of research) by individuals with amygdalar damage may simply be a function of these individuals' failure to examine the eye region (which represents the *most important* feature for the recognition of this particular emotion). Nevertheless, for patients with amygdalar dysfunction, the mouth may represent a most *practical* region to focus on so as to make the more salient, and arguably more important, distinction between positive and negative expressions (Adolphs et al., 2005).

The second alternative explanation for why much research shows greater sensitivity of the amygdala to negative emotions relies on the fact that, as mentioned earlier, threatening stimuli tend to be associated with greater intensity of arousal. Interestingly, levels of intensity, regardless of valence, appear to determine the degree to which the amygdala is activated (Cunningham, Raye, & Johnson, 2004). In line with this reasoning, more recent studies have examined highly intense positive stimuli such as smiling baby faces. These studies have demonstrated that the amygdala does process emotional stimuli that are *positive* (Burgdorf & Panksepp, 2006; Hamann & Mao, 2002; Lee et al., 2004; Liberzon, Phan, Decker, & Taylor, 2003) and plays a role in appetitive conditioning and reward learning (Baxter & Murray, 2002; Everitt, Cardinal, Parkinsons, & Robbins, 2003).[8]

Hemispheric Asymmetry. One way of potentially reconciling the inconsistencies in the literature regarding which types of stimuli are processed by the amygdala is to examine the differences between the processing that takes place in the left *versus* the right hemisphere. Although most imaging studies that have utilized only negative stimuli have generally found more prominent left, *not* right, amygdalar activation (Baas, Aleman, & Kahn, 2004), other research that has pitted different types of stimuli against one another has not been consistent with those findings. Some of the most recent studies that tackled this question are summarized in Table 3.2. Of note, recent research with high-resolution fMRI has found *bilateral* amygdalar activation in response to five basic emotions, including both positive and negative stimuli (Derntl et al., 2009).

In summary, the amygdala plays a crucial role in the detection and processing of affectively loaded positive and negative stimuli, and in triggering an array of reflexive responses (covered in detail in Chapter 4). Additionally, in conjunction with the hippocampus and the orbitofrontal cortex, the amygdala links emotionally neutral stimuli and contexts with emotionally significant outcomes (whether through personal or vicarious experience), allowing emotional conditioning of neutral stimuli to occur.

TABLE 3.2 Review of Research on the Specificity and Laterality of the Amygdala's Role in Triggering Emotional Responses

Left	Right	References
Positive	Negative	Pourtois, de Gelder, Bol, & Crommelick (2005)
Imagined anticipated, symbolically expressed	Personally experienced	Funayama, Grillon, Davis, & Phelps (2001)
Verbal	Visual	Anderson & Phelps (2001); Benuzzi et al. (2004); Johnstone, van Reekum, Oakes, & Davidson (2006)
Retrieval (memories)	Encoding (memories)	Sergerie, Lepage, & Armony (2006)
Cognitive evaluation	Autonomic activation	Glascher & Adolphs (2003); Skuse, Morris, & Dolan (2005)

Homeostasis and the Hypothalamus

Despite the overwhelming evidence for the role of the amygdala in triggering emotional responses, patients with bilateral amygdalar damage still experience variations in autonomic activation and express a range of emotional responses in their daily life (Anderson & Phelps, 2002). In other words, although such patients experience certain emotional situations differently than healthy individuals do (Tranel, Gullickson, Koch, & Adolphs, 2006), they are nevertheless *not* emotionally bereft. Clearly, then, while the amygdala appears necessary for rapid detection of emotion-evoking stimuli in the environment and the subsequent rapid triggering of an emotional response, other trigger mechanisms must exist for at least some aspects of a person's emotional life. This is particularly true for the maintenance of homeostasis.

In order to maintain homeostasis, an organism needs to be able to detect signals from within that provide information about abnormal internal states, such as increases or decreases in internal temperature, changes in the levels of hydration, and drops in glucose concentration in the bloodstream. Information about these internal fluctuations is detected by the hypothalamus, which contains receptors for neurochemical indicators of these internal states (Elmquist, Zigman, Lutter, & Tamminga, 2006). Because these internal states can be altered via corrective behavioral actions, they are invariably associated with emotional arousal, so as to facilitate initiation and maintenance of such actions. However, in addition to emotional arousal, such actions require motivation. These mechanisms are addressed in detail in Part III of this book.

Interplay with Cognition

Up to this point, we have focused on understanding the construct, and the neurobiological underpinnings, of the emotional trigger mechanism. However, it is also important to consider the degree to which the emotional trigger interacts with other aspects of neural processing. A number of studies have demonstrated that appropriate sensitivity to emotionally significant stimuli benefits some aspects of cognition, most notably (1) attention, (2) psychomotor speed, and (3) memory.

Attention

As should be abundantly evident from the yellow-jacket example provided at the beginning of this chapter, emotionally significant stimuli capture our attention without much, if any, goal-directed effort on our part. In fact, not only do emotional stimuli capture our attention effortlessly, they also seem capable of capturing our attention even when our attentional resources are depleted by other effortful cognitive activities. This latter principle has been demonstrated with an experimental paradigm called the *attentional blink* task (Raymond, Shapiro, & Arnell, 1992). In this task, participants watch a series of words presented on the computer screen in a rapid succession, such that it is not possible to perceive them all. Participants are asked to identify only those words that are printed in a different color ink (say, green, as opposed to the rapid string of stimuli printed in black). Although it is possible for participants to extract these different-colored stimuli from the otherwise unintelligible blur of a streaming black print, allocation of attentional resources to such targets causes the attentional resources to be momentarily depleted, a phenomenon known as the attentional blink. Thus, if such a target word is immediately followed by a second target word (i.e., a second word printed in green ink), the second word is generally not detected. However, if the second target word carries some emotional significance, the attentional blink is attenuated and participants are able to correctly identify the second word. Importantly, however, patients with amygdalar damage, particularly if involving the left hemisphere, do *not* benefit from the emotional content interjected among the otherwise neutral stimuli. In other words, they are unable to overcome the attentional blink, even if presented with stimuli that are emotionally significant (Anderson & Phelps, 2001).

The above example demonstrates that although effortful attention is a taxing process that fatigues and/or becomes depleted relatively easily, fewer resources appear to be needed when attending to emotionally significant stimuli. This mechanism not only has a clear survival value, but also likely allows one to conserve attentional resources in daily life.

Psychomotor Speed

With respect to psychomotor speed, the *snake in the grass* task (Ohman, Flykt, & Esteves, 2001) has been used to show that people respond faster to emotional, as compared to nonemotional, stimuli (Flykt, 2006). In this task, participants view a series of 3 × 3 matrices containing nine pictures of flowers, mushrooms, spiders, and snakes. In some matrices, all nine pictures are from a single category. In others, one of the nine pictures comes from a different category. Participants are required to make judgments as to whether all pictures in a given matrix come from the same category (i.e., are they all flowers, mushrooms, etc.).

In this task, participants reliably respond faster to a single snake or spider against the background of flowers or mushrooms, as compared to a single flower or a mushroom against the backdrop of snakes or spiders (Flykt, 2006; LoBue & DeLoache, 2008; Ohman et al., 2001; South et al., 2008). This faster response time has been interpreted as reflecting greater motor readiness when responding to emotional and/or threatening stimuli, and event-related potential (ERP) research has shown that this greater motor readiness can*not* be fully explained by greater allocation of attentional resources to such stimuli (Flykt & Caldara, 2006). In other words, it appears that the simple act of anticipating an emotional stimulus primes one's motor system to respond faster.

Memory

As mentioned earlier, the amygdala modulates the functioning of the hippocampus by facilitating episodic memories that have emotionally salient content (Frank & Tomaz, 2000; Gasbarri et al., 2005). This enhanced episodic memory (which is dependent on the hippocampal system) is thought to result from an increased activation in the perceptual cortical areas (mediated by the amygdala), which influences perception of emotionally salient stimuli and alters the priority with which the hippocampus *encodes* episodic events (Phelps, 2004). Additionally, following the initial encoding, the amygdala is thought to play a role in the subsequent *consolidation* of memories. In particular, following the initial exposure to, and encoding of, a stimulus, a favorable, unfavorable, or neutral outcome takes place. The relative survival value of a given outcome is thought to lead to differential amygdalar activation, which in turn determines the priority with which the hippocampus consolidates different events (Phelps, 2004). Predictably, individuals with amygdalar damage or dysfunction do not demonstrate the same memory facilitation by emotional content (Buchanan, Denburg, Tranel, & Adolphs, 2001; Dolan & Fullam, 2010; Phelps et al., 1998).

INTEGRATING THEORY AND PRACTICE

Understanding how the emotional trigger mechanism works, where it is located in the brain, and how it affects cognitive performances on various experimental tasks is one thing. It is a whole different matter, however, to know when, how, and in which populations these various issues matter to us as clinicians.

Assessment

Overactive Trigger

Because an overactive trigger mechanism mediated by the amygdala and the hippocampus has been shown to play a role in anxiety disorders (Hasler et al., 2007; van den Heuvel, Groenewegen, Witter, Veltman, & Sanfelippo, 2005; van den Heuvel, Veltman, et al., 2005), readers may consider a trigger mechanism that is overly active or sensitive to be the primary liability with respect to cognitive assessment. After all, anxiety is a common clinical confound, one that clinicians need to routinely consider when interpreting neuropsychological data. An overactive trigger can lead a patient to be excessively attentive to potential threats in the environment, and each time a threat is detected, a flood of stress hormones may overwhelm the system, interfering with the ability to focus on the cognitive task at hand (van den Heuvel, Veltman, et al., 2005). An anxious patient is more likely to remember a child crying in the hallway or a car backfiring in the street than a list of furniture or vegetable items. In fact, amygdalar activation has been shown to correlate with retrieval of emotionally relevant information (Cahill, 1996; Hamann, Ely, Grafton, & Kilts, 1999), and it is well known that exposure to emotionally relevant stimuli leads to a narrowing of attention, such that stimuli peripheral to the emotional content are *not* attended to or remembered (Christianson, 1992).

Underactive Trigger

Given the potentially deleterious effects of anxiety on test performance, one might consider that an emotional trigger that is somewhat underactive may be an advantage in a testing situation. However, recall the different ways in which emotionally significant stimuli can facilitate cognition. If such stimuli are actually contained *within* the testing materials, then, presumably, they could lead to an improvement in performance. This, in fact, appears to be the case. Consider, for example, the emotional significance of the ordeal that Anna Thompson[9] had to go through, as compared to the emotionally benign evening of Joe Garcia. The notion that the Anna Thompson story should be easier to remember due to its emotional significance is not just a clinical lore or an interpretive leap, but has been supported by empirical research (Crouse, 2005). Importantly, better memory for emotional, as compared to neutral, stories has also been demonstrated among patients with Alzheimer's dementia (Kazui et al., 2000; Moayeri, Cahill, Jin, & Potkin, 2000), and a failure to benefit from emotional story content has been shown in patients with bilateral amygdalar damage (Adolphs, Cahill, Schul, & Babinsky, 1997).

A few additional everyday examples of tests that contain emotionally significant stimuli include the Picture Arrangement subtest from the Wechsler series and the various reading comprehension tests that require matching of written and pictorial content. Although the intensity levels of the stimuli that make up these tests appear relatively minimal overall, there are likely idiosyncratic ways in which patients, based on their past life experiences, react emotionally to such testing materials. In other words, most patients likely get occasional slight boosts in performance due to either overt, or covert, emotional content of some testing materials, and such boosts may, cumulatively, yield an overall result that is slightly better than it would have been otherwise. Admittedly, with the exception of the one study, mentioned above, that examined the Anna Thompson story (Crouse, 2005), the degree to which emotional stimuli in extant clinical instruments differentially impact performance is not well understood and has, for the most part, not been empirically examined.

Everyday Functioning

As clinicians, we need to understand not only how a given emotional deficit affects test performance, but also how it affects daily functioning. With respect to the function and structure of the amygdala, the impact on daily functioning is mixed. On the one hand, amygdala damage has *not* been linked to intellectual declines (Amat et al., 2008; Pol et al., 2006), and, for the most part, emotional trigger deficits are not associated with readily noticeable cognitive impairments. On the other hand, discrete deficits in emotional memory do exist among patients with bilateral amygdalar damage. For example, a patient may recall the cities that he and his family visited during a vacation, but not recall any personally or emotionally significant autobiographical episodes that are readily recalled by other family members (Wiest, Lehner-Baumgartner, & Baumgartner, 2006). Such memory failures can understandably be confusing or frustrating to patients and their loved ones, primarily because they occur in the context of essentially normal recall of semantic or factual information. Thus, education of patients and their families about this discrete deficit is important and may ameliorate strain on interpersonal relationships.

In addition to insidious memory difficulties, patients with bilateral amygdalar damage may exhibit failures to learn from negative consequences, to respond appropriately to social cues, or to identify threats in the environment. Such failures may be misinterpreted as deficits in executive functioning, including as lapses in judgment, reasoning, and attention, or as apparent increases in callousness, marked by absence of emotional arousal in response to the distress of others (Huebner et al., 2008; Marsh et al., 2008). Relatedly, deficits in decision making, particularly in ambiguous situations when one might need to rely on one's "gut" reactions to the available options, can also be present in these patient populations (Weller, 2007).[10]

Lastly, it should be noted that, despite declines in episodic memory with age, normal aging does *not* appear to decrease the normal memory facilitation that is conferred by emotional content (Denburg, Buchanan, Tranel, & Adolphs, 2003). Thus, among older adults, such facilitation may represent an important aspect of daily functioning.

Clinical Signs and Syndromes

This chapter has thus far focused on the role of the amygdala in triggering emotional responses, and on the discrete deficits in the trigger mechanism associated with amygdalar damage. However, damage to the amygdala in conjunction with surrounding brain tissue, or the disconnection of the amygdala from other brain regions, can sometimes lead to syndromes in which the discrete deficit in trigger mechanism is obscured by much more blatant, and odd, behavioral manifestations. The two most prominent examples of this phenomenon are human Klüver–Bucy syndrome and Capgras syndrome.

Human Klüver–Bucy Syndrome

Klüver–Bucy syndrome is a result of bilateral destruction of the amygdala as well as damage to the surrounding cortical tissue. It was first described in the first half of the 20th century (Klüver & Bucy, 1937) in monkeys that had undergone bilateral anterior lobectomies (see Chapter 2). It has since been described in human patients suffering from a wide array of neuropathologies, including neurodegenerative disorders (Mendez & Perryman, 2002; Okuda, Harada, Mizutani, & Hamanaka, 1998), left or bilateral temporal lobe epilepsy (Janszky, Fogarasi, Magalova, Tuxhorn, & Ebner, 2005), multiple sclerosis (Lopez-Meza, Corona-Vazquez, Ruano-Calderon, & Ranirez-Bermudez, 2005), and traumatic brain injury (Slaughter, Bobo,

& Childers, 1999). In humans, the most common symptoms of the syndrome include hyperorality and hyperphasia, inappropriate and excessive sexual behaviors, and visual agnosia (Gaul, Jordan, Wustmann, & Preuss, 2007; Lilly et al., 1983; Okuda et al., 1998). In some cases, hyperorality may be particularly severe, even leading to accidental choking and death (Mendez & Foti, 1997).

Capgras Syndrome

Capgras syndrome (CS), also known as the imposter syndrome or the delusional misidentification syndrome, was first described by the French psychiatrist Jean Marie Joseph Capgras. CS presents with a bizarre delusional belief that a significant person in the patient's life, such as a spouse, a child, or a close friend, has been replaced by an impostor. In general, this belief is limited to the encounters with the familiar person's face (i.e., the delusion is *not* present during phone conversations), although rare cases in which the delusion was triggered by a voice have also been reported (Lewis, Sherwood, Moselhy, & Ellis, 2001). It is interesting that even though some deficiencies in face and voice recognition are often associated with CS, these deficiencies are not sufficient to account for the syndrome, nor are they of the same magnitude as those seen in patients with frank prosopagnosia (Dietl, Herr, Brunner, & Friess, 2003; Oyebode, Edelstyn, Patel, & Riddoch, 1996).

From a theoretical standpoint, CS is believed to be a result of a failure to *feel* the normal emotional response one typically experiences when in the presence of a familiar person. This absence of feeling presumably occurs due to a disconnection between the explicit, conscious processing of facial information and the implicit, unconscious orienting response to familiar faces, which tends to be associated with emotional and autonomic activation (Breen, Caine, & Coltheart, 2000; Ellis & Young, 1990; Young & Cleeremans, 2003). That this unconscious orienting response exists has been reliably demonstrated in patients with prosopagnosia, who experience autonomic activation in response to familiar faces even in the absence of the ability to recognize them (Tranel & Damasio, 1988; Tranel, Damasio, & Damasio, 1995). In contrast, patients with CS fail to exhibit such increases in autonomic activation when presented with familiar faces,[11] despite the fact that they have no difficulty recognizing them (Ellis, Lewis, Moselhy, & Young, 2000). Put in the context of this chapter, it appears that in CS the aspect of the trigger mechanism specific to recognition of familiar people is either disconnected or damaged. For an in-depth theoretical discussion of the literature, see Breen and colleagues (2000).

Although this explanation of CS is consistent with research findings and is generally accepted, the specific neuroanatomic substrate of such disconnection is not yet understood. Additionally, it is not fully clear why this disorder is not present among patients with bilateral amygdalar damage, since such patients also fail to react emotionally to family and friends. One possible explanation is that the disorder requires that there be a *discrepancy* between the emotional experience associated with strangers and that associated with loved ones. In other words, patients with CS (who have a normally functioning amygdala) do experience normal emotions in response to faces in general, while *not* experiencing the expected stronger emotional responses when interacting with friends and family. Another factor is that in order for patients to seriously consider the possibility that their loved ones have been replaced by an imposter, such patients must also have some additional cognitive deficits that negatively impact their ability to think critically and rationally and to maintain a strong grasp on reality.

Consistent with the notion that CS is unlikely a result of a circumscribed single lesion causing a circumscribed deficit, patients with CS tend to have relatively extensive brain damage, often involving both cerebral hemispheres (Edelstyn & Oyebode, 1999). With unilateral lesions, the damage is more often on the right than on the left (Edelstyn & Oyebode, 1999; Eren, Civi, & Yildiz, 2005), often involving the frontal and/or the temporal lobe (Signer, 1992). Additionally, some studies have found that CS is most often associated with neurodegenerative disorders, particularly dementia with Lewy bodies, which affects both hemispheres as well as multiple brain regions (Josephs, 2007). Lastly, CS has also been reported as a symptom of general decline in functional status and cognition among some older adults (Harwood, Barker, Ownby, & Duara, 1999).

Clinical Populations

In this next section, we briefly review clinical populations that either present with the syndromes reviewed above or are characterized by other types of amygdalar dysfunction. Note that most of the disorders listed below also present with other emotional abnormalities and, as such, are revisited in future chapters.

Neurodevelopmental Disorders

AUTISM

Among the neurodevelopmental disorders characterized by amygdalar abnormalities, *autism* is probably the one most commonly encountered by neuropsychology practitioners. Amygdalar abnormalities in autism have been demonstrated in neuroimaging studies (Munson et al., 2006), and the role of the amygdala in the phenomenology of autism has been implicated by a number of autistic characteristics, including impaired processing of affect in faces (Boelte & Poustka, 2003) and speech (Boucher, Lewis, & Collis, 2000). However, recent research suggests that amygdalar abnormalities among autistic individuals may be limited to the processing of socially relevant content, as people with autism appear to exhibit normal facilitation of attentional, perceptual, and learning processes by emotionally significant *non*social stimuli (South et al., 2008). Relatedly, individuals with autism appear to exhibit normal fear potentiation of a startle reflex (Bernier, Dawson, Panagiotides, & Webb, 2005).

FRAGILE X SYNDROME

Fragile X syndrome is the most common heritable cause of mental retardation. Individuals with this syndrome exhibit a number of cognitive and emotional abnormalities, with abnormal eye gaze and avoidance of eye contact being particularly relevant here (Watson, Hoeft, Garrett, Hall, & Reiss, 2008). Importantly, children and adults with fragile X syndrome exhibit enlarged hippocampal and amygdalar volumes (Hessl, Rivera, & Reiss, 2004) and increased left amygdalar (Watson et al., 2008) and left hippocampal (Dalton, Holsen, Abbeduto, & Davidson, 2008) activation in response to eye contact. There are some inconsistencies in the literature as to whether individuals with fragile X syndrome exhibit deficits in understanding emotional facial cues (Hagan, Hoeft, Mackey, Mobbs, & Reiss, 2008; Turk & Cornish, 1998).

TURNER SYNDROME

Turner syndrome is a chromosomal disorder in which all or part of one of the two X chromosomes is missing (i.e., X monosomy). Girls and women with Turner syndrome exhibit certain physical abnormalities, such as short stature, webbed neck, and gonadal dysfunction. In addition, Turner syndrome is associated with structural and functional brain abnormalities that are in turn associated with weaknesses in visuospatial and executive functioning (Brown et al., 2002; Tamm, Menon, & Reiss, 2003).

Women with Turner syndrome also exhibit structural abnormalities in the amygdala and the hippocampus (Geuze, Vermetten, & Bremner, 2005; Kesler et al., 2004). These abnormalities are associated with difficulties in recognizing facial affect (Lawrence, Kuntsi, Coleman, Campbell, & Skuse, 2003; Mazzola et al., 2006; Skuse, Morris, & Dolan, 2005), particularly when only the eye region of the face is available to them (Lawrence, Campbell, et al., 2003). It has been suggested that these weaknesses in affective processing may be partly responsible for interpersonal and social difficulties experienced by this population (McCauley, Kay, Ito, & Treder, 1987).

Neurodegenerative Disorders

DEMENTIAS OF OLD AGE

Neurodegenerative disorders have been associated with both Klüver–Bucy syndrome and Capgras syndrome. Most notably, Klüver–Bucy syndrome has been reported in up to 20% of patients with frontotemporal-lobar degeneration (FTD) (Mendez & Perryman, 2002), and even more commonly in a familial variant of FTD that is associated with a specific mutation in the presenilin1 gene (Tang-Wai et al., 2002). Additionally, patients with Alzheimer's disease (AD) may sometimes present with Klüver–Bucy syndrome in what has been described as the "amygdaloid variant" of AD (Kile, Ellis, Olichney, Farias, & DeCarli, 2009).

In addition to Klüver–Bucy syndrome, Capgras syndrome is also sometimes present in dementia, including dementia with Lewy bodies (Josephs, 2007), vascular dementia (Oyebode et al., 1996), and AD (Harwood et al., 1999). Lastly, Capgras syndrome can be seen among stroke patients, particularly following infarctions in the right frontal or temporal regions (Edelstyn & Oyebode, 1999; Edelstyn, Oyebode, & Barrett, 2001; Eren et al., 2005).

FRAGILE X–ASSOCIATED TREMOR/ATAXIA SYNDROME

Fragile X–associated tremor/ataxia syndrome (FXTAS) is a recently discovered neurodegenerative disorder that affects carriers (primarily males) of the fragile X gene and is characterized by intention tremor, gait ataxia, and dementia, among other symptoms (Hagerman & Hagerman, 2004; Hagerman et al., 2001). Although these individuals do not present with a full-blown fragile X syndrome in childhood, they nevertheless exhibit social and emotional deficits starting early in life (Bacalman et al., 2006). From among several brain abnormalities have been identified among FXTAS individuals, the one most relevant here is a volume reduction in the amygdala. Consequently, FXTAS individuals lack startle potentiation, and they exhibit reduced activation in the amygdala and reduced galvanic skin response (GSR) in anxiety-producing situations (Hessl et al., 2007). Thus, their daily lives may be marked by some of the difficulties in daily functioning described earlier in this chapter.

Other Neurological Disorders

SEIZURE DISORDER

The most common cause of acquired amygdalar damage is *seizure disorder.* Prolonged febrile seizures in childhood have been associated with amygdalar gliosis (Gloor & Aggleton, 1992) and volume reduction by 10–30% (Cendes, Andermann, Dubeau, et al., 1993; Cendes, Andermann, Gloor, et al., 1993). Most typically, this damage is unilateral, and there is some evidence that the type of deficits observed in patients may depend on which side of the brain is affected (see Table 3.2). Additionally, about 3% of patients with epilepsy exhibit multiple symptoms of Klüver–Bucy syndrome, particularly hyperorality. This is particularly true for patients with bilateral seizures, or patients with left temporal lobe epilepsy (Janszky et al., 2005).

Lastly, patients with pharmacologically intractable epilepsy may opt for elective amygdalectomy. When counseling these patients, clinicians need to consider not only the extensively studied array of cognitive morbidities, but also the different types of emotional sequelae that can result from amygdalar, hippocampal, and anterior temporal (i.e., amygdalar and hippocampal) resections, as reviewed earlier in this chapter.

URBACH–WIETHE DISEASE

Another cause of amygdalar damage is Urbach–Wiethe disease (also known as lipoid proteinosis). It is a rare autosomal (recessive) disorder that is characterized by hyaline deposits on skin and other tissues. In about 50% of cases, *bilateral* calcification of the amygdala also takes place, usually in the second half of life. As discussed earlier, bilateral amygdalar involvement is associated with deficits in emotional processing, as well as memory deficits that are specific to emotional content, or autobiographical memories. However, aside from mild memory problems, these patients seem generally less symptomatic (particularly when it comes to facial affect recognition) than those with neurodevelopmental amygdalar dysfunction. This is likely due to the opportunity to acquire semantic understanding of emotions before amygdalar abnormalities occur in the latter half of life, and thereby the availability of compensatory mechanisms (Siebert et al., 2003).

Neuropsychiatric Disorders

PSYCHOPATHY

Psychopathy is a disorder characterized by a pervasive pattern of antisocial behaviors and a failure to relate to others, as well as pervasive callousness and shallow affect (Cleckley, 1976). In North America, psychopaths account for approximately 30% of incarcerated criminals (Cooke, Michie, Hart, & Hare, 1999), and as such may represent a typical "client" of a clinical neuropsychologist practicing within correctional or forensic/criminal settings. Psychopaths are characterized by, among other things, a smaller amygdalar volume (Weber, Habel, Amunts, & Schneider, 2008), impaired fear conditioning (Birbaumer et al., 2005), deficits in recognizing facial affect (Kosson, Suchy, Mayer, & Libby, 2002; Suchy, Whittaker, Strassberg, & Eastvold, 2009), and deficits in memory for emotional content (Dolan & Fullam, 2010). Additionally, youth with psychopathic traits exhibit reduced amygdalar responsiveness to fearful expressions (Marsh et al., 2008). These abnormalities in the structure and function of the amygdala are consistent with the clinical presentation of this disorder, which includes callousness toward others and a failure to learn from negative consequences. These abnormalities also offer an explanation for why psychopaths are among the most intractable and most recidivistic of criminals (Harris, Rice, & Cormier, 1991).

ANXIETY DISORDERS

Unlike the disorders in which amygdalar functioning and activity are reduced, there are disorders in which the amygdala becomes hypertrophic or overactive. Most notably, chronic exposure to uncontrollable stress can lead to *hyper*trophy in the amygdala (Vyas, Mitra, Rao, & Chattarji, 2002), which in turn leads to excessive sensitivity to emotional stimuli. Additionally, chronic stress is associated with atrophy of the hippocampus (McEwen, 1999), leading to deficits in memory for contexts. Consequently, chronic stress is associated not only with an overactive emotional trigger, but also with the inability of the hippocampus to appropriately moderate amygdalar activation in contexts that are safe. This is particularly true in the case of posttraumatic stress disorder (PTSD) (Damsa, Maris, & Pull, 2005). More detailed discussion on the effects of stress on the structure and function of the brain can be found in Chapter 10.

Interestingly, there is growing evidence that other anxiety disorders, including generalized anxiety and panic disorders, appear to be characterized by *smaller* amygdalar volume (Hayano et al., 2009; Milham et al., 2005), in conjunction with perhaps even smaller hippocampi (MacMillan et al., 2003). Despite the smaller size, however, the amygdala of anxious individuals exhibits hyperreactivity to anxiety-provoking stimuli (McClure et al., 2007).

General Population

The above discussion of clinical populations needs to be considered in the context of base rates of amygdalar dysfunction in the general population. In particular, research has shown that close to 9% of healthy men show abnormalities in amygdalar processing that are similar to those seen in individuals with acquired amygdalar damage (no data exist for women) (Corden, Critchley, Skuse, & Dolan, 2006).

SUMMARY AND CONCLUSIONS

As can be seen from the above section, amygdalar dysfunction can be found in a variety of clinical populations, including neurodevelopmental, neurodegenative, neuropsychiatric, and other neurological disorders. With the exception of Klüver–Bucy and Capgras syndromes, which can be rather dramatic, the deficits seen among patients are relatively subtle, presenting as personality changes, Axis I psychopathology, or personality disorders. However, some mild cognitive weaknesses, particularly with respect to memory, attention, and executive functioning, may also be present, primarily due to patients' failures to benefit from the facilitation of cognitive processing that is normally conferred by emotionally significant material. In everyday life, these weaknesses can present as potentially confusing discrepancies between, for example, normal memory for factual information in the context of impaired memory for emotionally salient content. Patients and family members need to be educated about these potentially frustrating cognitive anomalies.

NOTES

1. Normal individual differences in trigger sensitivity among humans contribute to what makes each of us unique, providing a foundation for our temperaments and personalities (also see Chapter 11). However, trigger variability outside of the normal range—in other words, a trigger mechanism that is too sensitive or not sensitive enough—can be a source of emotional or cognitive problems. The impact of such abnormalities is discussed in more detail in the sections on clinical implications later on in this chapter.
2. Admittedly, the brief summary of the literature on the role of the amygdala in triggering an emotional response does not begin to do justice to the literally thousands of amygdala studies conducted to date. For an exhaustive review, the reader is directed to textbooks that specifically focus on the amygdala alone (Aggleton, 2000; Whalen & Phelps, 2009).
3. Species-specific motor and visceromotor responses are covered in more detail in Chapter 4.
4. If the reader doubts that saving maybe a hundred milliseconds via this crude "mindless" process may have any practical impact on the movement of large muscle groups and actual behavioral outcomes, consider this: At the 2008 Summer Olympics in Beijing, China, Michael Phelps won the gold medal in the 100m butterfly by "out-touching" Milorad Cavic by a mere *10 milliseconds.*
5. Demonstrating that the amygdala is *sufficient* to produce a reflexive response is not a realistic quest, given the complexity of the networks involved in such responses (see Chapter 4).

6. Interestingly, patients with bilateral amygdala damage also exhibit deficits in learning associations between visual stimuli and odors (Siebert et al., 2003).
7. More extensive discussion of the role of the orbitofrontal cortex in emotional learning can be found in Chapter 9.
8. Recent studies have found that although the amygdala responds to both positive and negative valence, there are individual differences in the *relative sensitivity* to positive versus negative stimuli (Baeken et al., 2009; Haas et al., 2009; Keightley, Chiew, Winocur, & Grady, 2007).
9. Anna Thompson and Joe Garcia are characters in the story recall subtests of the Wechsler Memory Scale, 3rd edition (Psychological Corporation, 1997).
10. Emotional decision making is covered in more detail in Chapter 9.
11. And, rarely, voices (Lewis et al., 2001).

CHAPTER 4

Reflexive Emotional Responses

Let us recall for a moment the scenario introduced in the previous chapter. You were at a summer picnic, not a care, not a worry in the world. As you were taking in the picnic scene—the the terra cotta flower pots, the gentle breeze, the delicious scent of scorching meat—all of your attentional resources, abruptly and without warning, shifted away from the summer picnic and toward a yellow-jacket zigzagging about your face. Imagine your next reactions: You let out an audible gasp; your arms, legs, and torso stiffen; your elbows press tight against your ribcage; your shoulders pull up and the base of your skull presses down into your spinal column as if trying to turn the axis of your body inside out. Simultaneously, while your skeletal muscles go into contractive overdrive, the smooth muscles of your body—those lining your internal organs, your digestive tract, even your blood vessels and hair follicles—abruptly reverse their actions, producing an array of ominous sensations: the hairs on the back of your neck standing up on end; the moisture collecting on the palms of your hands; the unexpected ripple through your belly as digestion stops in its rhythmic tracks.

All this happens automatically, without any conscious effort on your part. These two reflexive processes—that is, the synchronized contraction of the skeletal muscles and the complex physiological response—are the primary focus of this chapter.

THEORETICAL BACKGROUND

Defining the Constructs

As already implied by Friedrich Golz and Philip Bard at the end of the 19th and the beginning of the 20th centuries (see Chapter 2), the initial stage of an emotional response can essentially be reduced to a *reflexive motor output*. To be sure, this motor output is not the same as the motor activity in which we can engage at will. Rather, the motor system that controls emotional responses reacts automatically and involuntarily. It consists of two branches: skeletal and endocrine. See Figure 4.1 for the location of these two branches within the larger motor system hierarchy.

Involuntary Skeletal Response

Involuntary skeletal response, that is, a response subserved by the emotional skeletal motor system, refers to an array of species-specific behavioral displays that involve rapid, reflexive, nonvolitional changes in facial expressions, vocalizations, posture, and bodily movements that occur for the purpose of the survival of an individual as well as an entire social group. Examples of such involuntary reflexive responses include a dog's tail-wagging or growling, a cat's purring or hissing, and a human's laughing or crying.

As already alluded to above, such overt emotional displays should *not* be confused with *voluntary* displays of emotions that represent learned, as

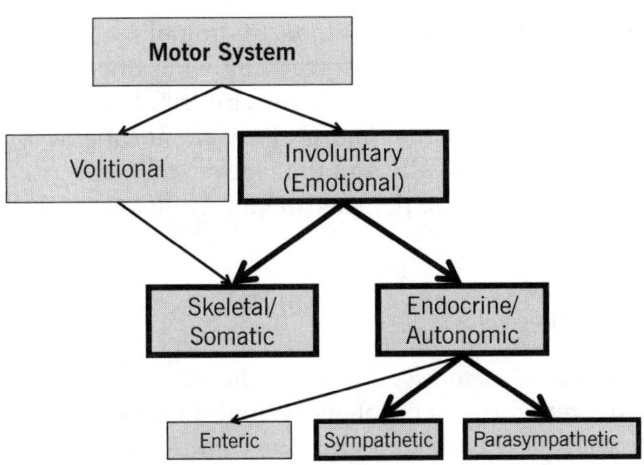

FIGURE 4.1. Two branches of the motor system. As can be seen, skeletal responses can be volitional or involuntary. The components of the motor system discussed in this chapter appear in bolded boxes.

opposed to hard-wired and fully automatic, behaviors (Miles, Johnston, Fletcher-Flinn, & Haberman, 2006). For example, it is possible for one to produce a smile voluntarily, based purely on one's understanding of the one primary characteristic of a smile, that is, the corners of the mouth go up. However, such a smile is likely to lack important hallmarks of a genuine smile, such as the contraction of the orbicularis oculi muscle that raises the cheeks, thus forming the characteristic wrinkling of the skin around the eyes (Duchenne, 1990). In other words, genuine smiles can be generated only by the involuntary motor system, which has the capacity to orchestrate a uniquely synchronized contraction of 12 different facial muscles needed for the production of such a smile.[1]

The dissociation between involuntary and volitional skeletal motor systems is supported by the clinical literature. For example, case studies have been reported in which damage to the primary motor cortex (Hopf, Mueller-Forell, & Hopf, 1992) or the basal ganglia (Kluger & Heilman, 2007) prevented a patient from generating a smile volitionally, whereas the ability to generate a smile involuntarily as a reflection of a genuine emotion was still preserved. Conversely, damage to the networks that control the involuntary emotional motor system rendered patients unable to generate natural, genuine smiles, a condition known as *facial emotional paresis*, although their ability to generate a smile volitionally was still preserved (Hopf et al., 1992).

Importantly, although one cannot voluntarily command the emotional motor system to generate emotional expressions, it is nevertheless possible to partially suppress, or delay, the release of a genuine emotional response. In fact, as humans, we rely on this ability on a daily basis, as we suppress laughter when a speaker makes an embarrassing blunder, an angry expression when our boss tells us to do something we do not feel like doing, or signs of fear when we want to protect our children from feeling distressed. However, research tells us that most of us are incapable of suppressing genuine emotional displays fully and that subtle, telltale signs of underlying emotions can nevertheless be detected by an intuitive, or skilled, observer (Ekman, 2009).

Autonomic/Endocrine Response

Autonomic/endocrine response refers to the physiological and hormonal changes in the body that complement and facilitate the *fight-or-flight* response, on the one hand, and the *digest-and-repair* processes, on the other. The signals that initiate autonomic responses originate in the brain (primarily the hypothalamus, discussed in more detail below, in the section on neuroanatomic substrates) and are communicated in two ways: through the *autonomic nervous system*, which acts rapidly via direct neuronal control, and the *endocrine system*, which acts more slowly via various hormonal and metabolic cascades.

THE AUTONOMIC NERVOUS SYSTEM

The autonomic nervous system (ANS) is a branch of the peripheral nervous system that controls smooth muscles and is outside of conscious or volitional control (see Figure 4.1). It has three branches: sympathetic, parasympathetic, and the sometimes omitted enteric (which controls the muscles of the digestive track). The relative activation of the sympathetic versus parasympathetic branches of the ANS, reflecting aroused versus vegetative states of the body, is a universal, albeit somewhat nonspecific, indicator of an emotional response. The overall effects of the two systems on various bodily organs can be found in Table 4.1.

In an older conceptualization, the sympathetic and parasympathetic branches of the ANS were viewed as opponent processors (with one, and *only one*, being always active). However, this view is being replaced by a newer conceptualization, in which the sympathetic nervous system is always maintaining an active tone, with more phasic activation of the parasympathetic nervous system providing a "brake" that periodically suppresses the sympathetic effect on bodily organs (Porges, 2007). This newer view provides a more viable explanation for complex interactions between the two systems, as well as for the speed with which the sympathetic response can occur.

THE ENDOCRINE SYSTEM

The endocrine system, which is primarily controlled by the pituitary (also known as the "master") gland, is a system of glands that release hormones, which in turn control the homeostasis of the body and augment the actions of the ANS. Although many aspects of the endocrine system are unrelated to emotions (e.g., the control of the salt and water balance in the body), some aspects (e.g., the release of adrenaline by the adrenal gland) are an integral part of the reflexive emotional response.

FEEDBACK MECHANISMS

In addition to the top-down control of autonomic/endocrine responses, there are bottom-up feedback mechanisms that deliver homeostatic information from the periphery to the brain. The pathways for the delivery of such signals are neural (e.g., the sensory branch of the vagus nerve), neurochemial (e.g., hormones from the endocrine system, cytokines from the immune system, gherin from the digestive system), or physicochemical (e.g.,

TABLE 4.1. The Effects of the Sympathetic and Parasympathetic Autonomic Nervous System on Bodily Organs

Organ	Sympathetic branch	Parasympathetic branch
Adrenal gland	Adrenaline into bloodstream	N/A
Arrector pili muscles	Contraction and erection of hairs	N/A
Blood vessels in the skin	Constriction	N/A
Blood vessels in the muscles	Dilation	N/A
Bronchi	Dilation	Constriction
Eye	Dilation	Constriction
Heart contraction	Increase	Decrease
Heart rate	Increase	Decrease
Kidneys	Decrease in urine production	Increase in urine production
Liver	Breakdown of glycogen	N/A
Reproductive system	Ejaculation/glandular secretions	Erection of penis/clitoris
Respiratory rate	Increase	Decrease
Salivary glands	Mucous, low enzyme	Watery, high enzyme
Stomach and intestines	Inhibition of peristalsis	Increased peristalsis
Sweat glands	Increased secretion	N/A
Tear glands	N/A	Increased secretion
Urinary bladder	Constriction of sphincter and relaxation of bladder	Constriction of bladder and relaxation of sphincter

Note. Based on Jaenig (2003).

blood glucose) (Jaenig, 2003). Glucocorticoids released by the cortex of the adrenal gland, as well as adrenaline, are among the key hormones that provide feedback to the brain (see Chapter 10 for a more detailed discussion of this latter feedback mechanism).

PATTERNS OF AUTONOMIC/ENDOCRINE RESPONSE

Whether or not the particular patterns of physiological responses generated by an emotional arousal are specific to individual emotions has been a source of controversy since William James (see Chapter 1). Recently, in his polyvagal theory, S. W. Porges (2007) proposed a hierarchically organized system of autonomic control, in which two different branches of the vagus nerve (i.e., the 10th cranial nerve, which is part of the parasympathetic nervous system) play different roles in inhibiting sympathetic activation. In particular, while the phylogeneticaly *older* branch inhibits sympathetic activation in a manner that facilitates phylogenetically older behaviors such as freezing or playing dead, the phylogenetically *newer* branch facilitates phylogenetically newer behaviors such as prosocial approach. Although this theory offers a mechanism for some specificity in physiological responses, such specificity does not address the larger number of emotional reactions a human being may experience.

Unfortunately, studies that *have* examined the psychophysiological specificity of more discrete emotional states have generally yielded inconsistent results, depending on the paradigms used and the intensity of emotions studied, as well as likely other, not fully understood factors. As an example of such inconsistencies, Table 4.2 presents profiles of two autonomic indices (i.e., heart rate and skin conductance) associated with the six basic human emotions found in two different studies (Hamm, Schupp, & Weike, 2003; Levenson, Ekman, Heider, & Friesen, 1992).

Neuroanatomic Substrates

Given that species-specific emotional displays and autonomic responses are present in all vertebrates and occur automatically, it follows that the majority of the substrates that control these processes would be located in phylogenetically older parts of the brain. Although this is particularly true for species-specific skeletal responses, the control of autonomic responses is distributed throughout the central nervous system, including the diencephalon, the midbrain, the lower brainstem, as well as the cerebral cortex. We examine these regions in turn below, discussing each area's role in both emotional–skeletal and autonomic/endocrine motor control. See Figure 4.2 for a stylized overview of the relative neuroanatomic locations of the relevant subcortical structures.

TABLE 4.2. Profile of Autonomic Changes Assessed by Two Indices across Six Basic Emotions in Humans

	Heart rate decreases		Skin conductance increases	
	Levenson et al. (1992)	Hamm et al. (2003)	Levenson et al. (1992)	Hamm et al. (2003)
Happiness	Middle	Low	Low	Middle
Sadness	High	Middle	High	Low
Fear	High	Middle	High	High
Anger	High	High	Middle	Low
Disgust	Low	High	High	High
Surprise	Middle	High	Low	High

Note. Based on Levenson et al. (1992) and Hamm et al. (2003).

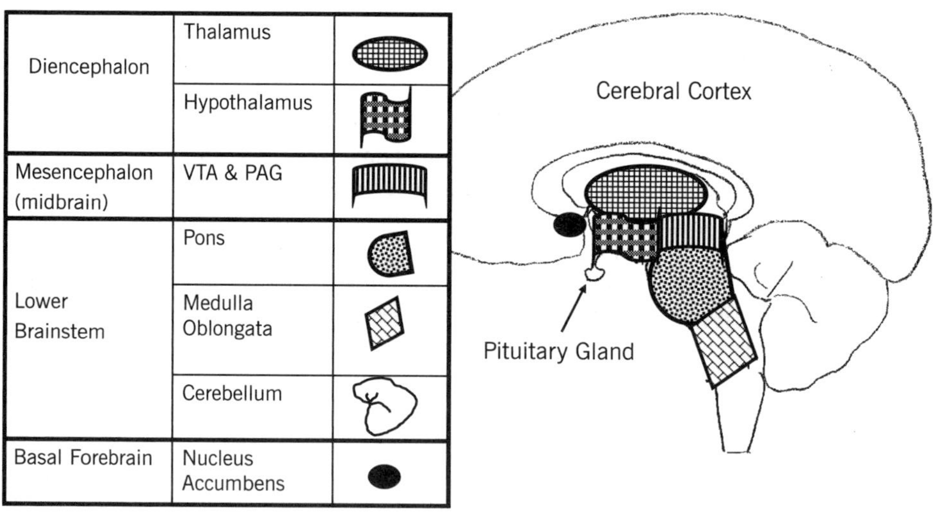

FIGURE 4.2. The general location of structures important for species-specific emotional responses within primary brain subdivisions. *VTA* stands for *ventral tegmental area* and *PAG* stands for *periaqueductal gray matter*, both of which are located in the mesencephalon.

Hypothalamus as the Emotional Relay

The hypothalamus is ideally located in the center of the brain for receiving information from the principal emotional trigger, that is, the amygdala. Also, as discussed in Chapter 3, it contains triggers within itself in the form of receptors for substances (e.g., hormones, neuropeptides, neurotransmitters) that provide specific information about various aspects of homeostasis. See Table 4.3 for an overview of the many hypothalamic nuclei and their role in homeostasis.

After receiving a message from an emotional trigger, the hypothalamus orchestrates a well-synchronized behavioral and autonomic response, which includes (1) activation of affective motor nuclei (located in the midbrain and the lower brainstem) that control species-specific involuntary

TABLE 4.3. The Primary Functions of Hypothalamic Nuclei

Hypothalamic nuclei	Function
Dorsomedial nucleus	Gastrointestinal stimulation
Posterior hypothalamus	Increased blood pressure Pupilary dilation Shivering
Perifornical nucleus	Hunger Increased blood pressure Rage
Ventromedial nucleus	Satiety Neuroendocrine control
Mammillary bodies	Feeding reflexes
Arcuate nucleus and periventricular zone	Neuroendocrine control
Lateral hypothalamic area	Thirst and hunger
Paraventricular nucleus	Oxytocin release Water conservation
Medial preoptic area	Bladder contraction Decreased heart rate and blood pressure
Posterior preoptic area and anterior hypothalamic areas	Body temperature, sweating, panting Thyrotropin inhibition
Supraoptic nucleus	Vasopressin release

Note. For a more detailed review of the functions subserved by various hypothalamic nuclei, see Guyton and Hall (2005).

skeletal motor responses, (2) sympathetic activation via a cascade of hormonal releases by the hypothalamus and the pituitary gland, and (3) direct sympathetic or parasympathetic activation via synapses within the autonomic nuclei in the brainstem and the spinal cord (e.g., the dorsal motor vagus nucleus, nucleus ambiguous, and superior salivary nucleus located in the brainstem; and the preganglionic sympathetic neurons located in the spinal cord). A more detailed discussion of the target structures that play key roles in reflexive motor responses follows.

Mesencephalon

AGGRESSION

Aggression is an example of a species-specific response that is often among the most stereotyped and recognizable. Two main classes of aggressive behavior have been consistently dissociated with respect to both neuroanatomic networks and autonomic and behavioral responses. These are (1) *predatory aggression*, which some authors prefer calling predatory "attack," and (2) *affective aggression*, which includes defensive aggression as well as aggression motivated by competition for resources, such as sexual mates, territory, or social dominance.

Predatory aggression and affective aggression rely on somewhat different brain circuitry and are autonomically and behaviorally mutually incompatible. In particular, predatory aggression is associated with calm, goal-directed behavioral actions designed for successful stalking or hunting of a prey. Typically, there is no vocalization or other behaviors that would warn the prey of the predator's presence, and there is minimal sympathetic activation, except for a dilation of pupils. In contrast, affective aggression is associated with frantic behavioral response designed to maximize one's presence and thus intimidate the competitor. As such, affective aggression tends to be associated with loud vocalization, aggressive posturing, and much sympathetic activation, including piloerection, increased cardiac output, constriction of surface blood vessels, increased blood flow to skeletal muscles and the brain, and decreased flow to the gastrointestinal tract (Folkow, 1993).

Because of the mutually incompatible nature of the behavioral and autonomic responses associated with the two types of aggression, each type is associated with a distinct neuroanatomic network in the periaqueductal gray (PAG) matter and the ventral tegmental area (VTA), both of which are located within the mesencephalon. To prevent occurrences of both predatory and affective responses at the same time, each network receives afferents from a different nucleus in the hypothalamus (i.e., the medial vs. the lateral hypothalamus). The two nuclei in turn communicate with each other via reciprocal inhibitory interneurons, making it impossible for both networks to be activated simultaneously (Bhatt, Bhatt, Zalcman, & Siegel, 2008; Siegel & Shaikh, 1997). Once activated, the respective networks then communicate with the brainstem nuclei, which control appropriate autonomic responses.

In addition to aggressive responses, the mesencepahlon also plays a role in defensive nonaggressive behaviors, such as freezing or escape. The networks that control these responses overlap with the networks that control defensive aggression, and the neuroanatomic dissociation of the specific behavioral responses (i.e., defensive aggression vs. escape) are not well understood. See Table 4.4 for the primary components of these networks.

APPETITIVE BEHAVIORS

In addition to being involved in aggression, the VTA is the source of the mesolimbic dopaminergic system, which projects along the medial fore-

TABLE 4.4. Hypothalamic Networks Involved in Basic Species-Specific Behaviors

Species-specific behaviors	Hypothalamic nuclei	Other brain structures
Flight	Ventromedial Dorsal premammillary	Dorsal PAG
Defensive aggression	Ventromedial Dorsal premammillary	Dorsolateral PAG
Predatory aggression	Perifornical lateral	Ventrolateral PAG VTA
Feeding	Lateral hypothalamic area Arcuate nucleus Paraventricular	VTA Nucleus accumbens Anterior cingulate Ventromedial prefrontal cortex Striatum Ventral pallidum Temporal cortex Cerebellum Area postrema
Sexual behavior	Ventromedial Anterior lateral Paraventricular Medial preoptic area	Olfactory bulb Nucleus accumbens Cerebellum Nucleus paragigantocellularis

Note. VTA, ventral tegmental area; PAG, periaqueductal gray matter. See Guyton and Hall (2005) for more extensive review.

brain bundle and synapses in the nucleus accumbens (NAc), ventral pallidum (VP), and ventral prefrontal cortex (Palmiter, 2007). This system contributes to reward and motivation networks that are necessary for normal appetitive behaviors such as feeding and mating (Kippin, Sotiropoulos, Badih, & Pfaus, 2004). In fact, in animal studies, complete blockage of mesolimbic dopamine leads to starvation (Faure, Reynolds, Richard, & Berridge, 2008) and a failure to engage in mating (Kippin et al., 2004). However, the mesolimbic dopamine system itself is only responsible for motivating these behaviors (see Chapter 9), whereas the *execution* of the behaviors relies on more complex motor and autonomic networks (Arendash & Gorski, 2007; Coolen, Allard, Truitt, & McKenna, 2004; Edmonds & Edwards, 1998; Schmahmann, 2001). See Table 4.4 for summary of known components of these networks.

Lower Brainstem

PONS

In addition to the complex behavioral responses associated with aggression and various appetitive behaviors, certain discrete species-specific vocalizations, such as laughter and crying, are controlled by the lateral pontine reticular formation. Within this general area, there appears to be a functional division between the dorsal structures, which play a role in nonvolitional vocalizations, and ventral structures, which seem to be important for volitional, nonemotional production of laughing or crying sounds. As a consequence, strategically located pontine lesions in the ventral region of the pons can result in a paresis of volitionally generated vocalizations, while the nonvolitional responses remain intact. In contrast, lesions in the dorsal region can result in muted genuine emotional vocal expressions, accompanied by a normal ability to vocalize volitionally (Wild, Rodden, Grodd, & Ruch, 2003).

MEDULLA OBLONGATA

The lower brainstem, in general, and the medulla oblongata, in particular, are the locations of important motor nuclei that receive afferents from the hypothalamus and from the mesencephalic structures and send efferents to organs and glands that control the basic vegetative functions of the body. The most notable among these are the nucleus ambiguous, salivary nucleus, and the dorsal motor nucleus. Disruption of the normal function of these nuclei can lead to abnormal physiological reactivity in the context of emotional responding. Importantly, damage to these nuclei results in disconnection of the central control of the bodily functions that are crucial for survival, with potentially lethal consequences (Guyton & Hall, 2005).

CEREBELLUM

Although traditionally the cerebellum has been viewed as primarily a motor structure, it is now well understood that it contributes, in important ways, to many cognitive processes as well. Additionally, direct reciprocal connections between the cerebellum and the hypothalamus have been discovered. These are hypothesized to play a role in cerebellar involvement in feeding behavior and autonomic control (Schmahmann, 2001; Zhu, Yung, Chow, Chan, & Wang, 2006).

Cerebral Cortex

ANTERIOR CINGULATE CORTEX AND AUTONOMIC REGULATION

In recent years, increasing evidence points to the role of the frontal lobes in autonomic regulation. This research does not refer to the conscious, effortful, top-down regulation of emotions that is discussed in Chapter 7 of this book. Rather, it refers to unconscious regulation of basic autonomic processes.

In particular, the anterior cingulate cortex (ACC), possibly via its connections with the hypothalamus, PAG, and pontine gray matter, has been shown to play a role in the sympathetic regulation of cardiac functions in both humans and laboratory animals (Critchley, Elliott, Mathias, & Dolan, 2000; Critchley et al., 2003; Loewy & Holstege, 1991; Ter Horst, Hautvast, De Jongste, & Korf, 1996), with ACC damage leading to blunted sympathetic activation (Critchley et al., 2003).

HEMISPHERIC ASYMMETRY AND AUTONOMIC REGULATION

Several lines of research have demonstrated hemispheric asymmetry with respect to autonomic control. In particular, there is evidence that the right hemisphere contributes to the control of the sympathetic branch of the ANS, whereas the left hemisphere contributes to the control of the parasympathetic branch (Hugdahl, 1996; Spence, Shapiro, & Zaidel, 1996; Wittling, Block, Schweiger, & Genzel, 1998; Yoon, Morillo, Cechetto, & Hachinski, 1997). This hemispheric asymmetry is consistent with lateralized control of cardiac functions. For example, a respiratory heart rate variability, known to be controlled by the parasympathetic branch, appears to decrease following left-hemisphere lesions (Yoon et al., 1997). In contrast, myocardial contractibility, known to be controlled primarily via the sympathetic branch of the ANS, appears to be under the control of the right cerebral hemisphere (Wittling, 1997). Consistent with this division of control, stimulation of the left insular cortex has been shown to lead to bradycardia, whereas stimulation of the right insular cortex leads to tachycardia (Oppenheimer, 1992). Finally, patients with right-hemisphere lesions, irrespective of etiology (e.g., traumatic brain injury or cardiovascular accident), have been shown to exhibit sympathetic hypoactivation as compared to patients with left-hemisphere lesions (Andersson & Finset, 1998).[2]

Interplay with Cognition

Although a deficit in generating nonvolitional skeletal motor responses is unlikely to have an impact on cognition, *autonomic* dysregulation can affect cognition considerably. Recall the inverted U of the Yerkes–Dodson law (Yerkes & Dodson, 1908), which shows that optimal performance requires optimal (i.e., neither too high nor too low) levels of autonomic arousal. Of course the importance of arousal for attentional and executive control is well recognized. In fact, there is evidence that the simple act of goal-oriented thinking facilitates sympathetic activation; in other words, goal *setting* facilitates autonomic arousal, which in turn optimizes the executive and attentional control processes needed for goal *attainment* (Gellatly & Meyer, 1992).

In light of the evidence that the ACC and the right hemisphere are crucial for maintenance of sympathetic activation, one might wonder to what extent the well-known role of these substrates in attention is, in fact, secondary to their role in arousal. For example, the virtually ubiquitous activation of the anterior cingulate gyrus in fMRI research is typically attributed to the attentional demands of a task (Osaka, Komori, Morishita, & Osaka, 2007; Weiss et al., 2007), but could, in reality, reflect an activation of the sympathetic nervous system that is needed for task performance.

Lastly, generalized right-hemisphere dysfunction, which can be evident by poorer performances on visuospatial measures, has been shown to be predictive of greater long-term mortality rates among healthy older adults, presumably due to its correlation with poorer sympathetic control (Royall, Chiodo, Mouton, & Polk, 2007).

INTEGRATING THEORY AND PRACTICE

Dysregulation of the reflexive emotional response (whether skeletal or autonomic/endocrine) can have several implications for clinical neuropsychological practice. In this next section, we first review syndromes that directly stem from a dysfunction within the skeletal and autonomic/endocrine branches of the reflexive emotional response system. Second, we examine clinical populations that are at risk for manifesting such syndromes. Lastly, we examine assessment implications.

Clinical Signs and Syndromes

Skeletal Branch

PSEUDOBULBAR AFFECT

Pseudobulbar affect (PBA) is a disorder characterized by episodes of uncontrollable laughing and crying that tend to be incongruent with the patients' emotional experience. It represents one of the most dramatic examples of the dissociation between the voluntary motor system and the emotional motor system. This disorder is a consequence of a neurological insult that interferes with downward regulation of emotional responses via cortico-hypothalamic or corticobulbar tracts. Thus, PBA has been associated with bilateral or unilateral lesions in frontal cortical and subcortical structures, as well as the brainstem (Achari & Colover, 1976; Kim, Choi, Kwon, & Seo, 2002; Rosen & Cummings, 2007). Common etiologies include stroke, amyotrophic lateral sclerosis (ALS), multiple sclerosis (MS), degenerative illness such as Alzheimer's disease, and traumatic brain injury (Rosen & Cummings, 2007).

The uncontrollable nature of PBA often leads patients to curtail social and recreational activities so as to avoid public embarrassment, resulting in a considerable decline in quality of life. Although there are no currently approved Food and Drug Administration (FDA) therapies for PBA, a number of pharmaceuticals have proven helpful in ameliorating symptoms, including antidepressants (tricyclic and selective serotonin reuptake inhibitors) as well as agents containing dextromethorphan and quinidine, particularly if combined and particularly for patients suffering from ALS or MS (Iannaccone & Ferini-Strambi, 1996; Miller & Panitch, 2007).

GELASTIC SEIZURES

Gelastic seizures (GS) are characterized by brief periods of laughter (up to 30 seconds) that can be difficult to distinguish from natural laughter, and as such can go undiagnosed for some time (Daly & Mulder, 1957). In some cases, however, the laughing episodes can last longer, and cases of gelastic status epilepticus have also been described (Glassman, Dryer, & McCartney, 1986). GS can occur in the context of a number of different types of seizures, including partial seizures with motor symptoms, generalized convulsive seizures, and petit mal absences (Loiseau, Cohadon, & Cohadon, 1971), and are characteristic of hypothalamic hamartoma (see the "Clinical Populations" section below).

FOU RIRE PRODROMIQUE

Fou rire prodromique (FRP) is another type of inappropriate laughter, sometimes followed by giggling or crying. It occurs for a relatively circumscribed period of time (approximately 30 minutes) and typically represents the first symptom of a cerebral vascular accident. As the stroke evolves, the laughter is replaced by more typical neurological signs of an infarction. This extremely rare syndrome has been associated with a variety of lesion locations, including ventral brainstem, frontal cortex, temporal lobe structures, and the thalamus and hypothalamus (Uzunca, Utku, Asil, & Celik, 2005; Wild et al., 2003).

FOIX–CHAVANY–MARIE SYNDROME

Foix–Chavany–Marie (FCM) syndrome, also known as *frontal opercular syndrome*, is characterized by dysarthria and paresis of cranial nerves, resulting in the inability to generate facial expressions volitionally. However, nonvolitional reflexive emotional displays are intact. This disorder is typically associated with cerebrovascular accidents (Wild et al., 2003).

FACIAL EMOTIONAL PARESIS

Facial emotional paresis (FEP) is a condition in which there is damage to the networks that control the involuntary emotional motor system, rendering patients unable to generate natural, genuine emotional expressions, although their ability to generate a smile volitionally is still preserved (Hopf et al., 1992). Because the condition typically affects the inferior facial muscles, the ability to generate a genuine smile is the most impaired. This condition has been described in conjunction with a variety of lesion locations, including descending pyramidal tracts, the posterior limb of the internal capsule, the mesencephalon, the pons, and the upper medulla oblongata (Cerrato et al., 2003; Hopf et al., 1992; Hopf, Fitzek, Marx, Urban, & Thoemke, 2000).

Autonomic/Endocrine Branch

AUTONOMIC (OR VISCERAL) SEIZURES AND AURAS

Autonomic seizures are typically associated with temporal lobe epilepsy and are characterized by autonomic ictal signs or auras. Epigastric or abdominal auras are among the most common symptoms of partial seizures, and can sometimes include nausea and vomiting (Sekimoto, Kato, Kaneko, & Onuma, 2007). Other symptoms include cardiovascular, respiratory, pupillary, genital, urinary, and pilomotor symptoms (Devinsky, 2004; Fogarasi, Janszky, & Tuxhorn, 2006). Ictal sympathetic activation (including tachycardia) is very common and may occur in as many as 85% of cases of complex partial and tonic–clonic seizures (Devinsky, 2004). Autonomic postictal dysregulation, particularly when affecting cardiac and pulmonary functions, is thought to be the cause of the sudden unexplained death in epilepsy patients (SUDEP) syndrome (Devinsky, 2004).

AUTONOMIC FAILURE

Autonomic failure (AF) refers to autonomic dysregulation caused by an imbalance between the sympathetic and parasympathetic branches of the ANS. Typically, both branches are affected, with the exception of the selective sympathetic disturbance of postural orthostatic tachycardia syndrome (POTS), which presents with excessive heart rate increases upon assuming an upright posture. Symptoms of AF include nausea, dizziness, fainting, syncope, visual disturbance, chest pain, fatigue, sexual dysfunction, and constipation and urinary retention, as well as dysregulation of blood pressure, heart rate, and respiration. Orthostatic hypotension can interfere with functional independence, and it has been suggested that the so-called standing time (i.e., time a person can stand without needing to sit down again[3]) can be used to determine the degree of functional disability (Robertson, 2008).

Usually, AF is associated with a disease of the central nervous system, such as Parkinson's disease, progressive supranuclear palsy, dementia with Lewy bodies, multiple system atrophy, or a cerebrovascular accident (Benarroch et al., 2005; Mabuchi et al., 2005; O'Sullivan et al., 2008; Wallner et al., 2007). In disorders that affect only the peripheral branches of the ANS, such as autoimmune autonomic neuropathy (AAN), the condition is referred to as pure autonomic failure (PAF). AF can also occur secondary to systemic diseases, such as diabetes (Pajouhi, Shaban, & Mohajeri, 2007).

PAROXYSMAL AUTONOMIC INSTABILITY WITH DYSTONIA

Paroxysmal autonomic instability with dystonia (PAID) is a relatively common condition typically associated with severe brain injury due to trauma or anoxia (Blackman, Patrick, Buck, & Rust, 2004). It is characterized by paroxysmal increases in at least five of seven clinical features, including heart rate, respiratory rate, temperature, blood pressure, perspiration, dystonia, and decerebrate posturing (Baguley, Heriseanu, Felmingham,

& Cameron, 2006; Baguley et al., 2007; De Tanti, Gasperini, & Rossini, 2005). It is thought to be caused by disruption of normal communication between the diencephalon and the cortical, subcortical, and brainstem controls of the autonomic nervous system. It can mimic, or mask, potentially life-threatening conditions such as sepsis, impending transtentorial herniation, or status epilepticus, and as such represents a serious and clinically challenging complication during acute and post-acute phases of traumatic brain injury (TBI) recovery (Blackman et al., 2004).

SEROTONIN SYNDROME

Adverse drug reaction to serotonin agonists (e.g., selective serotonin reuptake inhibitors [SSRIs]) caused typically by drug overdose or by interaction of multiple serotonergic agents, has been termed the serotonin syndrome. This is a potentially life-threatening condition, characterized by an autonomic hyperactivity that includes tachycardia, altered mental status, and neuromuscular hyperactivity, including tremor, myoclonus, and hyperreflexia (Dvir & Smallwood, 2008).

Clinical Populations

Because of the relatively large number of syndromes characterized by abnormalities in the reflexive emotional response, as well as the relative nonspecificity of these syndromes' etiologies, the association between the above-described syndromes and the neurological disorders described below has been cross-tabulated and is presented in Table 4.5.

Neurodevelopmental Disorders

ATTENTION-DEFICIT/HYPERACTIVITY DISORDER

Attention-deficit/hyperactivity disorder (ADHD) is a neurodevelopmental disorder of attention affecting approximately 3–5% of children. It is characterized by inattentive, hyperactive, and impulsive features. ADHD has been linked to a dysfunction in the right cerebral hemisphere (Casey, Castellanos, Giedd, & Marsh, 1997; Garcia-Sanchez, Estevez-Gonzalez, Suarez-Romero, & Junque, 1997) and the anterior cingulate gyrus (Colla et al., 2008; O'Connell et al., 2009; Smith, Taylor, Brammer, Halari, & Rubia, 2008). Consistent with the notion that these two brain regions also play a role in sympathetic control, research has demonstrated sympathetic *hypo*activation among children with ADHD (Crowell et al., 2006; Lazzaro et al., 1999). Importantly, individuals with ADHD who used biofeedback training to increase their autonomic arousal exhibited not only greater

TABLE 4.5. Summary of Symptoms Associated with Neurological Disorders That Affect the Autonomic/Endocrine and Skeletal–Motor Components of Reflexive Emotional Responses

Disorder	Autonomic/endocrine abnormalities	Skeletal–motor abnormalities
ADHD	Autonomic hypoactivation	N/A
ALS	Mild autonomic dysregulation	PBA
CVA	AF; increased death from cardiac events following right CVA	FRP, FCM, PBA
Epilepsy	Autonomic seizures and auras (primarily temporal lobe epilepsy)	GS
Hypothalamic lesions/tumors	Appetite abnormalities AF Endocrine abnormalities	GS (HH)
MS	AF	FRP, PBA
Neurodegenerative disorders	AF (PD, LBD, MSA)	PBA (LBD, PSP, AD)
Brain injury (trauma or anoxia)	PAID	PBA

Note. AD, Alzheimer's disease; ADHD, attention-deficit/hyperactivity disorder; AF, autonomic failure; ALS, amyotrophic lateral sclerosis; CVA, cerebral vascular accident; FCM, Foix–Chavany–Marie syndrome; FRP, fou rire prodromique; GS, gelastic seizures; HH, hypothalamic hamartoma; LBD, dementia with Lewy bodies; MS, multiple sclerosis; MSA, multiple system atrophy; PAID, paroxysmal autonomic instability with dystonia; PBA, pseudobulbar affect; PD, Parkinson's disease; PSP, progressive supranuclear palsy.

sympathetic activation, but also improved performance on a continuous performance test (O'Connell et al., 2008).

HYPOTHALAMIC HAMARTOMA

Hypothalamic hamartoma (HH) is a rare benign tumor that is located on or near the hypothalamus and often begins to develop during the first trimester of gestation. It tends to be associated with gelastic seizures that begin in infancy. In the first several years of life, the seizures tend to be brief and may go unnoticed. In the second half of the first decade, seizures become more prominent and frequent (Striano, Striano, Sarappa, & Boccella, 2005). Cognition in this population varies, with a large proportion of patients showing severe cognitive impairment (Prigatano et al., 2008;

Quiske, Frings, Wagner, Unterrainer, & Schulze-Bonhage, 2006), as well as severe behavioral problems and aggression (Berkovic et al., 2003). Occasionally, seizure onset does not occur until adulthood (Pearce, 2004).

The seizures associated with HH tend to be pharmacologically intractable, and because of the location of HH, they have traditionally been difficult to treat surgically. However, in recent years, a new minimally invasive surgical intervention has been developed that has shown much promise both with respect to seizure control and to minimal neurological and neurocognitive side effects (Quigg & Barbaro, 2008; Schulze-Bonhage et al., 2008).

In addition to HH, other types of lesions in the third ventricle/hypothalamus (mostly secondary to other types of tumors) can also occur and are usually characterized by appetite disorders and endocrine and autonomic disruptions with or without gelastic seizures, and only rarely personality or social/emotional problems (Weddell, 1994).

Neurodegenerative Disorders

AMYOTROPHIC LATERAL SCLEROSIS

Amyotrophic lateral sclerosis (ALS), also known as Lou Gehrig's disease, is a relatively rare terminal disease characterized by the gradual degeneration of the upper motor neurons. Symptoms include progressive muscle weakness and atrophy throughout the body. Because of the decreased downregulation of affective motor nuclei in the brainstem, pseudobulbar affect is a common symptom. Recently, the efficacy of quinine sulfate for controlling pseudobulbar affect in this population has been demonstrated, with patients exhibiting improvement not only in symptoms but also in quality of life and quality of relationships (Brooks et al., 2004).

In addition to pseudobulbar affect, patients with ALS have been shown to exhibit mild, subclinical autonomic dysregulation, suggesting the involvement of the ANS in addition to the skeletal motor system (Dettmers, Fatepour, Faust, & Jerusalem, 1993).

MULTIPLE SCLEROSIS

Multiple sclerosis (MS) is an autoimmune disorder that affects CNS myelin. Autonomic dysfunction is common in MS and tends to become more frequent with longer disease duration (Gunal, Afsar, Tanridag, & Aktan, 2002). Prevalence of autonomic dysregulation varies, with some studies reporting as high as 90% of patients (Gunal et al., 2002), while others reporting lower percentages (e.g., approximately 30% showing sympathetic dysregulation and approximately 20% showing parasympathetic abnormalities; Kodounis, Stamboulis, Constantinidis, & Liolios, 2005). Sympathetic dysregulation, particularly the failure to increase blood pressure to meet the demands of a task, has been shown to correlate with reports of fatigue (Flachenecker et al., 2003; Lebre, Mendes, Tilbery, Almeida, & Neto, 2007).

MULTIPLE SYSTEM ATROPHY

Multiple system atrophy (MSA) is an umbrella term for striatonigral degeneration, Shy–Drager syndrome, and olivopontocerebellar atrophies, all of which were found to be histopathologically related. All of these are progressive degenerative disorders affecting the basal ganglia, cerebellum, pons, and medulla oblongata, as well as autonomic neurons in the brainstem and spinal cord. MSA is characterized by autonomic failure, parkinsonism, and ataxia. Autonomic failure in MSA is typically caused by the depletion of sympathetic *pre*ganglionic neurons in the spinal column (which differentiates it from Parkinson's disease, see below), and a dysfunction of the medullary serotonergic system involved in regulation of cardiovascular and respiratory functions (Tada et al., 2009). Patients who present with autonomic failure early in the course of the disease and who exhibit medullary dysfunction are more likely to show shorter disease duration and are at risk for sudden death (O'Sullivan et al., 2008; Tada et al., 2009).

PARKINSON'S DISEASE

Parkinson's disease (PD) is a neurodegenative condition characterized by degeneration of the substantia nigra, leading to a profound depletion of dopamine and a dysfunction of motor control. In addition, patients with PD exhibit what is known as "masked" faces—that is, a face that is bereft of the normal range of emotional expressiveness produced spontaneously among healthy individuals.

It has previously been suggested that patients with PD are able to produce facial expressions volitionally, despite their difficulties with spontaneous, involuntary facial expressiveness (Rinn, 2007). A recent study challenged this notion, demonstrating that volitional facial expressions are reduced and slowed among patients with PD as compared to controls (Bowers et al., 2006). However, this study also confirmed that patients with PD do *not* exhibit facial paralysis. Thus, the degree to which this patient population represents an example of a dissociation between volitional and emotional motor systems remains unclear.

Additionally, PD can be associated with autonomic dysfunction, with prevalence reports ranging from 14 to 80%, depending on methodology. Autonomic symptoms can make PD difficult to differentiate from MSA, although recent research has identified markers that can differentiate the two disorders. In particular, in PD, *post*ganglionic sympathetic lesions (e.g., cardiosympathetic denervation) are a common cause of autonomic dysfunction; importantly, such lesions are thought to be absent in MSA (recall that *pre*ganglionic lesions are typical for MSA). Lastly, in PD, a secondary dysautonomia (particularly orthostatic hypotension) is common due to medication side effects. For a review, see Ziemssen and Reichmann (2010). See Table 4.6 for an overview of autonomic presentation in MSA and PD.

Other Neurological Disorders

SEIZURE DISORDER

As already described above, *temporal lobe epilepsy* can be associated with autonomic seizures. Given the presumed lateralization of the ANS, the question arises whether such signs may be used to aid in seizure lateralization. In a study that examined 416 patients with pharmacoresistant temporal lobe epilepsies who subsequently underwent a neurosurgical intervention, 16 patients presented with parasympathetic signs, such as cold shivers or goosebumps, as part of their aura or ictal presentation. Of the 16, 13 patients had seizures lateralized to the left hemisphere (Stefan, Pauli, Kerling, Schwarz, & Koebnick, 2002), consistent with the notion that the left hemisphere controls the parasympathetic branch of the ANS. Although one

TABLE 4.6. Comparison of Autonomic Failure Patterns in Multiple System Atrophy and Parkinson's Disease with Autonomic Failure

	MSA	PD with AF
Causes of AF	Degeneration of preganglionic neurons Medullary dysfunction	Degeneration of postganglionic neurons
Subjective AF complaints	Present	Present
AF symptom progression	Fast	Slow
Objective AF symptoms		
Orthostatic hypotension	Almost invariably present	Common
Anhidrosis (inability to sweat)	Diffuse	Absent or distal regions of limbs (fingers, toes)

Note. AF, autonomic failure; MSA, multiple system atrophy; PD, Parkinson's disease. Note that a wide range of AF symptoms can be seen in both populations. The table presents only select characteristics that can be useful for differential diagnosis. Based on Lipp et al. (2009).

other study did *not* find lateralized effects of autonomic seizures, in that study, shivers and piloerection were not examined (Fogarasi et al., 2006).

CEREBRAL VASCULAR ACCIDENTS

Because the symptoms associated with cerebral vascular accidents (CVAs) depend on the location of the infarction in the brain, there is of course great variability in the clinical presentations seen among patients with CVAs. Nevertheless, given the complexity and wide distribution of the networks that control reflexive emotional responses, a relatively large proportion of ischemic and hemorrhagic infarcts is associated with the syndromes described earlier in this chapter.

Most notably, sympathetic cardiac dysregulation has been associated with lesions in the brainstem (Strittmatter et al., 2003) and anterior cingulate cortex (Critchley et al., 2003), and right insular strokes, in particular, have been linked to severe asystolia (Rey, Cereda, & Michel, 2008). In fact, patients with right-hemisphere strokes in general (Aszalos, Barsi, Vitrai, & Nagy, 2002) and right insular strokes in particular (Colivicchi, Bassi, Santini, & Caltagirone, 2004) have a poorer long-term prognosis and a greater rate of death from cardiac complications. Other symptoms associated with these types of lesions are fatigue and a lack of drive (Manes, Paradiso, & Robinson, 1999). Interestingly, right-hemisphere lesions have also been associated with parasympathetic dysregulation in some studies (Erciyas et al., 1999; Strittmatter et al., 2003). Importantly, autonomic cardiac dysregulation following a brain insult has been suspected in sudden cardiac deaths that occur in the absence of structural ischemic or coronary heart disease (Ozdemir & Hachinski, 2008).

In addition to sympathetic dysregulation, strokes can lead to pseudobulbar affect (PBA), particularly following lenticulocapsular, frontocortical, or brainstem lesions (Kim & Choi-Kwon, 2000; Miller & Panitch, 2007). Contrary to popular belief that bilateral involvement is needed for PBA presentations, patients with both bilateral and unilateral lesions have been found to exhibit PBA (Achari & Colover, 1976; Kim et al., 2002; Rosen & Cummings, 2007).

Assessment

Autonomic Arousal and Test Performance

As already alluded to above, the inability to achieve appropriate autonomic arousal can translate into poorer functioning in everyday life, including difficulties with goal attainment and poorer performances in assessment settings. In fact, research has shown that phasic autonomic changes during test performance improve speed and accuracy on a *Continuous Performance Test* (CPT; Barry, Clarke, McCarthy, Selikowitz, & Rushby, 2005) as well as on other, more challenging tasks (Melis & van Boxtel, 2007). Relatedly, biofeedback training that improves autonomic activation has been associated with improved CPT performance (O'Connell et al., 2008). Thus, clinicians need to consider the role of autonomic arousal in the etiology of attentional and executive deficits, as well as of behavioral problems that are characterized by failures to follow through and achieve goals. Rehabilitation interventions directed at "training" the attentional system may consider employing biofeedback for the purpose of improving the sympathetic tone.

Assessment of Skeletal Branch Dysfunction

The *Pathological Laughter and Crying Scale* (PLACS; Robinson, Parikh, Lipsey, & Starkstein, 1993) is an 18-item semistructured interview, with items scored on a 4-point scale from "rarely or not at all" to "frequently." The scale was developed specifically for the purpose of differentiating between pseudobulbar affect (PBA) and major depression or a bipolar disorder, as making a differential diagnosis may sometimes be difficult (Husain, 2005). The PLACS has now been validated with several clinical populations (Robinson et al., 1993; Tateno, Jorge, & Robinson, 2004).

Assessment of Autonomic/Endocrine Branch Dysfunction

The *Composite Autonomic Symptom Scale* (COMPASS; Suarez et al., 1999) is a 169-item self-report scale, assessing problems in the areas of orthostatic and vasomotor (e.g., dizziness, cold clammy hands), secretomotor (e.g., sweating abnormalities, dry mouth), sexual (male only), urinary (e.g., urine leakage, difficulty passing urine), gastrointestinal (e.g., constipation), pupillomotor (e.g., inability to accommodate to light changes), and sleep (e.g., sleep apnea) functioning.

SUMMARY AND CONCLUSIONS

As can be seen from the above section, a dysfunction in the reflexive emotional response can be associated with a variety of brain lesions and neurological disorders. When such a dysfunction affects the emotional skeletal system, the principal concern is quality of life and social/interpersonal functioning. Additionally, in the absence of an existing diagnosis, abnormalities in emotional–skeletal responses can represent the first sign of a serious neurological illness.

In contrast, a dysfunction in the autonomic/endocrine system has implications for cognition and test performance, as well as for physical health and long-term survivor outcomes. Although assessment of autonomic functions is not, of course, under the purview of clinical neuropsychology, it is certainly appropriate for clinical neuropsychologists to recommend that such an evaluation be conducted, so as to help tease apart whether cognitive deficits (particularly in cases involving attentional/executive control) could be explained by poor sympathetic tone.

NOTES

1. The distinction between the two types of a smile has likely been intuitively recognized by people for millennia, but the anatomic distinction between the two was first empirically described in 1862 by a French neuroanatomist, Duchenne de Boulogne; since then, the natural, or genuine, smile has come to be known as the "Duchenne smile."
2. However, some inconsistencies in the literature exist, as some studies have found greater suppression of the parasympathetic branch after right-hemisphere lesions (Erciyas, Topalkara, Topaktas, Akyuz, & Dener, 1999; Strittmatter, Meyer, Fischer, Georg, & Schmitz, 2003). See Braun (2007) for review.
3. Standing time of 30 seconds or less is thought to be associated with significant impairment in functionality, whereas standing time of greater than 1 minute is thought to allow for independent functioning (Robertson, 2008).

CHAPTER 5

Awareness and Understanding of an Emotional Experience

Returning to the picnic scene from Chapters 3 and 4, recall the cascade of events: You were enjoying a pleasant, lazy afternoon at a summer picnic, not a care, not a worry in the world, until, with an abruptness of a lightning bolt out of a blue sky, all of your attentional and physiological resources were consumed by the darting presence of a yellow-jacket. You gasped loudly for air, then, squinting your eyes and baring your teeth, you stiffly backed away from the invader.

While your body acted on impulse and your mind stood still, one of your friends noticed your awkward retreat and ran to your rescue. With the palm of her hand, she swatted the yellow-jacket to the ground, then quickly pinned it with the tip of her shoe, grinding it into the lawn. What happens next?

Next, with the yellow-jacket's demise, your attention is drawn to your own body and mind. You revisualize your actions, from the initial gasp for air to the potentially grotesque retreat from the yellow-jacket's space. You begin to feel self-conscious, as others turn their heads to see what the commotion was all about. As your awareness of the situation increases, your cheeks begin to burn. You become aware of a thin stream of perspiration in the riverbed of your spine, now running downward and collecting above the belt of your jeans. You laugh—briefly, nervously—as you realize that the emotion you are experiencing now is no longer fear, but embarrassment. This ability to be aware of, and to understand, our own emotions is the topic of this chapter.

THEORETICAL BACKGROUND

Defining the Constructs

As is clear not only from the yellow-jacket example but also from some of the early debates and controversies discussed in Chapter 2, emotional experience is multifaceted. On the one hand, it includes our awareness of the skeletal and visceral responses that, frustratingly, take over our bodies without much, if any, volitional contribution from us. The mechanism that detects these responses and brings them into our awareness represents one aspect of emotional experience that we will call *interoceptive awareness*. On the other hand, once interoceptive awareness occurs, it becomes translated into emotional feelings, which in turn become translated into *feeling awareness*. We examine these two aspects of awareness separately below.

Interoceptive Awareness

Interoceptive awareness refers to our ability to detect the physiological responses that take place within our bodies. In other words, it refers to the ability to detect changes in our own heartbeat, breathing patterns, and peristaltic motion, as well as perspiration, temperature, and piloerection on our skin.

The notion that interoceptive awareness is important to the experience of emotions has a long history. It was first proposed by William James (James, 1884), who suggested that the feelings we experience are simply our interpretations of the physiological changes in our bodies (see Chapter 1). Although the James–Lange theory, in its purest form, has since been deemed untestable (Lindsley & Stevens, 1951), it has nevertheless been invoked with some regularity by modern-day researchers. For example, as was detailed in Chapter 1, Schachter and Singer demonstrated that physiological arousal enhances one's emotional experience (Schachter & Singer, 1962). More recent research complements those findings by showing that individuals who are better at *detecting* their own physiological arousal perceive emotional experiences as more intense (Pollatos, Kirsch, & Schandry, 2005b; Pollatos, Schandry, Auer, & Kaufmann, 2007). In contrast, patients with pure autonomic failure (PAF)[1]—that is, patients who are *un*able to generate normal autonomic reactions and who do not receive normal sensory feedback regarding such reactions—exhibit deficits in emotional attributions and subjective feeling states (Heims, Critchley, Dolan, Mathias, &

Cipolotti, 2004). In other words, the awareness of an emotional experience is diminished not only by the inability of the body to trigger (Chapter 3) and generate (Chapter 4) physiological arousal, but also by one's inability to *detect* that such an arousal has taken place.

Feeling Awareness

Feeling awareness refers to the ability to consciously *understand* emotions as well as the ability to *think about* emotions. People with good feeling awareness can discern how they and those around them feel, can label emotions correctly (i.e., anger as anger or happiness as happiness), and can distinguish between physiological arousal that occurs due to illness or physical exertion and arousal that is associated with emotions.

In contrast to people with normal feeling awareness, people with impaired feeling awareness exhibit difficulty identifying emotions not only in themselves but also in others (Mann, Wise, Trinidad, & Kohanski, 1994; Parker, Prkachin, & Prkachin, 2005), do not understand normal or expected emotional responses to various emotional situations (Lane, 1996), and generally underestimate the emotional seriousness of unsafe or interpersonally difficult situations (Luminet, Rime, Bagby, & Taylor, 2004; Vanman, Dawson, & Brennan, 1998). In fact, similar to patients with conversion disorders, people with poor feeling awareness tend to misinterpret physiological arousal in physical, rather than emotional, terms (De Berardis et al., 2007). As a result, they also tend to use fewer emotional words when describing various emotionally arousing situations (Luminet et al., 2004) and exhibit deficiencies in empathy (Guttman & Laporte, 2002; Moriguchi et al., 2007). Importantly, paucity of emotional ideation and expression in these individuals cannot be explained by an impairment in retrieval of emotional words, as they can normally generate emotional words out of the context of a specific emotional situation (Luminet et al., 2004). Last but not least, poor feeling awareness cannot be accounted for by deficits in the emotional trigger mechanism or abnormalities in reflexive emotional responding because people with impaired feeling awareness show normal startle response (Vanman et al., 1998), normal facial reactions to emotional stimuli (Luminet et al., 2004), normal baseline autonomic activity (Luminet et al., 2004; Stone & Nielson, 2001), and essentially normal autonomic arousal in emotional situations (Infrasca, 1997; Luminet et al., 2004).

The Relationship between Interoceptive and Feeling Awareness

Although healthy interoceptive awareness is *necessary* for healthy feeling awareness (Heims et al., 2004), it is certainly *not sufficient*. In other words, although for most healthy individuals interoceptive awareness correlates with feeling awareness (Pollatos, Schandry, et al., 2007), the two processes are separable, such that, at least for some people, keen interoceptive awareness does *not* necessarily translate into good awareness and understanding of their feelings (Winston, Dolan, Manstead, Frijda, & Fischer, 2004). In fact, paradoxically, patients who suffer from *alexithymia*, a disorder characterized by impaired feeling awareness, tend to be keenly aware of their bodily responses (Connelly & Denney, 2007); however, unlike healthy individuals, people with alexithymia perceive their physiological responses as *physical bodily discomfort* rather than as emotions (De Berardis et al., 2007).

The relationship between interoceptive and feeling awareness is depicted in Figure 5.1. Note that higher interoceptive awareness can be associated not only with alexithymia, but also with a greater frequency of anxiety symptoms. Ironically, this is true not only for normally aware individuals (Critchley, Wiens, Rotshtein, Ohman, & Dolan, 2004) but for people with alexithymia as well (De Berardis et al., 2007; Marchesi, Brusamonti, & Maggini, 2000).

Lastly, it has been suggested that feeling awareness benefits not only from interoceptive feedback, but also from feedback generated by the skin

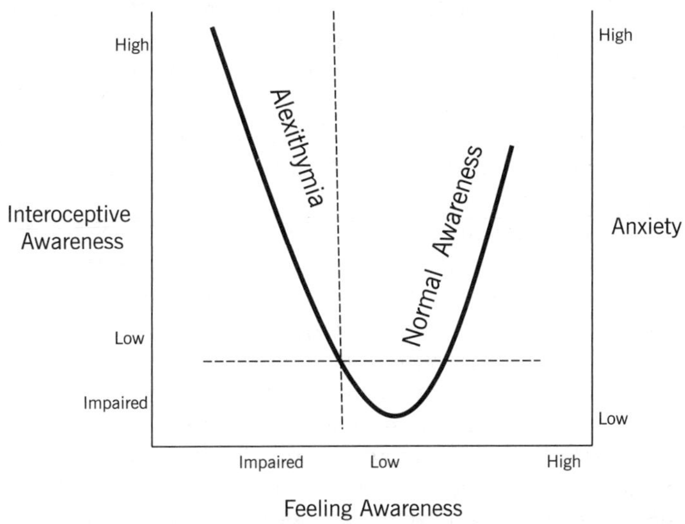

FIGURE 5.1. The relationship between feeling and interoceptive awareness. As can be seen, among normal individuals there is a positive linear relationship between these two constructs. However, among individuals with alexithymia, the opposite is true. Lastly, note that anxiety tends to be higher among individuals with high interoceptive awareness, regardless of their alexithymia status.

and musculature during one's own facial expressions. This latter notion has come to be known as the facial-feedback hypothesis (Izard, 1971; Tomkins, 1962, 1963). Although there is considerable evidence that facial feedback may contribute to the intensity of experienced emotions (Adelmann & Zajonc, 1989; Cappella, 1993; Davis, Senghas, & Ochsner, 2009), there is no clear evidence that it is either necessary or sufficient for good feeling awareness.

Neuroanatomic Substrates

Interoceptive Awareness

As already discussed in Chapter 4, the right cerebral hemisphere plays a crucial role in the regulation of the sympathetic nervous system. It is also the hemisphere that is dominant for somatosensory processing (Lezak, Howieson, & Loring, 2004). It would then follow that the right hemisphere would be dominant for the processing of interoceptive information as well. This, in fact, appears to be the case, as was elegantly shown in a recent series of studies using what is known as the *heartbeat perception paradigm.*

In the heartbeat perception paradigm, participants are typically asked either to attend to their own heartbeat or to judge the degree to which the pace of their heartbeat corresponds to some externally presented rhythm or pace. Studies that have used the heartbeat perception paradigm have demonstrated that people's ability to discern their own physiological states is related to functional and structural features of the right anterior insula and the right frontal operculum. Specifically, simply just *attending* to one's heartbeat activates the right anterior insula and the right operculum, along with the thalamus and somatosensory cortex (Pollatos, Schandry, et al., 2007). Furthermore, the *accuracy* of people's detection of their own heartbeat correlates with the *strength* of activation, of the right anterior insula and operculum (as indicated by an fMRI), as well as with the *volume* of the right anterior insula and operculum (Critchley et al., 2004). Interestingly, individual differences in opercular and insular volume may in part relate to differences in lifestyle, as individuals who practice mindfulness meditation (i.e., a practice that relies on keen perception of internal bodily states) also exhibit larger gray matter volume in the right anterior insula (Hoelzel et al., 2008). Lastly, given that people with alexithymia tend to experience *exaggerated* interoceptive awareness (see Figure 5.1), it should not be surprising that they show greater than normal activation in their right and anterior insula,[2] in response to emotionally significant stimuli (Moriguchi et al., 2007).

Interestingly, the right anterior insula also becomes activated during cardiovascular arousal (Pollatos, Gramann, & Schandry, 2007) and produces heartbeat-evoked potentials[3] (Pollatos, Kirsch, & Schandry, 2005a). However, the interoceptive abilities subserved by this region are *not* limited to heartbeat-related sensations. In fact, the right insula and operculum also appear to play a role in detection of fluctuations in electrodermal activity (Fredrikson et al., 1998), cardiovascular–respiratory activation (Cameron & Minoshima, 2002), and perception of skin temperature (Davis, Pope, Crawley, & Mikulis, 2004). These findings demonstrate that the right anterior insula and the right frontal operculum play a role in interoception in general, rather than in the interoception of only cardiac activity.

It should be noted that the heartbeat perception paradigm has also produced activation in other brain structures, primarily within the frontal lobes (Pollatos et al., 2005a). However, it has been suggested that such activation is more related to *feeling awareness* than to a simple awareness of internal physiological states (Critchley et al., 2004). This notion is discussed next.

Feeling Awareness

The study of the neuroanatomic substrates of feeling awareness has relied on two main approaches: first, the examination of structural and functional abnormalities among individuals with impaired feeling awareness, and second, the examination of functional activation patterns among normally aware individuals while they are experiencing, and are aware of experiencing, different emotional states. The former category relies almost exclusively on the study of alexithymia. We examine this line of research first.

ALEXITHYMIA

Although older theories of alexithymia proposed a variety of psychodynamic causes (McDougall, 1982), it is now clear that frank alexithymia is associated with abnormalities in brain structure and function. In particular, functional imaging studies have shown that individuals with alexithymia, when exposed to emotionally loaded material, exhibit less than normal activation in the dorsolateral prefrontal cortex, pons, and cerebellum (Moriguchi et al., 2007), as well as posterior (Mantani, Okamoto, Shirao, Okada, & Yamawaki, 2005) and anterior (Karlsson et al., 2008) cingulate gyrus. These findings are further buttressed by the association between the severity of alexithymia and the size and/or integrity of the right anterior cingulate gyrus (Guendel et al., 2004; Paradiso, Vaidya, McCormick, Jones, & Robinson, 2008; Schaefer et al., 2007). Furthermore, right-hemisphere abnormalities have also been associated with increased alexithymic symptomatology (Larsen, Brand, Bermond, & Hijman, 2003). Lastly, in addition to the abnormalities in *gray* matter volume or function, alexithymia has been linked to *white* matter dysfunction, most notably to slower interhemispheric transfer (Richter et al., 2006; Zeitlin, Lane, O'Leary, & Schrift, 1989)[4] as well as agenesis (Ernst, Key, & Koval, 1999; Paul et al., 2006) and atrophy (Habib et al., 2003) of the corpus callosum. Together, these findings demonstrate that feeling awareness relies on a complex cortical network, as well as a normal rate of information transfer between the two cerebral hemispheres.

NORMALLY AWARE INDIVIDUALS

The primary approach to the study of feeling awareness among normally aware individuals relies on induction of emotions in subjects undergoing some form of functional neuroimaging. Methods of inducing emotions can be divided into two main categories: (1) induction of emotion via exposure to emotionally salient stimuli, and (2) induction of emotion via the recall of emotional events from one's own life (Berthoz, Blair, Le Clec'h, & Martinot, 2002). Because the effectiveness of these methods, with respect to emotion elicitation, is generally verified by the participants' self-report (Gerrards-Hesse, Spies, & Hesse, 1994; Weiss, Salloum, & Schneider, 1999), it follows that such self-reports speak not only to the validity of the methodology, but, equally importantly, to the notion that emotion elicitation research essentially examines emotional awareness. However, it is important to note that the two methods described above appear to generate somewhat different patterns of brain activation (Gordon, 2003).

On the one hand, the *internally* generated emotions (i.e., recall of emotional events from one's life) are associated with anterior activation, primarily the anterior cingulate gyrus, anterior temporal poles, and orbitofrontal cortex. Because this induction method requires effortful focusing as the participants actively manipulate their own emotional experiences, these patterns of activation also likely relate to emotion regulation, discussed in more detail in Chapter 7. On the other hand, *externally* induced emotions are associated with widespread activation that appears to vary with the type of emotional experience (for reviews, see Berthoz et al., 2002; Reiman et al., 1997), most notably as a function of negative versus positive emotional valence[5] (Pelletier et al., 2003). Because emotional valence has specific implications for survival-related behaviors (i.e., approach vs. withdrawal from a stimulus), several theoretical models that consider the evolutionary importance of positive and negative emotions have been suggested. The two most prominent among these utilize vertical brain organization, on the one hand, and laterality, on the other.

With respect to *vertical* organization, it has been suggested that experience of *negative* emotions tends to rely on more primitive, or phylogenetically older, brain regions, such as the amygdala and the hippocampus, whereas experience of *positive* emotions tends to be associated with activation in phylogenetically newer limbic areas, such as the anterior superior insula, ventral stiatum, and inferior frontal gyrus (Heilman & Zaidel, 1994; Mitterschiffthaler, Fu, Dalton, Andrew, & Williams, 2007). However, these theoretical models are not fully consistent with the literature. In fact, some studies have found that the experience of negative emotions activates the presumed "positive" neural networks, including the insula, the ventral striatum, and ventral frontal cortex. Additionally, ventral frontal activation has been demonstrated during induction of both sad and happy emotions (for a review, see Berthoz et al., 2002).

With respect to *laterality*, it has been suggested that *positive*, prosocial, or approach emotions are more associated with phylogenetically newer cognitive abilities such as language and thus, by extension, the left hemisphere. In contrast, *negative*, self-preservation, or withdrawal emotions are thought to be associated with phylogenetically older functions such as attention and are thus subserved by the right hemisphere (see Borod, 2002, for review). Similar valence-related hemispheric differences have been described for mood and mood disorders; these are discussed in more detail in Chapter 8.

In addition to the presumably distinct networks for positive and negative emotions, there is considerable evidence showing that even individual emotions can be linked to discrete emotional networks. Among the most studied individual emotions are anger, fear, and disgust (see Table 5.1).[6] However, it is not yet clear which, if any, components of the networks are *necessary and sufficient* for the experience and awareness of the corresponding emotions.

In summary, the neuroanatomic substrates necessary for normal experience and awareness of emotions appear to rely, in the very least, on the right anterior insula and opereculum (which together subserve interoceptive awareness), and the right anterior cingulate gyrus and normal hemispheric transfer via the corpus callosum (which together appear important for feeling awareness). Other discrete substrates may be necessary for awareness of individual emotions, although this has been only inferred from research using exposure to different emotional stimuli.

Interplay with Cognition

Interoceptive Awareness

Not much is known about cognition among individuals with poor interoceptive awareness, although it has been suggested that such awareness is crucial for higher-order cognitive processes such as decision making (Ben-

TABLE 5.1. Functional MRI Activation Associated with Presentation of Emotional Stimuli

Activated brain regions	Emotion			References
	Anger	Disgust	Fear	
Amygdala	F	S	F, M, S	Carter & Pelphrey (2008); Hadjikhani & de Gelder (2003); LaBar et al. (2003); Schaefer, Schienle, & Vaitl (2005); Williams et al. (2005)
Anterior cingulate	F	P		Mataix-Cols et al. (2008); Williams et al. (2005)
Caudate nucleus		F		Sambataro et al. (2006)
Globus pallidus		F, P		Mataix-Cols et al. (2008)
Putamen		F		Mataix-Cols et al. (2008)
Superior temporal sulcus	F		F	Carter & Pelphrey (2008); LaBar et al. (2003); Simon, Craig, Miltner, & Rainville (2006)
Middle temporal gyrus	F		S	Carter & Pelphrey (2008); Schaefer et al. (2005)
Fusiform gyrus	F		F, M	Carter & Pelphrey (2008); Hadjikhani & de Gelder (2003); LaBar et al. (2003); Vuilleumier & Pourtois (2007)
Insula		F, P, S	S	Mataix-Cols et al. (2008); Sambataro et al. (2006); Schaefer et al. (2005); Schroeder et al. (2004); Williams et al. (2005); Wright, He, Shapira, Goodman, & Liu (2004)
Orbitofrontal cortex		F, P, S	F, S	Benuzzi et al. (2004); Mataix-Cols et al. (2008); Sambataro et al. (2006); Schaefer et al. (2005); Vuilleumier & Pourtois (2007)

Note. Stimulus types: F, faces; M, body movements; P, photos of objects or situations; S, scenes.

nett, 2009; Herbert & Pollatos, 2008). The principles behind this presumed association are addressed in more detail in Chapter 9.

Feeling Awareness

Research has repeatedly demonstrated that poor feeling awareness (i.e., alexithymia) is related to certain personality characteristics, most notably, higher neuroticism and lower openness to experiences, as assessed by the NEO Personality Inventory (Bagby, Taylor, & Parker, 1994; Luminet, Bagby, Wagner, Taylor, & Parker, 1999). Interestingly, high neuroticism and low openness to experience have also been shown to be related to poorer executive functioning (Williams, Suchy, & Kraybill, 2010). Additionally, research consistently shows that low openness to experience is related to lower intelligence (Chamorro-Premuzic & Furnham, 2008; Holland, Dollinger, Holland, & MacDonald, 1995; Wainwright, Wright, Luciano, Geffen, & Martin, 2008). Given these findings, it should not be surprising that alexithymia, too, tends to be associated with somewhat lower intellectual (Valdes, Jodar, Ojuel, & Sureda, 2001) and executive abilities (Xiong-Zhao, Xiao-Yan, & Ying, 2006), as well lower educational and occupational achievement (Chinet, Bolognini, Plancherel, Stephan, & Halfon, 1998; Jin, Mai, & Ding, 2001; Lunazzi de Jubany, 2000; Saarijarvi, Salminen, Tamminen, & Aarela, 1993; Salminen, Saarijarvi, Aarela, Toikka, & Kauhanen, 1999; S. S. Smith, 2006). With respect to other neurocognitive functions, research suggests that some individuals with alexithymia exhibit poor memory for emotional content, although memory for nonemotional material is thought to be normal (Luminet, Vermeulen, Demaret, Taylor, & Bagby, 2006; Vermeulen & Luminet, 2009).

INTEGRATING THEORY AND PRACTICE

Clinical Signs and Syndromes

Alexithymia

As already mentioned, alexithymia is a syndrome characterized by a deficit in the ability to consciously experience, identify, understand, and describe emotions (Taylor, 1984), in the context of normal (or even exaggerated) ability to exhibit, and be aware of, the physiological arousal stemming from encounters with emotionally salient stimuli (Infrasca, 1997; Luminet et al., 2004). Because people with alexithymia generally underestimate the seriousness of emotional situations (Luminet et al., 2004; Vanman et al., 1998) and have difficulty understanding emotions not only in themselves but also in others (Mann et al., 1994; Parker et al., 2005), it is not surprising that they also exhibit deficiencies in empathy (Guttman & Laporte, 2002; Moriguchi et al., 2007) and, consequently, poor interpersonal relations. In addition to problems with feeling awareness and empathy, individuals who are characterized by alexithymia also exhibit a number of other psychological symptoms (Taylor, 1984; Warnes, 1986), some of which may, to some extent, overlap with those seen among individuals with Asperger syndrome (Fitzgerald & Molyneux, 2004). A summary of symptoms shared by the two disorders can be seen in Table 5.2.

Alexithymia commonly occurs in conjunction with neurological illness and/or acquired brain lesions (Becerra, Amos, & Jongenelis, 2002; Henry, Phillips, Crawford, Theodorou, & Summers, 2006; Koponen et al., 2005; Schafer et al., 2007; Williams et al., 2001), and as such is commonly seen in populations undergoing neuropsychological evaluations. However, alexithymic tendencies can also be found in non-neurological populations and are then considered a personality trait. As such, they are often associated with an elevation on the Minnesota Multiphasic Personality Inventory (MMPI) Hypochondriasis Scale (Kauhanen, Julkunen, & Salonen, 1991), as well as higher Neuroticism and lower Extraversion and Openness to Experience on the NEO-Personality Inventory (Bagby, Taylor, & Parker, 1994; Luminet et al., 1999).

Given that alexithymia can be seen as a personality trait,[7] it should not be surprising that there are considerable individual differences among healthy individuals with respect to their feeling awareness. Although such variability can be partly accounted for by one's genetic and biological background, it is also partly a function of people's prior experiences and socialization, determined largely by familial and cultural norms (Fischer & Good,

TABLE 5.2. Select Set of Characteristics Exhibited by Patients with Alexithymia and Asperger Syndrome

Alexithymia[a]	Asperger syndrome[b]
Difficulty describing feelings to other people	A failure to share personal feelings and experiences with other people
Awkwardness in nonverbal behavior	Impairments in the use of nonverbal communication (e.g., facial expression, body posture, and gestures)
Constricted imagination and fantasy	Interest restricted to one or few topics
Externally oriented or stimulus-bound cognitive style	Preoccupation with parts of objects

[a]Bagby, Parker, and Taylor (1994).
[b]American Psychiatric Association (2000).

1997). In general, poorer feeling awareness among healthy individuals is associated with lower socioeconomic status, a lower level of education, and male gender (Salminen et al., 1999). With respect to male gender, some readers may be tempted to consider the notion that males have been reported to have smaller corpus callosums than females (de Lacoste-Utamsing & Holloway, 1982; Johnson, Pinkston, Bigler, & Blatter, 1996), which theoretically could account for their lower feeling awareness. However, this notion has been sharply criticized (Hamberg & Lee, 2005; Wallentin, 2009), and meta-analytic research has failed to support sex differences in the corpus callosum size (Dorion, Capron, & Duyme, 2001; Morton & Rafto, 2006). Nevertheless, some studies continue to find differences in brain morphology between males and females (Schneiderman et al., 2007), and the degree to which the sexes do, or do not, differ in terms of interhemispheric connectivity remains a topic of debate and controversy.

Everyday Functioning

Interoceptive Awareness

Interoceptive awareness has increasingly received the attention of health psychologists, as it appears to contribute to life satisfaction and success in everyday life. In particular, interoceptive awareness correlates positively with emotional intelligence (Schneider, Lyons, & Williams, 2005), which in turn relates to job satisfaction (Craig, 2008; Smith, Ciarrochi, & Heaven, 2008; Smith, Heaven, & Ciarrochi, 2008) and general sense of well-being (Extremera & Fernandez-Berrocal, 2002; Gallagher & Vella-Brodrick, 2008; Singh & Woods, 2008; van Heck, den Oudsten, Vingerhoets, Nykicek, & Denollet, 2008). Thus, interventions aimed at improvements of interoceptive awareness, such as engagement in mildfulness meditation, may be indicated for such individuals. Unfortunately, assessments of interoceptive awareness are currently conducted for research purposes only, with no direct clinical application yet available.

Feeling Awareness

Similar to interoceptive awareness, poor feeling awareness (i.e., alexithymia) has begun to figure prominently in behavioral medicine research due to its relationship with life satisfaction and success, as well as with physical and mental health. For example, alexithymia shows associations with poorer quality of life and increased rates of depression and anxiety. This has been demonstrated both in the general population (Henry, Phillips, Maylor, et al., 2006; Mangelli, Semprini, Sirri, Fava, & Sonino, 2006), as well as among patients with alexithymia and lung cancer (Zhou & Xu,

2005), breast cancer (Grassi, Rossi, Sabato, Cruciani, & Zambelli, 2004), renal failure (Fukunishi & Tsurata, 2001; Jin et al., 2001), inflammatory bowel syndrome (Verissimo, Mota-Cardoso, & Taylor, 1998), or substance dependence (Guilbaud et al., 2002). Additionally, even among nonclinical populations, individuals high in alexithymia are characterized by poorer health-related quality of life (Mattila et al., 2009).

Due to the increased rates of depression, anxiety, and stress among individuals with alexithymia, it has been proposed that alexithymia indirectly confers an increased risk for the development of chronic diseases (van Heck et al., 2008) and even an increased mortality (Kauhanen, Kaplan, Cohen, & Julkunen, 1996). Consistent with that notion, alexithymia occurs more commonly among medical populations than in the general public (Jin et al., 2001; Nordby, Ekeberg, Knardahl, & Os, 1995; Wise, Mann, Mitchell, & Hryvniak, 1990) and has been associated with higher rates of psychosomatic illness (Kauhanen et al., 1991). A variety of possible pathways for this association has been suggested, including the possibility that alexithymia may be associated with unhealthy behaviors or may be secondary to illness (Fukunishi & Tsurata, 2001; Lumley et al., 2008).

Assessment

Neurocognitive Assessment

Alexithymia, a disorder of deficient awareness and understanding of feelings, is associated with an increased tendency to experience bodily sensations, leading to panic attacks and anxiety. Thus, during assessment, individuals with alexithymia may experience cognitive problems that are similar to those with an "overactive trigger" described in Chapter 3—that is, becoming easily distracted by their own bodily sensations or narrowing their attention toward potentially threatening situations or stimuli. However, unlike other patients, people with alexithymia may deny feeling anxious and may instead overfocus on reporting unpleasant bodily symptoms such as shortness of breath. To mitigate these problems during assessment, clinicians may need to allow ample time for patients to become at ease, without necessarily labeling patients' reactions as anxiety.

Assessment of Alexithymia

Given the increasing evidence of alexithymia among neurological populations, as well as its association with somatoform illnesses (Bach & Bach, 1996; Stroebel, 1998), depression and anxiety (Henry, Phillips, Maylor, et al., 2006; Hintikka, Honkalampi, Lehtonen, & Viinamaeki, 2001; Mangelli et al., 2006), and poor quality of life (van Heck et al., 2008), there is increased interest in both clinical and research assessments of alexithymia.

Currently, the *Toronto Alexithymia Scale–20* (TAS-20; Bagby, Parker, & Taylor, 1994) represents the instrument of choice for assessment of alexithymia. The most recent version of this instrument has 20 self-report items that load on three factors: "difficulty identifying emotions" (DIE), "difficulty describing emotions" (DDE), and "externally oriented thinking" (EOT) (Bagby, Parker, & Taylor, 1994; Parker, Taylor, & Bagby, 2003; Taylor, Bagby, & Parker, 2003). The DIE factor is likely the most germane to the topic of this chapter, as it is thought to measure difficulties separating bodily sensations from emotions, as well as distinguishing among different types of emotions. In contrast, the DDE factor measures an inability to verbally express emotions, and as such may be more susceptible to cultural and familial norms (Fukunishi, Kawamura, Ishikawa, & Ago, 1997; Le, Berenbaum, & Raghavan, 2002). Finally, *EOT* refers to a cognitive style that is marked by a lack of introspection and fantasy, as well as paucity in thinking about emotions, and as such is characterized by a somewhat concrete style reminiscent of individuals with Asperger syndrome.

The TAS-20 has been normed and extensively validated (Bagby, Taylor, et al., 1994; Luminet et al., 1999; Parker, Bagby, Taylor, & Endler, 1993; Parker, Taylor, & Bagby, 1998; Simonsson-Sarnecki et al., 2000; Taylor, Parker, Bagby, & Bourke, 1996). Although scores on the TAS-20 generally correlate somewhat with depression and tend to decrease over time as depression decreases (Honkalampi, Hintikka, Laukkanen, Lehtonen, & Viinamaki, 2001; Saarijarvi, Salminen, & Toikka, 2001), the two constructs have nevertheless been successfully separated (Marchesi et al., 2000; Muller, Buhner, & Ellgring, 2003). Scores on the TAS-20 have been shown to be relatively stable over a 5-year period (Saarijarvi, Salminen, & Toikka, 2006). Instructions on how to order the TAS-20 can be found at *www.gtaylorpsychiatry.org/tas.htm.*

Clinical Populations

Neurodevelopmental Disorders

Agenesis of corpus callosum is a rare congenital defect in which all or parts of the corpus callosum fail to form functional connections between the two hemispheres. Cases studies (Buchanan, Waterhouse, & West, 1980; Ernst et al., 1999) as well as studies utilizing larger patient samples (Paul et al., 2006) have demonstrated that individuals with agenesis of the corpus callosum exhibit alexithymic symptoms. As is typical of alexithymia, these individuals tend to show normal or exaggerated physiological arousal in response to emotional stimuli, but poor feeling awareness. Misinterpretation of physiological reactions in physical terms, including reports of chronic pain, may also be present (Ernst et al., 1999).

Neurodegenerative Disorders

PARKINSON'S DISEASE

Patients with PD commonly exhibit symptoms of alexithymia, with prevalence rates of about 21%, as compared to about 15% among healthy elderly individuals (Costa, Peppe, Carlesimo, Pasqualetti, & Caltagirone, 2006). In this patient population, alexithymia was found to be a predictor of poorer performances on measures of visuospatial processing (Costa, Peppe, Carlesimo, Salamone, & Caltagirone, 2007) and showed a strong association with depression (Costa et al., 2006).

MULTIPLE SCLEROSIS

Among patients with MS, reports of alexithymia rates vary. For example, one study found a rate that was similar to that of the general population (13%) (Bodini et al., 2008), whereas another study found a prevalence rate of 43% (Chahraoui et al., 2008). Alexithymia symptom severity in this population increases with greater atrophy in the corpus callosum (Habib et al., 2003). Additionally, alexithymia among patients with MS contributes independently to the severity of symptoms of depression and fatigue (Bodini et al., 2008; Gay, Vrignaud, Garitte, & Meunier, 2010). The tendency to report more fatigue among patients with alexithymia is consistent with their general tendencies to overfocus on bodily sensations and to interpret emotions in physical terms.

Other Neurological Disorders

TRAUMATIC BRAIN INJURY

Given that TBI is commonly associated with contusions of the anterior temporal poles and inferior frontal cortex (two regions that have been implicated in feeling awareness), it should not be surprising that symptoms of alexithymia (including diminished empathy) represent common sequelae of TBI (Becerra et al., 2002; Henry, Phillips, Crawford, et al., 2006; Koponen et al., 2005; Schafer et al., 2007; Williams et al., 2001). Reports of prevalence of alexithymia among patients with TBI range between 31% (Koponen et al., 2005) and 57% (Wood & Williams, 2007). Interestingly, among patients with TBI, there appears to be no relationship between alexithymia and the severity of injury or cognitive deficits, with the exception of weaknesses in verbal fluency and sequencing (Henry, Phillips, Crawford, et al., 2006; Wood & Williams, 2007). Consistent with the broader alexithymia literature, alexithymic TBI patients experience poorer quality of life, even after depression and anxiety are accounted for (Henry, Phillips, Crawford, et al., 2006), and alexithymia in this population predicts somatization and emotional disturbance (Wood, Williams, & Kalyani, 2009). Although more research is needed, clinicians are encouraged to assess alexithymia in their patients who have TBI, especially given the high rates of poor physical and mental health, as well as the poor quality of life seen among individuals with alexithymia on the whole.

CEREBRAL VASCULAR ACCIDENT

Right-hemisphere lesions are associated with elevated prevalence (30%) of alexithymia, and patients who simultaneously exhibit both alexithymia and anosognosia tend to also exhibit deficits in executive functions (Spalletta et al., 2007).

Neuropsychiatric Disorders

Alexithymia is a common correlate of a variety of neuropsychiatric disorders, most notably major depression (Honkalampi et al., 2010), schizophrenia (van't Wout, Aleman, Bermond, & Kahn, 2007), PTSD (Spitzer, Vogel, Barnow, Freyberger, & Grabe, 2007), obsessive–compulsive disorder (Grabe et al., 2006), somatization (Mattila et al., 2008), chronic fatigue syndrome (van de Putte, Engelbert, Kuis, Kimpen, & Uiterwaal, 2007), psychopathy (Rogstad & Rogers, 2008), and insomnia (Kronholm, Partonen, Salminen, Mattila, & Joukamaa, 2007). Alexithymia is also associated with addictive disorders (Thorberg, Young, Sullivan, & Lyvers, 2009) and eating disorders (Mazzeo, Mitchell, & Williams, 2008; Ridout, Thom, & Wallis, 2010). Patients with dual diagnosis (e.g., alcohol abuse and depression) exhibit greater severity of alexithymia (Evren, Evren, & Dalbudak, 2009). It has been suggested that alexithymia represents a vulnerability for poor treatment outcome, a notion that has been supported by at least one study with patients who have an eating disorder (Speranza, Loas, Wallier, & Corcos, 2007).

Importantly, among individuals with schizophrenia, alexithymia does not appear to be related to the severity of negative symptoms, suggesting that it represents a distinct construct (Todarello, Porcelli, Grilletti, & Bellomo, 2005). It may, however, represent a vulnerability, as similarly elevated levels of alexithymia were found both among individuals with schizophrenia and their unaffected siblings (van't Wout et al., 2007).

SUMMARY AND CONCLUSIONS

Problems with emotional awareness can be seen in a variety of neurological, medical, and psychiatric populations. The most prominent syndrome is alexithymia, which, somewhat counterintuitively, tends to be associated with keen attention to one's internal physiological changes, as well as psychiatric symptoms such as depression, anxiety, and somatoform disorders. Individuals with alexithymia may be characterized by somewhat lower intellectual functioning, as well as mild weaknesses in executive functioning and emotional memory. Because of the relatively high prevalence of alexithymia in neurological populations, clinicians are encouraged to assess emotional awareness in their patients. Currently, the instrument of choice is the TAS-20, which has been normed for clinical use and extensively validated.

NOTES

1. See Chapter 4 for additional information about autonomic failure.
2. Among people with alexithymia, exposure to emotion-evoking stimuli has also been shown to activate the left anterior insula (Karlsson, Naaanen, & Stenman, 2008).
3. Heartbeat-evoked potential, or HEP, is a brain wave that is contingent on heartbeat.
4. At least one study, however, showed the opposite pattern of results (Grabe et al., 2004).
5. Because the terms *negative* and *positive* are fairly vague, other ways of classifying emotional valence have been suggested, such as "pleasant vs. unpleasant," "approach vs. withdrawal," or "prosocial vs. self-preservation" (for a review, see Borod, Bloom, Brickman, Nakhutina, & Curko, 2002).
6. Much of the research that studies individual emotions relies on simple viewing of affectively expressive human faces. This should not be a problem, as exposure to facial affect has been shown to be sufficient for elicitation of actual *experience and awareness* of the corresponding emotions (Wild, Erb, & Bartels, 2001).
7. Consistent with other personality traits, alexithymia has been shown to be dimensional rather than taxonomic (Parker, Keefer, Taylor, & Bagby, 2008).

CHAPTER 6

Emotional Communication

Now back to our picnic scene discussed in previous chapters: You have just gone through the emotional roller coaster of being affronted by a yellow-jacket, experiencing a flood of bodily and mental sensations, losing your cool in a panicky attempt to retreat, and finally being rescued by a friend who with the bare palm of her hand swatted the yellow-jacket to the ground. Now with the yellow-jacket gone, you become keenly aware that your strong reaction has attracted the attention of others, and that you just may have made a fool of yourself. What will you do next?

Undoubtedly, your next move is to scan the environment to assess the interpersonal damage. To your relief, most everyone is smiling. But not all the smiles are the same: Some appear amused, as if accompanied by a roll of the eye or an incredulous headshake, while others appear sympathetic, as if to say, "I do the same darn thing around yellow-jackets each and every time." You choose to make eye contact with the sympathetic, understanding smiles, telegraphing to them a sheepish, "I know I overreacted. Glad you are still my friend."

The abilities to detect and understand the subtleties of nonverbal emotional reactions of others, and to telegraph one's own reactions to them, are the topics of this chapter.

THEORETICAL BACKGROUND

Defining the Constructs

Emotional communication is a multifaceted construct that can be divided into categories based on (1) the mode of communication (i.e., linguistic vs. paralinguistic vs. situational), (2) the direction of the communication (i.e., receptive vs. expressive), and (3) volitional control. These are described separately below.

The Modes of Affective Communication

Emotional communication can be divided into three modes: (1) linguistic (also known as lexical), (2) paralinguistic, and (3) situational. It has been suggested that the linguistic and paralinguistic aspects of affective communication are contained within the *verbal* and *nonverbal affect lexicons* (Bowers, Bauer, & Heilman, 1993), respectively, and, at least with regard to receptive communication, have been found to correlate with one another (Borod, Pick, et al., 2000). In contrast, the situational mode, which reflects one's ability to understand the emotional contents of situations, has been inconsistently linked to the other modes, with some studies finding associations (e.g., Besel, 2007) and others not (e.g., Carr & Lutjemeier, 2005).

LINGUISTIC (LEXICAL) MODE

The *linguistic mode of affective communication* simply refers to the ability to understand emotional messages that are expressed by language. This does not necessarily mean that patients with deficits in the linguistic affective mode will not understand the meaning of affective words such as *happy*, *sad*, or *angry*. Rather, these individuals have difficulty understanding sentences or words that communicate affective content indirectly. As an example, the statement "he seems to have lost interest in her" communicates sadness or disappointment, without the use of the words *sad* or *disappointed* (Karow, Marquardt, & Marshall, 2001). This is arguably the least well-researched area of emotional communication within the field of affective neuroscience, with extant findings marked by many inconsistencies.

PARALINGUISTIC MODE

The paralinguistic mode of emotional communication simply informs words and grammar with the emotional undertones of what is being communicated. This can occur via a variety of channels (e.g., prosody, gestures, posture, and facial expressions) (Borod et al., 2002). In contrast to the linguistic mode, the paralinguistic mode arguably represents the most studied aspect of emotional communication to date.

Of note, some aspects of paralinguistic communication are nonaffective in nature, such as intonation denoting grammatical concepts (e.g., questions vs. statements), and are sometimes referred to as "linguistic intonation" or "propositional prosody." These nonaffective aspects of paralinguistic communication have been shown to rely on neuroanatomic networks that largely overlap with those of affective paralinguistic communication (Barrett, Pike, & Paus, 2004), except perhaps with a greater tendency to show bilateral involvement (Heilman, Bowers, Speedie, & Coslett, 1984). These nonemotional aspects of prosody are *not* considered further here.

SITUATIONAL MODE

The *situational mode of affective communication* refers to one's knowledge or understanding of the expected emotional correlates of various emotionally loaded situations. For example, seeing a lethal car accident, hearing about a friend's terminal illness, or reading about a devastating earthquake should evoke an understanding of the types of emotional reactions experienced by the victims of these events. Such understanding reflects the person's capacity for *empathy*, which has been conceptualized in two ways: (1) as *emotional empathy*, and (2) as *cognitive empathy*. The first component, emotional empathy, is the capacity to *experience* the feelings that are being experienced by others. It takes place intuitively and consists of a sense of having something in common with others. Emotional empathy is thought to be a product of an "emotional contagion," that is, an implicit mimicry of affective displays of others, which presumably plays a crucial role in "catching" other people's emotions (Doherty, 1997; Hatfield, Rapson, Greco, & Stenner, 2008). The second component, cognitive empathy, is the capacity to evaluate a given situation and arrive at a reasoned understanding of how others might feel. Cognitive empathy is thought to rely on the capacity for perspective taking also known as "theory of mind" (ToM; Premack & Woodruff, 1978).[1] The distinction, and the relationship, between cognitive and emotional empathy has been a topic of much research (A. Smith, 2006), and the dissociation between the two has been demonstrated in both clinical (Dziobek et al., 2008; Rankin, Kramer, & Miller, 2005; Shamay-Tsoory, Aharon-Peretz, & Perry, 2009; Shamay-Tsoory, Tomer, Yaniv, & Aharon-Peretz, 2002) and normal populations (Davis, Hull, Young, & Warren, 1987).

Direction of Affective Communication

Just as verbal communication relies on the ability both to comprehend and to express language, emotional communication reflects a person's ability both to comprehend and to express emotional messages. Comprehension of the emotional meaning behind facial expression, prosody, gestures, and so on, of others is referred to as *receptive* affective communication, and expression of one's own emotional states to others, via facial expression, prosody, gestures, and so on, is referred to as *expressive* affective communication. However, unlike the well-recognized dissociation of the receptive and expressive modules for spoken language, the degree to which receptive versus expressive paralinguistic abilities are dissociated is not clear. On the one hand, there appears to be a dissociation between comprehension versus expression of *prosodic* messages (Nakhutina, Borod, & Zgaljardic, 2006); on the other hand, expression and comprehension of *facial* affect appear closely linked. In fact, it has been suggested that the ability to comprehend facial affect in others relies, in part, on one's own affective expressiveness; in other words, by mimicking facial expressions of others, we presumably receive feedback from the muscles and skin of our own face, which in turn helps us decode the meanings of those expressions (Tomkins, 1962, 1963). Recent interest in the concept of "embodiment" and "embodied emotions" is in line with those earlier theories.

Briefly, according to the theory of embodied emotions, processing and understanding of a particular emotional stimulus is associated with emotional reexperiencing of prior encounters with similar stimuli. This reexperiencing involves not only reactivation of neural networks that were involved in processing of those prior encounters, but also activation of other bodily systems, including facial muscles. Thus, for example, when asked to classify words based on whether or not they were emotionally loaded, participants inadvertently activated facial muscles involved in the corresponding emotional expressions. However, when the same stimuli were classified based on other characteristics (i.e., capital vs. lowercase print), no systematic activation of facial muscles was found (Niedenthal, Winkielman, Mondillon, & Vermeulen, 2009). Based on these findings, it would then appear that *receptive* affective abilities would have to rely on normal *expressive* affective abilities, at least with regard to facial affect. Such a model, of course, is incomplete, since it leaves out the *mechanism* that is responsible for the activation of the relevant facial muscles or neural networks. Although the mirror neuron system, known to play a role in imitation, may be a good candidate for mimicry of facial expressions of others, it cannot explain generation of facial expressions in response to written words.

Importantly, while activation of facial muscles appears to coincide with the act of comprehending affective stimuli, it is not clear that this activation is *necessary* for comprehension to take place. For example, it has been shown that bilateral facial paralysis does *not* preclude one from discriminating the emotional expressions of others (Keillor, Barrett, Crucian, Kortenkamp, & Heilman, 2002). Nevertheless, it is still possible that comprehension of affective stimuli relies on feedback from *neuronal networks* (rather than the facial muscles themselves) that become activated in anticipation of a production of facial expressions, whether the expressions are actually generated or not. Functional imaging research provides additional support for this notion, showing that simple viewing of facial expressions generates a pattern of brain activation that overlaps with the patterns generated by production of facial expressions (van der Gaag, Minderaa, & Keysers, 2007).

Volitional Control: Genuine versus Posed versus Spontaneous Affect

As discussed in Chapters 3 and 4, tripping the emotional trigger leads to a variety of automatic responses, some of which are reflected in changes in one's internal environment (e.g., changes in blood pressure), whereas others are reflected in automatically released, externally observable behaviors. Quite obviously, many of the externally observable behaviors serve the purpose of communicating with others, whether it be sending threatening messages to potential predators, inviting messages to potential mating partners, or danger signals to members of one's social group. These rapid, reflexive behaviors clearly reflect a form of *non*volitional *expressive* paralinguistic communication. Similarly, the rapid, preconscious detection (see Chapter 3) of such hardwired emotional displays by the amygdala clearly represents a form of *non*volitional *receptive* paralinguistic communication.

Although the nonvolitional forms of affective communication undoubtedly contribute to daily emotional discourse, purely reflexive responses such as uncontrollable sobbing or laughter are fairly rare among adult humans. Rather, most of emotional communication that takes place on a daily basis is a function of an interaction between the reflexive, nonvolitional responses and the volitional affective communication system (see Figure 6.1). This is because some degree of top-down control over the nonvolitional emotional responding is virtually always present. Thus, to the extent that one volitionally *chooses to release* reflexive responses, it could be argued that such reflexive responses are, for all intents and purposes, volitional. However, as can be seen in Table 6.1, there are aspects of volitional communication that are distinct from the simple release of a reflexive response. In the remainder of this chapter, only these volitional forms of affective communication are considered.

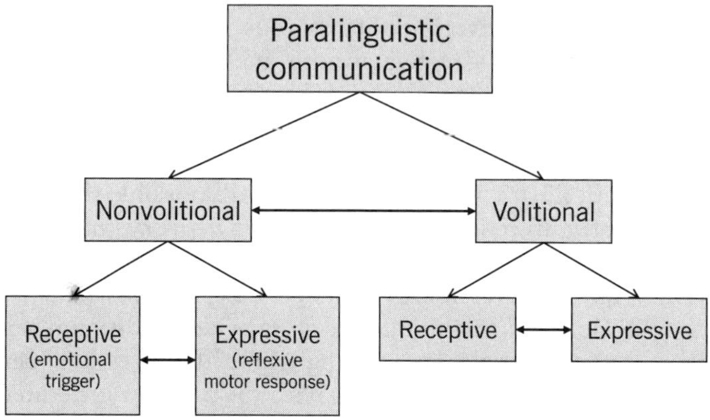

FIGURE 6.1. In their extremes, paralinguistic communications could be purely volitional or purely nonvolitional. However, in everyday life, the two systems interact: On the one hand, there is virtually always some top-down control of nonvolitional aspects of communication; on the other, the volitional aspects of communication rely on contributions from intuitive, unconscious processing of emotional stimuli, as well as reflexive, species-specific motor responses.

TABLE 6.1. Differences between Volitional and Nonvolitional Affective Communication

	Type of affective communication		
Dependent variable	Volitional (posed)	Nonvolitional (genuine)	References
Physiological arousal	Absent or minimal	Present	Boiten (1996)
Emotional experience	Absent or minimal	Present	Boiten (1996)
Facial symmetry	Less symmetric	More symmetric	Ekman, Hager, & Friesen (1981)
Ease of recognition by others	Easier	More difficult	Allen & Atkinson (1981); Gosselin & Kirouac (1995); LaRusso (1978)
Facial muscles	Somewhat different muscle groups engaged in each		Boiten (1996)

A related issue involves whether emotions are generated spontaneously or on command. For example, the *New York Emotion Battery* (Borod, Welkowitz, & Obler, 1992) is designed to assess both *spontaneous* emotional expressiveness (by surreptitiously rating examinees' expressiveness during the evaluation), as well as *posed* expression (by requiring that a person either volitionally mimic affective expressions of others, or generate affective expressions on verbal commands) (Borod et al., 1992). Note that this distinction does not necessarily address the *volitional* dimension.[2] In other words, whereas emotional expressions generated on command are more likely to be almost entirely posed in character (i.e., volitional), spontaneously generated emotional communications likely comprise a mixture of genuine and posed expressions, as is the case for all of our social interactions. Thus, although impairment in the ability to generate emotional expressions spontaneously may provide a clinician with an insight about barriers to a patient's interpersonal functioning, it does not necessarily implicate any particular discrete aspect of emotional processing.

Neuroanatomic Substrates

When considering the substrates of emotional communication, it is once again important to consider the mode (i.e., linguistic, paralinguistic, or situational) and the direction (i.e., receptive vs. expressive) of communication. Because of the complexity of the topic, the organization of the next section is depicted graphically in Figure 6.2. Please note that because the substrates for the purely reflexive affective communication have already been covered in Chapters 3 and 4, they are *not* covered here (i.e., only processes that are under volitional control are considered next).

Linguistic (or Lexical) Mode of Affective Communication

Although, as mentioned before, the linguistic mode of affective communication has received somewhat less attention from affective neuroscientists as compared to the paralinguistic mode, this is not to say that the literature in this area is scant. In fact, the neuroanatomic substrates of affective linguistic communication has drawn attention from several different disciplines, including affective neuroscience (Borod, Bloom, Haywood, Beeman, & Chiarello, 1998), neurolinguistics (Atchley, Stringer, Mathias, Ilardi, & Minatrea, 2007), and aphasiology (Sherratt, 2007). Consequently, there is a range of methodologies, theoretical viewpoints, and basic assumptions, with extant findings considerably inconsistent across studies. On the whole, the take-home message from the literature that is summarized below is that both hemispheres likely play a role in both expressive and receptive lexical affective abilities, with the exact networks not yet well understood.

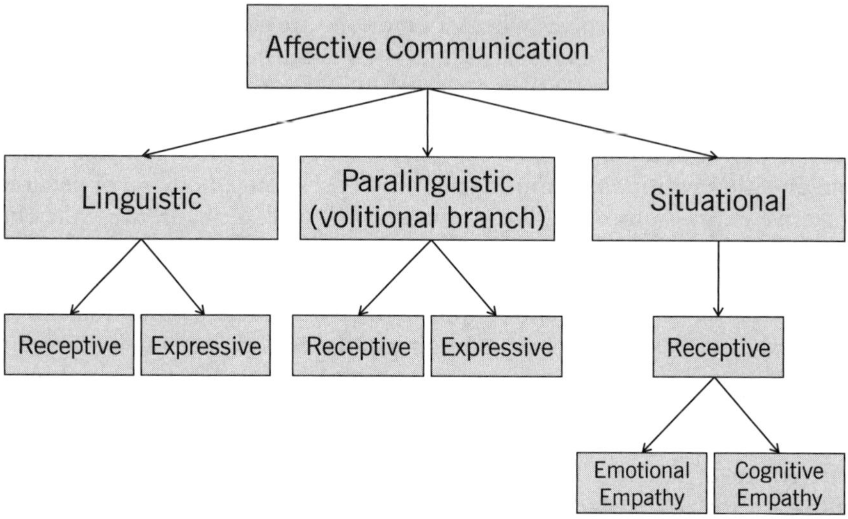

FIGURE 6.2. An overview of the types of affective communication covered in Chapter 6.

RECEPTIVE LINGUISTIC COMMUNICATION

Some research has reported that patients with right-hemisphere damage have greater difficulty comprehending emotional lexical content than normal controls or even than patients with left-hemisphere damage (Cicero et al., 1999). However, the opposite pattern (i.e., greater deficits among patients with left-hemisphere damage) has also been found, especially when affective cues such as prosody were removed (Karow et al., 2001) or when the content was positively valenced (Pick, 2002). Similarly, functional neuroimaging research has shown both left (Beaucousin et al., 2007) and bilateral (Dietrich, Hertrich, Alter, Ischebeck, & Ackermann, 2008) hemispheric activation (primarily in the superior temporal sulcus) in response to affective lexical statements. For additional review of the literature, see Borod et al. (2002).

EXPRESSIVE LINGUISTIC COMMUNICATION

The findings regarding the neuroanatomic underpinnings of expressive linguistic communication are mixed, in part due to highly variable assessment methods, and in part due to the lack of clarity regarding the construct of verbal expression of emotion (Sherratt, 2007). On the one hand, several studies by Borod and colleagues have found that patients with right-hemisphere damage exhibit a decreased output of emotional words as well as decreased spontaneous emotional expressiveness (for a review, see Borod et al., 2002). Additionally, decreases in emotional appraisals among patients with right-brain damage have also been found (Sherratt, 2007). In contrast, other research has shown a decrease in emotional verbal output (relative to the overall total verbal output) among patients with left-hemisphere damage (Blonder et al., 2005).

Paralinguistic Mode of Affective Communication

Among the most elegant theories of affective paralinguistic communication is that of Eliott Ross, who proposed that the frontal and temporal lobes of the right cerebral hemisphere contain areas that are structurally and functionally analogous to the Broca and Wernicke areas of the left hemisphere. According to this theory (Ross, 1981, 1984; Ross & Mesulam, 2000), these right-hemisphere areas represent the substrates for expressive and receptive paralinguistic abilities. In his early work, Ross proposed a system for assessing and classifying prosody disorders (i.e., aprosodias) that paralleled the assessment methods and the classification system of aphasias.[3]

Ross's theory was supported by his early work involving bedside clinical judgments (Gorelick & Ross, 1987), as well as by a recent, scientifically rigorous examination of a sample of patients with left- or right-hemisphere damage with or without aprosodia (Ross & Monnot, 2008). However, in face of scientific scrutiny from other laboratories, Ross's theory has failed to hold up fully. Firstly, the right hemisphere, although dominant for affective paralinguistic communication, nevertheless does not appear to accomplish the task alone. Second, although some distinctions between expressive and receptive networks of prosody have been identified, these do not always follow the anterior–posterior divide proposed by Ross. And lastly, the theory cannot be applied to other channels of paralinguistic communication because some neuroanatomic differences have been identified between facial versus prosodic channels, as well as among individual emotions, arguing against localized affect recognition and affect production modules. In fact, as mentioned earlier, there is some overlap between networks for expression versus recognition of facial affect (van der Gaag et al., 2007). Thus, in the final analysis, expression and comprehension of affect likely relies on networks that are, on the one hand, much more distributed and, on the other hand, much less unique than those originally proposed by Ross. This literature is reviewed in more detail below.

RECEPTIVE PARALINGUISTIC COMMUNICATION (A.K.A. "AFFECT RECOGNITION")

First, consistent with Ross's theory, much evidence confirms that damage to the right cerebral hemisphere is associated with deficits in affect recognition in both visual (Bowers, Bauer, Coslett, & Heilman, 1985) and auditory (Ross, Thompson, & Yenkosky, 1997; Shapiro & Danly, 1985; Tompkins & Flowers, 1985) channels. These deficits persist even after other relevant aspects of cognition, such as lower-order perceptual/attentional abilities, higher-order conceptual abilities, as well as the ability to experience or understand emotions, have been accounted for (Blonder, Burns, Bowers, Moore, & Heilman, 1993; Blonder et al., 2005; Borod, Cicero, et al., 1998; Bowers, Coslett, Bauer, & Speedie, 1987; Orbelo, Grim, Talbott, & Ross, 2005). Taken together, these findings suggest that the right hemisphere plays a dominant role in facial and prosodic affect recognition, and that such affect recognition deficits are *not* secondary to other cognitive or perceptual impairments.

However, the finding that the right hemisphere is dominant for receptive paralinguistic communication is not ubiquitous, especially when it comes to prosody comprehension (Buchanan et al., 2000; Van Lancker & Sidtis, 1992). In particular, whereas some aspects of prosody (e.g., pitch information) are processed primarily by the right hemisphere (Lattner, Meyer, & Friederici, 2005; Murayama, Kashiwagi, Kashiwagi, & Mimura, 2004), other prosodic cues such as rhythm (Platel et al., 1997) and emphasis (Pell, 1998) are processed primarily by the left. Consistent with this notion, Van Lancker and Sidtis (1992) found that although patients with left- and right-hemisphere damage performed equally poorly on a task of receptive prosody, the errors of patients with left-hemisphere damage were due to poor understanding of timing, whereas the errors of patients with right-hemisphere damage were due to poor understanding of pitch. Thus, depending on the exact nature of the stimuli or the study design, some research may find greater or lesser reliance on the left hemisphere. These findings may also explain why at least one study found that receptive affective deficits in the *prosodic* channel were more associated with left-hemisphere damage, whereas those in the *facial* channel tended to be associated with right-hemisphere damage (Karow et al., 2001).[4]

With respect to the localization of affect recognition *within* the cerebral hemispheres, anterior regions (*not* posterior, as Ross had suggested) appear to play the most critical role. In particular, most studies have localized facial and prosodic affect recognition to the orbitofrontal/frontal opercular and/or anterior cingulate cortex, primarily on the right (Blood, Zatorre, Bermudez, & Evans, 1999; Buchanan et al., 2000; Frey, Kostopoulos, & Petrides, 2000; Hornak et al., 2003; Kipps, Nestor, Acosta-Cabronero, Arnold, & Hodges, 2009), as well as the basal ganglia and/or the thalamus (Breitenstein, Daum, & Ackermann, 1998; Cancelliere & Kertesz, 1990; Ross & Monnot, 2008; Weddell, 1994). Furthermore, at least one study has shown that basal ganglia lesions are *necessary and sufficient* for a receptive impairment in paralinguistic processing (Karow et al., 2001). Additional regions that have been implicated include the temporoparietal cortex, bilateral frontal poles, right frontoparietal operculum, right temporal operculum, and left frontal operculum (Adolphs, Damasio, et al., 2002; Ross & Monnot, 2008; Starkstein, Federoff, Price, & Leiguarda, 1994), although these latter findings have not been robustly replicated.

It is also important to note that some investigations have found more discrete networks for recognition of specific emotions, although this line of research is marked by many inconsistencies across studies and is beyond the scope of this chapter.[5] One finding, however, that tends to be fairly consistent is that recognition of disgust requires normal integrity of the basal ganglia and the insula (Adolphs, 2002). Thus, for example, patients with Huntington's chorea tend to be impaired specifically on recognition of this emotion (Hayes, Stevenson, & Coltheart, 2007). In contrast, patients with Alzheimer's disease, whose basal ganglia structures are relatively spared, show normal recognition of facial disgust, while exhibiting deficits in recognition of other emotional expressions (Henry et al., 2008).

Lastly, there is considerable evidence that both age (Calder et al., 2003; Gunning-Dixon et al., 2003; Tessitore et al., 2005) and gender (Lee, Liu, Chan, Fang, & Gao, 2005; Marumo, Takizawa, Kawakubo, Onitsuka, & Kasai, 2009) mediate the size and location of the networks that are involved in affect recognition. These demographic effects are also undoubtedly responsible for some of the inconsistencies in the literature.

In summary, it appears that the networks that subserve affect recognition vary somewhat as a function of the channel (i.e., visual vs. auditory), the particular components of auditory processing (e.g., pitch vs. stress), age, and gender, as well as the specific types of emotions. Regardless of those differences, the majority of the findings implicate the right cerebral hemisphere in general and the right frontal lobe (including the basal ganglia) in particular. The fact that affect recognition would be localized in the anterior regions of the brain may, at first blush, appear counterintuitive, given that visual, auditory, somatosensory, and language reception are all localized posteriorly. To understand this anomaly, one needs to consider the possibility that comprehension of emotional communication may be accompanied by an *experience* of the communicated emotion. For example, recall from the previous chapter that simply just being exposed to affective facial expressions is sufficient for generation of subjective emotional feelings (Wild et al., 2001). This notion is also consistent with the theories of embodied emotions discussed earlier in this chapter (Niedenthal, 2007). In other words, it is possible that interpretation of affective displays of others may, in part, rely on fluctuations in subjective emotional experiences and, consequently, neuroanatomic networks that overlap with such experiences. Such networks, although varied as a function of specific emotions and/or emotional valence, tend to involve the frontal lobes, with considerable implication of the right anterior cingulate gyrus (see Chapter 5 for more detailed discussion).

EXPRESSIVE PARALINGUISTIC COMMUNICATION

With respect to the expression of emotion, some research has provided support for the right frontal lobe hypothesis proposed by Ross (1981). In particular, expression of *prosody* has been found to be impaired following lesions in the right hemisphere in general (Blonder et al., 2005; Wertz, Henschel, Auther, Ashford, & Kirshner, 1998) and the right frontal lobe (Nakhutina et al., 2006) in particular. Within the right frontal lobe, studies have found expressive prosody deficits following lesions in the right basal ganglia and the right medial frontal lobe (Cancelliere & Kertesz, 1990; Heilman, Leon, & Rosenbek, 2004; Karow et al., 2001), as well as large lesions involving and extending beyond the right frontal operculum (Ross & Monnot, 2008). Of note, several studies found *no* differences in prosody production between patients with left- and right-hemisphere damage (Baum & Pell, 1999; Bradvik, Dravins, Holtas, & Rosen, 1991; Cancelliere & Kertesz, 1990; Ross et al., 1997). However, it has been suggested that deficits in prosody production among patients with left-hemisphere lesions are a result of midcallosal disconnection between the left and the right hemispheres, making the integration of spoken language with the production of prosody impossible (Ross & Monnot, 2008).

Similarly, decreased spontaneous *facial affect* has been found among patients with right-, as compared to left-, hemisphere damage (Blonder et al., 1993, 2005; Montreys & Borod, 1998), consistent with the notion that much of the affective intensity in facial expressions is present on the left side of the face, which is controlled by the right hemisphere (Borod, Koff, Yecker, Santschi, & Schmidt, 1998). Lastly, imitating emotional expressions has been shown to enhance activation within the right inferior frontal gyrus (Lee, Josephs, Dolan, & Critchley, 2006).

Situational Mode of Affective Communication: Empathy Networks

Before proceeding, readers may wish to reorient themselves to the hierarchical organization of this section by briefly perusing Figure 6.2. As can be seen in the figure, whereas linguistic and paralinguistic modes of communication have an expressive and receptive direction of communication, the situational mode is only receptive. As mentioned earlier, one way of conceptualizing situational communication is to think of it as empathy. As discussed in Chapter 5, empathy is a correlate of alexithymia, and as such, has some overlap with the networks that have been implicated in alexithymia. However, because empathy consists of at least two distinct components (i.e., emotional empathy and cognitive empathy) that have been shown to be neuroanatomically dissociable (Shamay-Tsoory, Aharon-Peretz, et al., 2009), the networks subserving each of the two empathy types are considered separately below.[6]

EMOTIONAL EMPATHY

Emotional empathy is the capacity to feel what others feel, presumably resulting from implicit mimicry of emotional displays of others. As such, emotional empathy is thought to rely on the "mirror neuron system" (MNS), a network of neurons that plays a role in imitation of motor behavior and abstract intentions, as well as social interactions and shared emotional states. The MNS in humans has been shown to include the inferior frontal gyrus and the somatosensory cortex. The strength of activation in this network correlates with self-report measures of empathy (Carr, Iacoboni, Dubeau, Mazziotta, & Lenzi, 2003; Schulte-Ruether, Markowitsch, Fink, & Piefke, 2007), although lesion studies suggest that only the inferior frontal gyrus aspect of this network is *necessary* for emotional empathy to occur (Shamay-Tsoory, Aharon-Peretz, et al., 2009).

COGNITIVE EMPATHY

Cognitive empathy relies on the affective aspect of the ToM. Functional imaging research has demonstrated that a variety of ToM paradigms fairly reliably activate the medial prefrontal and medial orbitofrontal cortices, and, to a lesser degree, the anterior paracingulate cortex, superior temporal lobe, and temporal–parietal juncture (Carrington & Bailey, 2009; Gallagher & Frith, 2003). Components of this network, most notably the medial prefrontal and anterior temporal cortices, also become activated during empathy tasks (Schulte-Ruether et al., 2007). However, there are some inconsistencies in findings, as cognitive empathy that occurs in the absence of emotional empathy has also been shown to activate the inferior temporal and fusiform gyri (Preston et al., 2007), and at least some cognitive empathy paradigms also recruit parts of the MNS networks (Hooker, Verosky, Germine, Knight, & D'Esposito, 2010). Although these findings suggest that cognitive empathy may rely on regions above and beyond those implicated in ToM, at least one lesion study has shown that the medial orbitofrontal (or ventromedial) prefrontal cortex is the *only* region that is

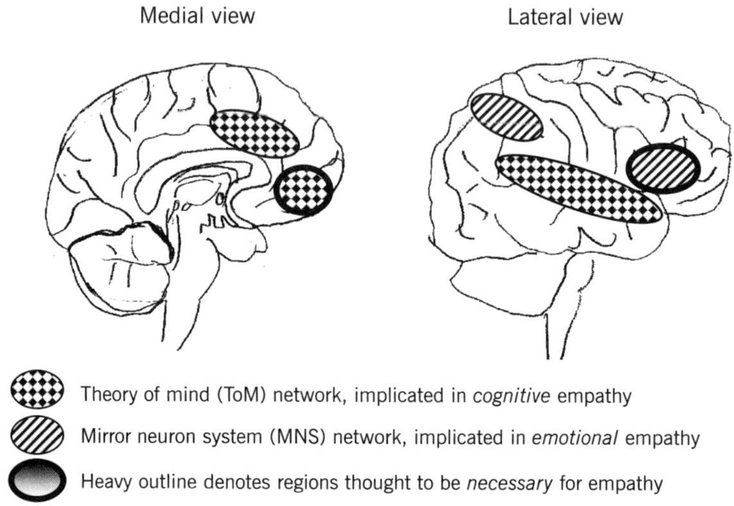

FIGURE 6.3. A general summary of the functional imaging findings on the theory of mind (ToM) and mirror neuron system (MNS) networks, as they correspond to cognitive and emotional empathy, respectively. Lesion research indicates that only portions of these networks (heavy black outline) are *necessary* for empathic responses.

necessary for cognitive empathy to take place (Shamay-Tsoory, Aharon-Peretz, et al., 2009). See Figure 6.3.

Summary

In summary, there is considerable evidence that affective communication in all modes and domains relies on distributed networks that are partly a function of mode, direction, and channel of communication; partly a function of particular characteristics of a given stimulus; and partly a function of demographic characteristics such as age and gender. However, there also appears to be considerable overlap among such networks, generally involving the right frontal lobe, the MNS, and the networks that subserve perspective taking. Interestingly, both expressive and receptive affective communication relies, at least in part, on more anterior regions of the brain, consistent with several related theoretical accounts of affect recognition, including the facial-feedback hypothesis (Tomkins, 1962, 1963), embodied emotions (Niedenthal et al., 2009), and the emotional contagion model (Doherty, 1997; Hatfield et al., 2008).

Interplay with Cognition

Facial and Prosodic Affect Recognition

Given the well-documented association between the right hemisphere and affect recognition, it is not surprising that, even among non-neurological populations (i.e., in the absence of a right-hemisphere injury), affect recognition deficits are sometimes associated with weaknesses in visual–spatial (i.e., right-hemisphere) functions. For example, individuals with nonverbal learning disability are typically characterized both by affect recognition deficits (Dimitrovsky, Spector, & Levy-Shiff, 2000; Dimitrovsky, Spector, Levy-Shiff, & Vakil, 1998) and by visual–spatial deficits (Forrest, 2004; Worling, Humphries, & Tannock, 1999). Similarly, among patients with bipolar disorder, poor affect recognition has been found to correlate with poor performance on visual recognition memory (Summers, Papadopoulou, Bruno, Cipolotti, & Ron, 2006), and among patients with schizophrenia, poor affect recognition correlates with visual–spatial skills and visual–spatial scanning (Bozikas, Kosmidis, Anezoulaki, Giannakou, & Karavatos, 2004; Summers et al., 2006), as well as visual recognition memory (Whittaker, Deakin, & Tomenson, 2001) and visual learning (Sachs, Steger-Wuchse, Kryspin-Exner, Gur, & Katschnig, 2004).

However, there are other (i.e., *not* visual–spatial) weaknesses in cognition that have been associated with poor affect recognition. For example, among patients with schizophrenia, poor affect recognition appears to be related to poor performance on measures of executive functioning as well as vocabulary and learning (Bozikas et al., 2004; Sachs et al., 2004; Whittaker et al., 2001). Such deficits are difficult to explain as stemming from a general right-hemisphere dysfunction, and have instead been explained as perhaps reflecting more general cognitive dysfunction such as low intelligence (Bozikas et al., 2004; Whittaker et al., 2001). However, this interpretation has been questioned, as the association between affect recognition deficits and poor test performance on verbal measures has been observed even after intelligence and educational background have been accounted for (Suchy, Rau, Whittaker, Eastvold, & Strassberg, 2009). Clinical implications of these associations are discussed in the "Assessment" section later in this chapter.

Empathy

Empathy, particularly cognitive empathy, has been found to correlate with cognitive flexibility (Shamay-Tsoory, Harari, et al., 2009; Shamay-Tsoory, Tomer, Goldsher, Berger, & Aharon-Peretz, 2004), which in turn has been shown to correlate with performance on ToM tasks (Milders, Ietswaart,

Crawford, & Currie, 2008). It has even been suggested that cognitive empathy and cognitive flexibility share the same neuroanatomic networks (Grattan & Eslinger, 1989). Thus, patients with poor cognitive flexibility may also be characterized by impairments in cognitive empathy.

INTEGRATING THEORY AND PRACTICE

Affective communication, perhaps due to its reliance on complex neuroanatomic networks, represents an area of impairment that is extremely common among many clinical populations. Such impairment can be present congenitally, may develop in the course of a neurodegenerative disorder, or may result from a brain injury. Regardless of the etiology, deficits in affective communication, as discussed above, appear to go hand in hand with cognitive weaknesses or poorer test performance. Additionally, given that affective communication involves not only the ability to accurately convey or receive information, but also the ability to feel and express empathy for others, it is key for healthy interpersonal functioning at all levels, from successful interactions with coworkers to successful development and maintenance of intimate relationships. Consequently, clinical neuropsychologists need to consider the possibility that deficits in affective communication are responsible for patients' problems in everyday life, to the same or perhaps even greater degree than deficits in other, more typically assessed, neurocognitive domains. This section reviews the most representative clinical populations that are characterized by deficits in affective communications, as well as various assessment issues.

Signs and Syndromes

Problems with affective communication mirror the tree diagram of affective communication abilities presented in Figure 6.2. For that reason, providing a detailed description of these deficits here would be redundant. The reader is reminded, however, that deficits may be present only for a particular type of an emotion. Additionally, with respect to paralinguistic communication, one or multiple channels may be affected (e.g., prosody, gestures, posture, and facial expressions).

Clinical Populations

Neurodevelopmental, Neuropsychiatric, and Neurodegenerative Disorders

Deficits in emotional communication observed in various patient populations are in some cases fairly global, including all aspects of affective communication, while in others, they are fairly circumscribed. However, research findings need to be interpreted with caution. In perusing the literature, readers should be aware that the majority of research has focused on facial affect recognition (FAR); consequently, not enough is known about how, or whether, other aspects of affective communication are impaired in a given population. Because of the frequency with which deficits in emotional communication occur in a variety of neurodevelopmental, neuropsychiatric, and neurodegenerative disorders, a full review of the literature is beyond the scope of this chapter. Tables 6.2, 6.3, and 6.4 summarize the main findings in this area of research and provide select references.

Other Populations Not Included in the Tables

ACQUIRED BRAIN INJURY

As already discussed in the section on neuroanatomic substrates earlier in this chapter, aside from amygdalar lesions (i.e., dysfunctional trigger), lesions in the right hemisphere in general and in the right frontal lobe (including the basal ganglia) in particular can lead to deficits in affective communication. Such lesions are most commonly a result of cerebral-vascular accidents, tumors, or epilepsy surgeries. Additionally, survivors of TBI have been shown to have deficits in FAR (Radice-Neumann, Zupan, Babbage, & Willer, 2007), as well as deficits in cognitive and emotional empathy, particularly if characterized by lesions in the ventral and medial prefrontal areas or the right parietal lobe (Shamay-Tsoory et al., 2004).

CRIMINAL OFFENDING

It has been suggested that criminal populations, in particular violent, aggressive, or sadistic criminals, are capable of committing heinous crimes primarily due to their inability to recognize emotional expressions of others, or due to an impairment in empathy (Kirsch & Becker, 2007). FAR deficits have, in fact, been demonstrated in a variety of criminal offenders (Carr et al., 2003; Dolan & Fullam, 2006; Hastings, Tangney, & Stuewig, 2008; Kosson et al., 2002; McCown, Johnson, & Austin, 1986, 1988; Suchy et al., 2008).

Some evidence for deficits in recognition of specific emotions has also emerged, showing facial *fear* recognition problems among individuals with antisocial personality disorder (Dolan & Fullam, 2006), and a greater tendency to mislabel other emotions as *anger* among individuals with aggressive (Matheson & Jahoda, 2005), psychopathic (Kosson et al., 2002;

(text resumes on page 131)

TABLE 6.2. Neurodevelopmental Disorders and Affective Communication

Population	Deficits in affective communication	Discrete emotions	Comments	References
Autism	FAR; prosody; cognitive empathy	Fear, happiness, disgust, sadness, anger	Not due to lower-level perceptual deficit or IQ limitations; emerges by age 3 years; emotional empathy appears normal.	Dawson, Webb, & McPartland (2005); Dziobek et al. (2008); Hubbard & Trauner (2007); Humphreys, Minshew, Leonard, & Behrmanna (2007); Smith (2009); Zaja & Rojahn (2008)
ADHD	FAR; prosody; situational cues	All, but primarily fear and disgust	Deficits are hypothesized to be related to right-hemisphere dysfunction in ADHD	Boakes, Chapman, Houghton, & West (2008); Cadesky et al. (2000); Corbett & Glidden (2000); Da Fonseca, Seguier, Santos, Poinso, & Deruelle (2009); Williams et al. (2008)
Children with Down syndrome	FAR	All, but primarily fear	Comparable to controls up to age 3 years; poorer after age 4 years.	Kasari, Freeman, & Hughes (2001); Wishart, Cebula, Willis, & Pitcairn (2007)
Adults with Down syndrome	FAR	Primarily surprise; greater tendency to judge expressions more positively than controls	Related to receptive vocabulary and impulsivity, but not nonverbal reasoning.	Barisnikov, Hippolyte, & Van der Linden (2008)
Fetal alcohol syndrome	Prosody comprehension	N/A	Impairment is present in the context of normal cognition.	Monnot et al. (2001)

Note. FAR, facial affect recognition; ADHD, attention-deficit/hyperactivity disorder.

TABLE 6.3. Neurodegenerative Disorders and Affective Communication

Population	Deficits in affective communication	Discrete emotions	Comments	References
Alzheimer's dementia (including mild)	FAR; empathy	All emotions; some studies show spared disgust.	Correlates with MMSE, interpersonal behavior problems, and/or progression of illness.	Lavenu & Pasquier (2004); Rankin, Baldwin, et al. (2005); Shimokawa et al. (2000, 2003); Spoletini et al. (2008)
ALS, bulbar variant	FAR; some prosody	All emotions	Not related to depressive symptoms or dementia.	Zimmerman, Eslinger, Simmons, & Barrett (2007)
Frontotemporal-lobar degeneration	FAR; receptive prosody; cognitive empathy	All emotions, but primarily negative emotions (fear, anger, disgust)	Greater impairment in the frontal than in the temporal variant, although both are affected.	Fernandez-Duque & Black (2005); Keane, Calder, Hodges, & Young (2002); Lavenu & Pasquier (2004); Lough et al. (2006); Rankin, Kramer, et al. (2005); Rosen et al. (2004); Snowden et al. (2008)
Huntington's dementia	FAR	Primarily disgust; also possibly fear and anger	Presumably due to the reliance of disgust on the putamen.	Hennenlotter et al. (2004); Snowden et al. (2008)
Mild cognitive impairment	FAR	Low-intensity fear only	N/A	Spoletini et al. (2008)
Parkinson's dementia	FAR; receptive and expressive prosody	All emotions, but primarily disgust and anger	Early in the disease, unrelated to motor symptoms; greater deficits in unmedicated patients.	Dujardin et al. (2004); Goberman, Coelho, & Robb (2005); Gray & Tickle-Degnen (2010); Kan, Kawamura, Hasegawa, Mochizuki, & Nakamura (2002); Lawrence, Goerendt, & Brooks (2007); Pell & Leonard (2005); Sprengelmeyer et al. (2003)
Semantic dementia	Empathy (both emotional and cognitive)	N/A	N/A	Rankin, Baldwin, et al. (2005)
Vascular dementia	FAR	All emotions	Not related to MMSE; poorer than AD patients.	Shimokawa et al. (2000, 2003)

Note. FAR, facial affect recognition; MMSE, Mini-Mental State Exam; AD, Alzheimer's disease.

TABLE 6.4. Neuropsychiatric Disorders and Affective Communication

Population	Deficits in affective communication	Discrete emotions	Comments	References
Bipolar disorder	FAR	All	Comparable deficits also among youth at risk for bipolar disorder and patients in remissions.	Bozikas, Tonia, Fokas, Karavatos, & Kosmidis (2006); Brotman et al. (2008); Schenkel, Pavuluri, Herbener, Harral, & Sweeney (2007)
Major depression	FAR; FA expression (to command)	All	Only mild deficits that resolve when patients in remission; expression deficits primarily for positive emotions.	Jaeger, Borod, & Peselow (1986); Weniger, Lange, Rather, & Irle (2004)
Schizophrenia	FAR; spontaneous prosody; prosodic recognition; prosodic repetition; linguistic emotional content comprehension; empathy	All, but more prominently fear and disgust	Some studies show deficits only on posed, but not genuine, emotions.	Addington & Addington (1998); Bediou et al. (2005); Bozikas et al. (2004, 2006); Davis & Gibson (2000); Leentjens, Wielaert, van Harskamp, & Wilmink (1998); Scholten, Aleman, & Kahn (2008); Shamay-Tsoory, Shur, Harari, & Levkovitz (2007)

Note. FAR, facial affect recognition.

Suchy, Whittaker, Strassberg, & Eastvold, 2009), or conduct disorders (Cadesky, Mota, & Schachar, 2000). Lastly, criminals with psychopathy appear to have difficulty with lexical affective abilities, in particular with understanding metaphorical or indirectly stated emotional content in spoken language (Herve, Hayes, & Hare, 2003).

In addition to deficits in affect recognition, criminal offending in general and psychopathy in particular is associated with deficits in empathy. However, the literature is somewhat inconsistent with respect to which type of empathy (i.e., cognitive or affective) is impaired in this population. On the one hand, both cognitive and emotional empathy deficits have been found in children with psychopathic traits, with cognitive empathy improving during puberty, which presumably allows people with psychopathy to manipulate and deceive others (Dadds et al., 2009). On the other hand, ventromedial prefrontal cortex, thought to subserve cognitive empathy, has been shown to be dysfunctional in people with psychopathy (Shamay-Tsoory, Harari, Aharon-Peretz, & Levkovitz, 2010). Additionally, there is new emerging evidence that empathy deficits are different for males and females with psychopathy, with females *not* exhibiting affective empathy deficits (Dadds et al., 2009) and exhibiting smaller deficits in cognitive empathy (Rogstad & Rogers, 2008).

SUBSTANCE ABUSE

There is a considerable overlap between substance abuse, psychopathy, criminal offending, and aggression. Thus, it should not be surprising that individuals who abuse substances exhibit deficits in affective communication that are similar to those seen in criminal populations (Foisy et al., 2005; Kornreich et al., 2001; Monnot, Lovallo, Nixon, & Ross, 2002; Monnot, Nixon, Lovallo, & Ross, 2001; Philippot et al., 1999; Uekermann, Daum, Schlebusch, & Trenckmann, 2005).

Assessment

Cognitive Test Performance

As discussed above, many neuropsychiatric, neurodevelopmental, and neurodegenerative conditions are associated with some degree of affect recognition deficits. It has also already been stated earlier that poor affect recognition is potentially associated with an array of verbal and nonverbal weaknesses. Although the relationship between affective communication and visual–spatial or executive functions can be explained by the reliance of these processes on common neural networks, the mechanism behind the association with verbal abilities is not understood. One possibility is that poor performances on some cognitive measures may represent *the effect*, rather than just a correlate, of deficits in affective processing. For example, patients with affect recognition deficits may have difficulties relating to the examiner, identifying aspects of instructions that are important, or even relating appropriately to certain test stimuli that inadvertently contain emotionally laden material. Consequently, affective communication problems may simply *mimic* deficits in other, apparently unrelated (i.e., verbal), cognitive domains. This, in fact, was found in a recent study showing that affect recognition abilities were related to performances on cognitive measures that contained emotionally significant content, but *not* to measures that were emotionally neutral (Suchy, Rau, et al., 2009). This relationship held even after accounting for education, intelligence, and vocabulary skills. However, we know of no other studies that have examined this question, and more work in this area is clearly needed. In the meantime, clinicians may consider that the use of pictorial stimuli that include affectively loaded scenes may potentially lead to poor test performance among patients with affect recognition deficits or deficits in understanding emotional scenes.

Assessment of Affective Communication

The clinical utility of assessing affective communication abilities has been demonstrated. For example, the *Ekman 60 Faces Test* has been shown to discriminate patients with mild frontotemporal-lobar degeneration (FTD) from healthy controls with 94% sensitivity and 100% specificity (Diehl-Schmid et al., 2007). However, despite the large body of research on affective communication and the relatively large number of excellent experimental stimuli and batteries,[7] until relatively recently, no commercial instruments have been widely available for clinical use. The few that exist are relatively obscure and have not yet been widely incorporated into a typical clinical practice.

The *Awareness of Social Inference Test* (TASIT; McDonald, Flanagan, & Rollins, 2002) is an Australian measure for assessment of deficit in social perception. It consists of three parts: (1) the Emotion Evaluation Test, (2) the Social Inference Test—Minimal, and (3) the Social Inference Test—Enriched. Together, the three tests assess the individual's ability to understand prosody, facial affect, gestures, and situational cues. Stimuli are videotaped vignettes enacted by professional actors. Norms are available for the adult lifespan (14–60 years).

With the publication of the fourth edition of the Wechsler series for assessment of intelligence and memory (Wechsler, 2008), the test publisher (NCS Pearson, Inc.) introduced the Advanced Clinical Solutions (ACS) supplement (Pearson, 2009). This supplement includes a *Social Cognition Test*, designed to assess the patients' understanding of facial expression, social interactions, and prosody. The test contains both booklet and audio stimuli. The battery has high-quality demographically stratified norms for the adult lifespan (16–90 years) that are co-normed with the Wechsler Adult Intelligence Scale—Fourth Edition/Wechsler Memory Scale—Fourth Edition (WAIS-IV/WMS-IV; Wechsler, 2008).

SUMMARY AND CONCLUSIONS

Deficient affective communication represents a fairly common disorder in a variety of neurological populations, and as such may be a common etiology of interpersonal problems experienced by patients and their families. While deficient affective communication is typically associated with poorer performances on measures of visual–spatial, verbal, and executive abilities, it is not clear whether these poorer performances reflect true cognitive weaknesses. In fact, at least some evidence suggests that individuals with poor receptive affective communication may have difficulty with comprehending the affective content that is inadvertently present within some assessment materials.

Several clinical batteries for assessment of affective communication exist, but have not yet entered the mainstream of neuropsychological assessment. Incorporating an assessment of affective communication should be a priority in the field for two reasons: (1) documentation of affective communication deficits can facilitate patient management, and (2) affective communication deficits may represent important hallmark symptoms of some clinical populations, such as, for example, FTD, and as such may help with differential diagnosis.

NOTES

1. Theory of mind (ToM) is a nonunitary construct, which can be divided into a cognitive and an affective component. Counterintuitively, it is the affective component of ToM that is believed to generate cognitive empathy.
2. However, in some studies, the term *spontaneous* is used to denote *genuine*.
3. The analogue with Wernicke's area of the left hemisphere was further echoed by the suggestion that the right hemisphere contained the so-called "nonverbal affect lexicon" (Bowers et al., 1993).
4. Functional imaging research also found specific patterns of activation for prosodic and facial affect recognition, such that recognition of *facial* affect uniquely (i.e., above and beyond the common areas discussed above) recruited

the right frontoparietal cortex (i.e., somatosensory areas) and the left temporal pole, whereas recognition of *prosody* uniquely recruited the right temporal pole (Adolphs, Damasio, & Tranel, 2002).

5. For a review, see Adolphs (2002).
6. Most studies of empathy have not differentiated between cognitive and emotional empathy, leading to inconsistencies in findings.
7. Prominent examples include the New York Emotion Battery (NYEB; Borod, Welkowitz, & Obler, 1992) and the Florida Affect Battery (FAB; Bowers, Blonder, & Heilman, 1999). For an excellent review of experimental batteries, see Borod, Tabert, Santschi, and Strauss (2000).

CHAPTER 7

Emotion Regulation

For the last time, let us recall the by-now intimately familiar face-off between you and the yellow-jacket described in prior chapters: After having experienced an array of physiological upsets and reflexive posturing, which all seem rather silly to you now with the yellow-jacket finally out of the picture, you look around and see the reactions of the other picnic attendees. Some flash smiles that seem understanding, even empathic, but others shake their heads and roll their eyes, at best amused and quite possibly annoyed by all the commotion you have caused. Feeling uncomfortable for having become the center of attention, you now have the task before you to select a coping strategy that would best alleviate your growing distress.

You might consider acting as if nothing had happened, as though you didn't feel at all embarrassed—in other words, the stiff-upper-lip approach. Or you might seek the support of others by engaging them in a conversation about your prior yellow-jacket experiences, justifying your reaction not only to them, but to yourself as well. Or you may just accept the situation for what it is, recognizing that this is not even remotely the end of the world and treating yourself to a kind thought: "How lucky I didn't get stung! And how fortunate to have friends who understand!" The ability to control one's own feelings in the face of emotional upsets—that is, emotion regulation—is the topic of this chapter.

THEORETICAL BACKGROUND

Defining the Constructs

Emotions can be viewed as a double-edge sword of sorts. On the one hand, they facilitate our survival by allowing us to attend to relevant stimuli (Chapter 3), providing us with adequate physiological arousal for dealing with the world's challenges (Chapter 4), helping us make sense of the world (Chapter 5), and facilitating communication with others (Chapter 6). On the other hand, as was suspected as far back as antiquity (see Introduction to Part 1) and is now supported by an enormous body of research, prolonged emotional distress is deleterious to our health (Denollet, Nyklicek, Vingerhoets, & Vingerhoets, 2008; Myers et al., 2008). Consequently, the ability to utilize the beneficial properties of emotions, on the one hand, and the ability to turn off, or at least turn down, the unhealthy emotional intensity, on the other, are key for a healthy, well-balanced life. The latter ability is referred to as *emotion regulation* (or coping) and, if employed successfully, leads to decreases in amygdalar and insular activation, which in turn lead to a reduction in unhealthy or prolonged autonomic arousal (Ohira et al., 2006).

As can be seen in Figure 7.1, there are different ways in which emotion regulation can be accomplished. In general, one can act *proactively*,

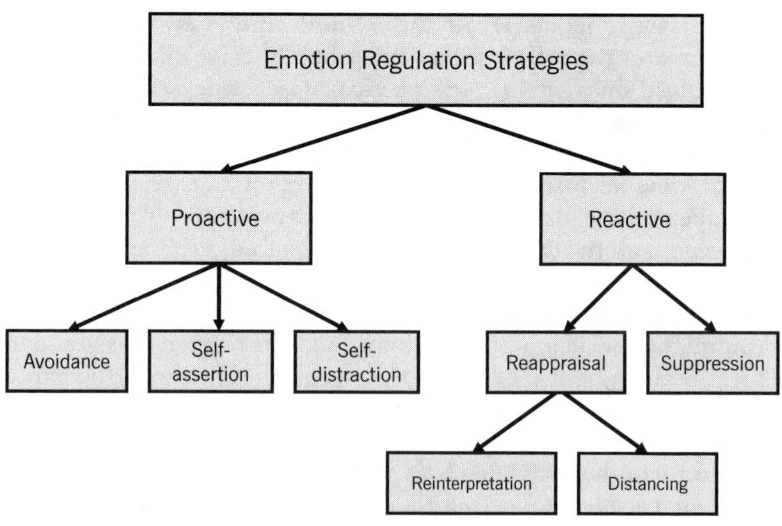

FIGURE 7.1. Overview of coping strategies according to the Gross et al. (2006) and Ochsner and Gross (2008) models.

so as to minimize the triggering of negative emotions, or *reactively*, so as to down-regulate those emotions internally, once they have occurred, as well as to suppress or modify one's overt emotional behavior. Arguably, among the most comprehensive theoretical accounts of emotion regulation strategies is that described by Gross and colleagues (2006). According to this model, management of one's emotional experiences takes place via (1) deliberate avoidance of stressful or emotionally unpleasant situations; (2) self-assertion and active modification of an emotionally arousing situation; (3) deliberate self-distraction away from the emotionally salient aspects of a situation, such as by engaging in a distracting activity; (4) cognitive reappraisal; and (5) suppression of overt affective responses. From among these, cognitive reappraisal and suppression have been studied the most, proving to be not only independent of each other (Moore, Zoellner, & Mollenholt, 2008), but also differentially related to quality of life (Haga, Kraft, & Corby, 2009), psychopathology (Aldao, Nolen-Hoeksema, & Schweizer, 2010), health (Denollet et al., 2008), and cognition (Egloff, Schmukle, Burns, & Schwerdtfeger, 2006; Jing & Jiamei, 2007).

Cognitive Reappraisal

Cognitive reappraisal refers to the ability to view a given situation in a new, more positive light. According to Gross's model (Ochsner & Gross, 2008), two ways in which cognitive reappraisal can be accomplished are by *reinterpretation* and by *distancing*. Specifically, one can *reinterpret* a given situation, as if rewriting the story of what had happened—or, put differently, by looking for the silver lining. Alternatively, one can *distance* oneself by adopting a removed, depersonalized perspective, such as considering how trivial our daily human strivings are in the context of the infinity of the universe and time. Although the utility of distancing in decreasing emotional and autonomic arousal is still questionable (Fontana & McLaughlin, 1998), cognitive reinterpretation has been found to be the most effective way of down-regulating emotions because it adjusts the *internal* context of the emotional experience (John & Gross, 2004) while at the same time decreasing the intensity of external emotional displays (Goldin, McRae, Ramel, & Gross, 2008). Importantly, reinterpretation has been associated with better psychological functioning (John & Gross, 2004), better physical health (for a review, see Denollet et al., 2008), and better interpersonal relationships (Gross & John, 2003) than suppression. However, a recent large meta-analytic study suggests that these better outcomes may be not so much a function of the salubrious effects of cognitive reappraisal, but rather a function of the deleterious effects of suppression (Aldao et al., 2010).

Suppression

Suppression refers to the ability to consciously inhibit the behavioral manifestation of an emotion. Suppression is commonly used in everyday life, and is quite appropriate in many situations. For example, suppression is what keeps us from losing our temper with a difficult customer, laughing when a coworker makes an embarrassing blunder, or crying when disappointed by not winning a contest. However, suppression of overt emotional displays does not appear to be effective or beneficial when it comes to regulation of one's *internal* emotional experience. In fact, it has been shown that whereas reappraisal has the effect of *reducing* amygdalar activation, suppression of an overt emotional response leads to an *increase* in amygdalar (and therefore also autonomic) activity over time (Ohira et al., 2006), as well as *increases* in the negative experience of emotions (Dalgleish, Yiend, Schweizer, & Dunn, 2009). Thus, although suppression affords the overt appearance of healthy emotion regulation and coping, individuals who overrely on this strategy usually continue to experience negative feelings, rumination,[1] or autonomic arousal—which, in the long run, can have adverse effects on physical and mental health (Aldao et al., 2010; Denollet et al., 2008; Moore et al., 2008; Myers et al., 2008).

Other Conceptualizations

The classification of coping strategies introduced in Gross's model is by no means universally accepted. For example, it has been suggested that self-distraction may mediate both suppression and cognitive reappraisal (Kalisch, Wiech, Herrmann, & Dolan, 2006), and some researchers have used the terms *self-distraction* and *suppression* interchangeably (Kalisch et al., 2006). Similarly, in an excellent fMRI study, Phan and colleagues (2005) refer to cognitive reappraisal as "suppression of negative affect." Consequently, readers are encouraged to carefully read the method sections of studies on emotion regulation, rather than rely on terminology used by a given author.

Neuroanatomic Substrates

Functional Imaging Research

Because of the growing evidence that effective down-regulation of emotion is crucial for both mental and physical health (for a review, see Williams, Suchy, & Rau, 2009), recent years have witnessed an increase in the investigation of the neurophysiological and neuroanatomic underpinnings of these regulatory processes. Much of this research has taken advantage of functional neuroimaging methodologies, typically examining regulation of emotional responses to emotion-evoking images or films or down-regulation of anticipatory anxiety. The types of emotion regulation strategies that have been most studied include reappraisal and suppression.

COMMON NETWORKS FOR EMOTION REGULATION

Before examining the finer distinctions among different types of coping, let us first review the general emotion regulation networks that have been identified. In particular, regardless of the type of emotion regulation mechanism or the specific paradigms used, most studies have shown prefrontal activation, often involving the anterior cingulate cortex (or different subregions thereof), dorsolateral prefrontal cortex (left, right, or bilateral, depending on the paradigm), and ventral prefrontal cortex (Ochsner & Gross, 2008). In general, the strength of prefrontal activation correlates with the decreases or increases in amygdalar activation, depending on whether the goal of participants' regulatory strategy was to decrease or increase (respectively) a given emotional experience (Goldin et al., 2008; Kent et al., 2005; Ochsner, Bunge, Gross, & Gabrieli, 2002; Phan et al., 2005; Urry et al., 2006). These patterns of coactivation demonstrate that the prefrontal cortex exerts some degree of control over the emotional trigger, thereby also up- or down-regulating the reflexive emotional responses discussed in Chapter 4.

STRATEGY-SPECIFIC NETWORKS FOR EMOTION REGULATION

In addition to identifying the substrates for coping in general, recent research has begun to identify some differences in the networks associated with different types of emotion regulation. This research has suggested that behavioral affective suppression (as opposed to reappraisal) relies primarily on the ventral (as opposed to the dorsal) prefrontal cortex (Ohira et al., 2006), whereas reappraisal appears to be related to dorsolateral (usually left or bilateral) prefrontal activation (Ochsner & Gross, 2008). Consistent with these findings, participants who habitually rely on suppression and only minimally utilize cognitive reappraisal exhibit greater regional cerebral blood flow (rCBF) in the ventral medial prefrontal cortex, as compared to those with the opposite pattern of coping strategies (Abler, Hofer, & Viviani, 2008). Interestingly, while reappraisal is associated with a virtually instantaneous prefrontal activation, prefrontal activation associated with suppression exhibits a 10-second (approximately) delay (Goldin et al., 2008).

In addition, Ochsner and Gross (2008) aimed to identify the neuroanatomic correlates of the two subtypes of reappraisal strategies: reinterpretation and distancing. Based on their review of the functional imaging literature, they concluded that reinterpretation abilities depend more on the *left* dorsolateral prefrontal cortex, presumably due to the requirements of language for constructing a new "story"; in contrast, distancing presumably requires greater attentional resources for directing attention *away* from the emotion-evoking stimuli, thus relying on the medial and *right* dorsolateral prefrontal cortex. However, another study found that the *right* prefrontal cortex is involved in reappraisal, and the *left* prefrontal cortex is involved in self-distraction (Kalisch et al., 2006). Note that the distinction between Kalisch's and Ochsner's studies is that the former examined the ability to regulate anxiety, whereas the latter examined the ability to regulate reactions to disturbing (potentially depressing?) images. Thus, it is possible that the laterality differences between the findings have less to do with the specific reappraisal strategy and more to do with the type of emotion that is being regulated.

Lastly, somewhat inconsistent with both the suppression and the reappraisal literature, research has also shown that simply labeling negative emotions leads to decreases in distress as well as deactivation in the amygdala. Interestingly, attaching labels to emotional stimuli has been shown to be related to the right ventrolateral prefrontal cortex (M. D. Lieberman et al., 2007), demonstrating the complexities of emotion regulation strategies. It is possible that this coping strategy explains why individuals who have good emotional awareness also have better emotional control and better physical and mental health, as compared to those with poorer self-awareness, that is, those who suffer from alexithymia (Chapter 5).

Lesion Studies

The findings of the functional imaging research reviewed above are consistent with what is generally well understood in clinical neuropsychology: that lesions in the prefrontal cortex or related circuitry can lead to emotional and behavioral dysregulation, personality changes, and an increase in psychopathology (Lezak et al., 2004). Lesions in the ventral frontal areas, in particular, are associated with irritability, aggression, emotional outbursts, and other overtly apparent problems with affective regulation, consistent with the notion that the ventral frontal areas are important for the suppression of overt affective displays (Duffy, Campbell, Salloway, & Malloy, 2001). Interestingly, lesions in the right orbitofrontal and ventromedial prefrontal areas are also sometimes associated with increased anxiety (Robinson, 1997; Tranel, Bechara, & Denburg, 2002), which in turn appears to be the motivating force behind aggressive acting out among brain-injured individuals (Falkenbach, Poythress, & Creevy, 2008; Skeem, Johansson, Andershed, Kerr, & Louden, 2007).

In contrast to individuals with ventral lesions, those with dorsolateral and frontopolar lesions tend to have more problems with *reinterpretation* rather than with *behavioral control*. The most notable among these are patients with prefrontal lesions in the *left* hemisphere, who are well known to have depressive tendencies (Narashima et al., 2003). In particular, if we accept that the left dorsolateral prefrontal cortex is necessary for the generation of a new story (i.e., reinterpreting) (Ochsner & Gross, 2008), then it follows that patients with left dorsolateral lesions would be characterized by the inability to abandon their initial negative interpretations of a given difficult situation, which would in turn lead to the maintenance of a depressed mood (Narashima, Kosier, & Robinson, 2003).

Summary

Taken together, lesion and functional imaging research consistently point to the reliance of suppression on the ventral frontal areas. With respect to reappraisal, dorsolateral and frontopolar cortices appear to play a role. However, a more complex picture emerges when laterality is considered, such that an interaction appears to exist between the exact type of reappraisal strategy employed and the type of emotion that is being regulated.

Interplay with Cognition

It is rather intuitive to assume that emotion regulation should be, at least in part, dependent on executive functioning (EF). In fact, the above section on neuroanatomic substrates reviewed evidence of a robust and clear relationship between emotion regulation and the prefrontal cortex, the presumed substrate of EF. Additionally, research has shown that (1) the ability to inhibit overt emotional displays correlates with EF (Schmeichel, Volokhov, & Demaree, 2008); (2) EF and emotion regulation begin to emerge together during early development (Carlson & Wang, 2007; Liebermann, Giesbrecht, & Maller, 2007); and (3) clinical populations with deficient attentional and EF systems also exhibit deficits in emotion regulation (Magar, Phillips, & Hosie, 2008; Martel, 2009).

However, the relationship between emotion regulation and EF has implications that reach beyond what is intuitively obvious. In particular, an increasing amount of evidence is beginning to show that the simple act of engaging in some form of emotion regulation can have taxing consequences on cognition in general and EF in particular. For example, emotional suppression decreases the amount of remembered material (Egloff, Schmukle, Burns, & Schwerdtfeger, 2006; Jing & Jiamei, 2007; Richards & Gross, 2000, 2006), and even the simple act of exaggerating or suppressing emotional facial expressions depletes executive resources (as reflected in poorer

EF test performance) to the same degree as engagement in executively taxing cognitive tasks (Schmeichel, 2007). Additionally, decision making (discussed in more detail in Chapter 9) becomes impaired as a function of engaging in emotion regulation (Heilman, Crisan, Houser, Miclea, & Miu, 2010).

INTEGRATING THEORY AND PRACTICE

Assessment

Emotion Regulation and Test Performance

STEREOTYPE THREAT

The recent evidence that engagement in emotion regulation depletes cognitive and executive resources serves as a reminder of the need for optimal rapport and testing conditions. For example, it is well recognized that when people perceive a threat of being negatively stereotyped (e.g., women and girls fearing that their math skills will be under scrutiny, African Americans fearing that their language skills will be under scrutiny, or a child who has been labeled as learning disabled fearing that his or her spelling performance will be under scrutiny), they perform less well on cognitive measures than when no such stereotype threat is present or perceived (Spencer, Steele, & Quinn, 1999; Steele, 1997; Steele & Aronson, 1995).

Recently, the mechanism behind these well-known effects has been examined, and the results suggest that poorer performance under stereotype threat conditions can be explained by the demands placed on emotion regulation resources during the testing situation. Specifically, individuals who fear that they may be perceived as less likely to succeed commit EF resources to emotion regulation (e.g., controlling one's facial and behavioral signs of anxiety), which in turn depletes EF reserves (Johns, Inzlicht, & Schmader, 2008). The same principle can explain the deleterious effects of anxiety, depression, bereavement, and so on, on test performance. Thus, this line of research also suggests that allowing patients to express their concerns about testing, to share their grief, or to reveal other uncomfortable feelings during the preassessment interview may be key to securing optimal performance during testing, as it may free up EF resources from the demands of emotion regulation.

RESPONSIVENESS TO FEEDBACK

There is some evidence that individuals who tend to rely on reappraisals for emotion regulation also tend to exhibit improvements in test performance when given negative feedback, whereas habitual suppressors are less likely to do so (Raftery & Bizer, 2009). It is unclear whether this effect is a function of depletion of cognitive resources associated with suppression, or whether it simply reflects a habitual failure to incorporate feedback cognitively. Regardless of the exact mechanism, these findings suggest that suppressors may fail to benefit from important feedback of their teachers, supervisors, or employers, perhaps even precluding them from realizing their full potential. This tendency may also translate into sub-par performance in neuropsychological assessment situations, if feedback on practice items is not fully incorporated. Although no research has thus far examined whether suppressors would also perform more poorly on measures for which negative feedback is an integral part of the test, such as the Wisconsin Card Sorting Test or the Category Test, this possibility must be considered and should be examined empirically in future research.

Assessment of Emotion Regulation Styles

The *Emotion Regulation Questionnaire* (ERQ; Gross & John, 2003) was developed specifically with the goal of distinguishing between two types of emotion regulation: reappraisal and suppression. The ERQ consists of 10 Likert scale items, with six loading on the reappraisal factor and four loading on the suppression factor. The scale has good reliability, with *r* values ranging from .73 to .79. Validity studies show that ERQ scores correlate in a theoretically consistent fashion with personality traits as well as with levels of experienced emotions (Gross & John, 2003). Reliability and validity results have been replicated with Italian (Balzarotti, John, & Gross, 2010), German (Abler & Kessler, 2009), and French (Christophe, Antoine, Leroy, & Delelis, 2009) versions of the scale, as well as with adolescents (Watson, 2008) and patients with MS (Phillips et al., 2009). The scale items and administration and scoring instruction can be found on the Stanford Psychophysiology Laboratory website (*www-psych.standord.edu/~psyphy/*).

Clinical Signs and Syndromes

It is intuitively obvious that psychopathology is virtually defined by impairments in emotion regulation. In other words, failures to control one's internal affective reactions can translate into depressed and anxious states, and failures to control one's external manifestations of such states translate into maladaptive behaviors that interfere with the achievement and maintenance of adult goals. To be sure, hormonal and neurotransmitter imbalances contribute to both psychopathology and impairments in emotion regulation. However, it is also the case that learning effective ways of regulating one's emotions, such as coping methods promoted by cognitive-behavioral therapy, actually changes brain chemistry and normalizes patterns of brain activation (Rabe, Zoellner, Beauducel, Maercker, & Karl, 2008; Roffman, Marci, Glick, Dougherty, & Rauch, 2005; Saxena et al., 2009). In other words, neurochemistry and coping skills likely interact in reciprocal ways. However, exploring the complexity of such interactions is beyond the scope of this book. Thus, for the purpose of this chapter, psychopathology is discussed from the standpoint of a breakdown in emotion regulation.

Secondary Depression

Among the most common syndromes associated with impaired emotion regulation is *secondary depression*, which can present as a full-blown major depression characterized by the same symptomatology as endogenous depression (Nicholl, Lincoln, Muncaster, & Thomas, 2002) and, at least in some populations, responds to similar interventions (see the section "Cerebral–Vascular Accident" below). Secondary depression is typically associated with lesions in the left frontal lobe, and the severity of depression tends to be related to the distance of the lesion from the frontal pole (i.e., the further anterior the lesion, the more severe the symptomatology) (Narashima et al., 2003; Robinson, 1983, 1985a, 1985b; Vataja et al., 2004).[2] The association of secondary depression with lesions in the left dorsolateral prefrontal cortex is consistent with the relative hypoactivation seen in the left prefrontal cortex among individuals suffering from primary depression (Henriques & Davidson, 1990, 1991). Although secondary depression is best recognized among patients with stroke (Starkstein & Lischinsky, 2002), left frontal pathology has been associated with depression in other neurological populations, including those with epilepsy (Suchy & Chelune, 2001), MS (Feinstein et al., 2004), complicated mild TBI (Busch & Alpern, 1998), and brain tumor (Starkstein & Migliorelli, 1993).

Secondary Mania and Bipolar Disorder

Unlike secondary depression, both secondary mania and secondary bipolar disorder tend to be associated with lesions in the right hemisphere, typically involving the ventral portions of the frontal and anterior temporal lobes for mania, and basal ganglia and thalamus for bipolar disorder (Bornke, Postert, Przuntek, & Buttner, 1998; Gafoor & O'Keane, 2003; Goyal, Sameer, & Chandrasekaran, 2006; Jorge, Robinson, Starkstein, & Arndt, 1993; Robinson, 1997; Starkstein & Robinson, 1997). However, lesions in other brain regions have also been reported, including the right temporoparietal (Celik, Erdogan, Tuglu, & Utku, 2004), right internal capsule (Nagaratnam, Wong, & Patel, 2006), and the left hemisphere (Fenn & George, 1999).

It has been suggested that secondary mania represents a point on a continuum that includes disinhibition syndrome, on one end, and mania with psychotic features, on the other (Nagaratnam et al., 2006). In fact, the same lesions that lead to disinhibition among most patients also seem to be associated with mania, although only if combined with family history of affective disorder and/or other genetic predisposition for psychopathology (Robinson, Boston, Starkstein, & Price, 1988). Despite the theoretical questions about how to classify secondary mania, manic symptoms secondary to neurological insults have been shown to respond to traditional pharmacological treatments (da Rocha, Correa, & Teixeira, 2008; Goyal et al., 2006).

Secondary mania and/or bipolar disorder most commonly occurs following TBIs (Jorge et al., 1993), but have also been described in patients with strokes (Bornke et al., 1998), brain tumors (Starkstein, Boston, & Robinson, 1988), renal disease (El-Mallakh, Shrader, & Widger, 1987; Wilson, 1998), HIV infection (Ellen, Judd, Mijch, & Cockram, 1999; Nakimuli-Mpungu, Musisi, Mpungu, & Katabira, 2006), MS (Miao, 2003), and epilepsy (Nishida et al., 2006).

Secondary Psychopathy (a.k.a. Acquired Sociopathy)

Secondary psychopathy describes individuals who, following a lesion to the frontal lobes, develop a personality characterized by diminished behavioral and affective control (e.g., increases in irritability and aggression), socially inappropriate behavior (e.g., unwanted sexual advances), decreases in empathy, and addictive and antisocial tendencies. These personality changes are generally related to lesions in the ventral portions of the frontal lobes, namely the orbitofrontal and ventromedial prefrontal cortices (Blair, 2001; Blair & Cipolotti, 2000). See Chapter 3 for a description of additional characteristics of primary psychopathy. Table 7.1 provides a review of empirically identified differences between primary and secondary psychopaths. Secondary psychopathy has been described primarily in relation to TBI (Blair & Cipolotti, 2000) and frontotemporal dementia (Mendez & Shapira, 2009).

Secondary Anxiety Disorders

One could argue that secondary anxiety disorders occur along the same continuum as pseudopsychopathic syndrome. As can be seen in Table 7.1, secondary psychopathy (in contrast to primary psychopathy) is characterized by high levels of anxiety, and anxiety may be the driving force behind some of the dysfunctional behaviors exhibited by secondary psychopaths. Anxiety of any type is, of course, a clear example of poor emotion regula-

TABLE 7.1. Characteristics Associated with Primary and Secondary Psychopathy

	Psychopathy type	
Characteristics	Primary	Secondary
Origin	Genetic	Environmental
Anxiety levels	Low	High
Aggression type	Predatory (instrumental)	Defensive (reactive)
Aggressive motivation	Personal gain	Anxiety and impulsivity
Impulsivity levels	Normal	High

Note. Based on Blair (2001); Newman, MacCoon, Vaughn, and Sadeh (2005); and Skeem et al. (2007).

tion. The literature on anxiety disorders following brain insult is inconsistent, although in general there is evidence of an increased risk for virtually all types of anxiety disorders (Hiott & Labbate, 2002; Moore, Terryberry-Spohr, & Hope, 2006; Williams & Evans, 2003). Among the most common etiologies are stroke (Robinson, 1997) and TBI (Chan, Parmenter, & Stancliffe, 2009; Horner, Selassie, Lineberry, Ferguson, & Labbate, 2008).

With respect to lesion location, evidence suggests that secondary anxiety may be associated with lesions to the orbitofrontal and ventromedial prefrontal areas, primarily on the right (Robinson, 1997; Tranel et al., 2002). This is consistent with research conducted with patients suffering from primary anxiety disorders. For example, patients with primary generalized anxiety disorder show less myelinated uncinate fasciculus (Phan et al., 2009), and patients with panic disorder show lesser activation in the orbitofrontal cortex in response to anxiety-inducing stimuli (Kent et al., 2005). In fact, abnormalities in the orbitofrontal cortex, particularly on the right, are shared by several different anxiety disorders (Rauch, Savage, Alpert, Fischman, & Jenike, 1997), consistent with the notion that keeping anxiety in check relies at least in part on down-regulation of the amygdala by the orbitofrontal cortex (Milad et al., 2007).[3]

Interestingly, however, one study found that in child survivors of TBI, greater damage in the orbitofrontal cortex was associated with *lower* levels of anxiety (Vasa et al., 2004). Although this finding seems at odds with the remainder of the literature, it is the only study that actually correlated anxiety with lesion size, as opposed to examining concordance of anxiety and orbitofrontal lesions. Because some research suggests that childhood brain injuries place one at risk for criminal offending in adulthood (Timonen et al., 2002), it is possible that when orbitofrontal injuries occur in childhood, the subsequent developmental disruption results in a more typical (and thus incorrectly assumed to be primary) psychopathic syndrome characterized by low levels of anxiety.

Clinical Populations

Neurodevelopmental Disorders

Among the most common neurodevelopmental disorders characterized by impaired emotion regulation is attention-deficit/hyperactivity disorder (ADHD). It has been argued that ADHD may be better, or at least as well, explained by emotional dysregulation than by cognitive impairments (Martel, 2009). For example, in one study, emotion regulation emerged as an independent predictor of ADHD, above and beyond impulsivity and attentional problems (Berlin, Bohlin, Nyberg, & Janols, 2004). In another study, emotion regulation proved to be a useful predictor of aggression among children with ADHD (Melnick & Hinshaw, 2000). Additionally, it has been suggested that emotion regulation deficits represent a common risk factor for the development of both conduct disorder and childhood depression, two disorders that are often comorbid with ADHD (Wolff & Ollendick, 2006).

Neurodegenerative Disorders

DEMENTIAS OF OLD AGE

Given the importance of the prefrontal cortex for emotion regulation, it is not surprising that emotion dysregulation is a common comorbidity of most dementing illnesses, as pathology in frontal–subcortical circuitry is common in dementias. The most frequent comorbidity is depression, occurring in approximately 50% of cases, but irritability and agitation are also frequently seen (Ritchie & Lovestone, 2002). Compared to other dementias, frontotemporal dementia is particularly associated with disinhibition and emotional–behavioral dysregulation (Engelborghs et al., 2005), undoubtedly due to considerable involvement of ventral frontal regions in this disorder. In contrast, vascular dementia is most often associated with depression (Lind, Edman, Sjogren, Wallin, & Karlsson, 2002), likely due to disconnection of the dorsolateral-basal ganglia circuitry. As compared to other dementias, AD is more often associated with verbal and physical aggression (Engelborghs et al., 2005), although the neuropathology of this presentation is not well understood. Lastly, relatively little work has been done on the relationship between dementias and anxiety disorders (Seignourel, Kunik, Snow, Wilson, & Stanley, 2008).

MULTIPLE SCLEROSIS

Patients with MS exhibit much higher rates of psychpathology in general and depression in particular when compared to the general population (Dalton & Heinrichs, 2005; Patten, Beck, Williams, Barbui, & Metz, 2003; Patten, Svenson, & Metz, 2005), as well as when compared to individuals suffering from other chronic illnesses (Patten et al., 2003). There is some evidence that greater lesion load in the left hemisphere predisposes patients with MS to depression (George, Kellner, Bernstein, & Goust, 1994). Specific lesion locations within the left hemisphere that appear to increase depression risk include the left arcuate fasciculus (Pujol et al., 2000; Pujol, Bello, Deus, Marta-Vilalta, & Capdevila, 1997) and the left anterior temporal gray matter and left ventral medial cortex (Feinstein et al., 2004). However, other studies have failed to find an association between lesion location and depression in MS (Moller, Wiedemann, Rohde, Backmund, & Sonntag, 1994), and still others have found associations between depression in MS and nonfrontal areas of the brain (Berg et al., 2000; Honer, Hurwitz, Li, Palmer, & Paty, 1987).

Other Neurological Disorders

TRAUMATIC BRAIN INJURY

TBI is often associated with psychiatric and behavioral symptoms that are likely secondary to deficiencies in emotion regulation. The most typical psychiatric problems include depression, anxiety, social inappropriateness, and irritability or aggression in response to slight provocation (American Psychiatric Association, 2000; Fann et al., 2004). Additionally, persistent behavioral problems have been identified among children with a history of TBI (L. Schwartz et al., 2003), and more serious psychiatric illnesses, such as mania, appear to be more common among TBI survivors as compared to the general population (Sagduyu, 2002).

The etiology of psychiatric and behavioral symptoms following a TBI has been a source of controversy, with some suspecting premorbid psychiatric or personality disorders, while others supporting neurogenic origins (Ruff, 2005). Evidence for the etiological contributions of both injury-related characteristics and premorbid psychopathology has been found (Fann et al., 2004; Rogers & Read, 2007; Ruff, 2005; L. Schwartz et al., 2003), and it is unlikely that either hypothesis alone can explain all symptoms of all patients. Rather, an interaction between the patient's premorbid emotion regulation style and injury location may play a role.

In particular, recall that there are individual differences in the use of emotion regulation strategies. In other words, some people overrely on behavioral suppression, whereas others are more prone to utilize cognitive reappraisal. Importantly, these two emotion regulation strategies are related to different brain circuits and different patterns of psychological functioning. That is, cognitive reappraisal appears to be subserved by the dorsolateral prefrontal cortex (Ochsner & Gross, 2007, 2008; Phan et al., 2005) and is associated with better emotional adjustment (Denollet et al., 2008) than suppression, which relies on the ventral prefrontal cortex (Abler et al., 2008; Phan et al., 2005; Ray et al., 2005) and is associated with greater experience of stress and interpersonal difficulties in everyday life (Denollet et al., 2008). Two conclusions can be drawn here.

First, given that (a) suppression is subserved by the ventral prefrontal cortex and (b) the ventral prefrontal cortex is among the brain areas most susceptible to injury in TBI, it would follow that individuals who were premorbid suppressors would also exhibit the greatest emotion regulation problems following a TBI. And second, given that suppressors (a) tend to have poorer premorbid psychological functioning (because of poor stress regulation) and (b) tend to have emotion regulation problems following a TBI (because of orbitofrontal damage), it would follow that the patients with postinjury adjustment issues also had premorbid issues. The important message is that, at least in this scenario, poor premorbid coping represents a correlate, not the cause, of poor postinjury adjustment. Thus, it may not be the psychiatric vulnerability alone that causes poor adjustment among these individuals following their TBI, but rather the fact that the brain area that subserves their preferred coping style—that is, the ventral frontal lobe—was damaged in their injury. See Figures 7.2a and 7.2b.

CEREBRAL–VASCULAR ACCIDENT

Secondary depression due to a cerebral–vascular accident (CVA) is often referred to as poststroke depression (PSD). It represents the most frequent psychiatric complication of CVA, with prevalence rate estimates ranging from 30 to 60% (Lenzi, Altieri, & Maestrini, 2008; Paolucci, 2008). PSD appears unrelated to prior personal or family history of depression (Lee, Tang, Yu, & Cheung, 2007); rather, as reviewed in the neuroanatomic substrates section above, PSD tends to be associated with infarcts affecting frontal-subcortical circuitry (primarily on the left), and is presumed to be at least in part caused by stroke-related executive dysfunction (Vataja et al., 2005). Although PSD tends to spontaneously decrease within the first several years following stroke (Morrison, Pollard, Johnston, & MacWalter, 2005), it is nevertheless associated with a number of serious adverse effects. These include poorer functional recovery (Paolucci, 2008), difficulties with activities of daily living (Narushima & Robinson, 2003), higher mortality

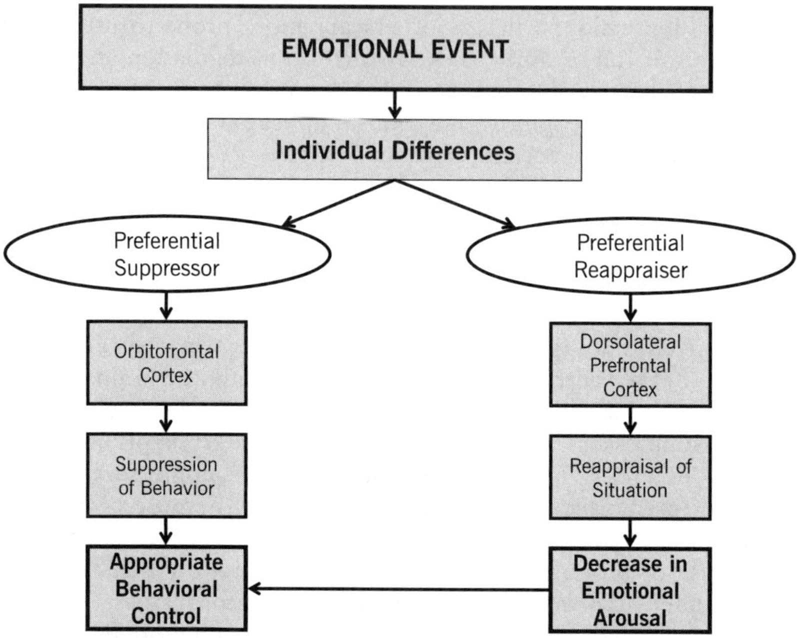

FIGURE 7.2a. Whether one prefers suppression or cognitive reappraisal as a coping strategy, behavioral control is achieved, only in different ways: Preferential suppressors cope by inhibiting external displays of emotions, a strategy that essentially equals behavioral control. In contrast, preferential reappraisers cope by altering the emotions they are experiencing. Once emotions are modified or diffused internally, inappropriate behavioral displays (as they relate to the given negative emotion) no longer need to be inhibited. Note that although both groups achieve behavioral control, only reappraisers achieve a decrease in emotional arousal and successful stress management, resulting in better mental health and better interpersonal relationships as compared to suppressors.

rates within the first decade following stroke (Jorge, Robinson, Arndt, & Starkstein, 2003; Williams, Ghose, & Swindle, 2004), and further exacerbation of cardiovascular disease (Thomas, Kalaria, & O'Brien, 2004).

PSD appears to be similar in its presentation to primary depression (Nicholl et al., 2002), and as such is presumed to respond to similar treatment methods. Pharmacological (Bhogal, Teasell, Foley, & Speechley, 2005; Turner-Stokes & Hassan, 2002), cognitive-behavioral (CBT) (Khan-Bourne & Brown, 2003), repetitive transcranial magnetic stimulation (rTMS) (Jorge et al., 2004), and high-intensity light (Sondergaard, Jarden, Martiny, Andersen, & Bech, 2006) treatments have all shown promise.

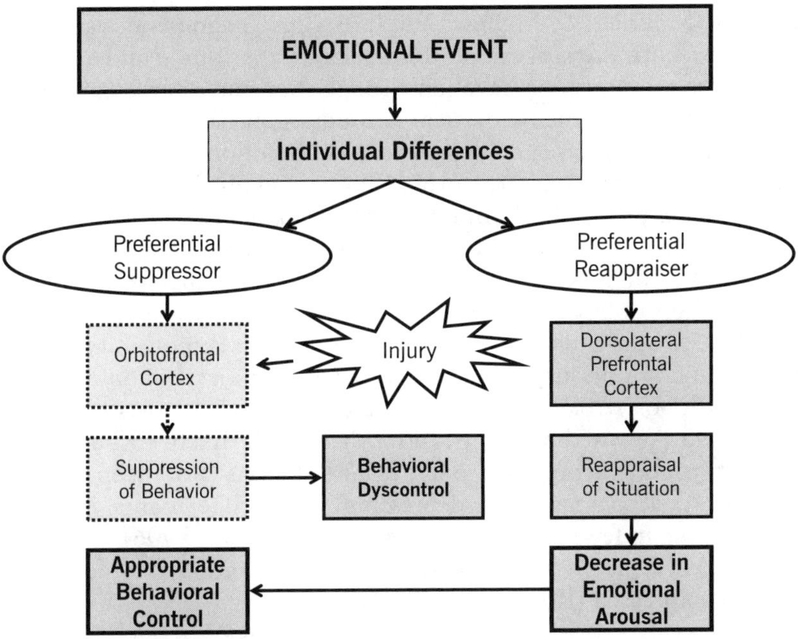

FIGURE 7.2b. Coping among individuals who have sustained an injury to the orbitofrontal cortex, resulting in compromised ability to inhibit behavioral manifestations of emotions (i.e., suppression). As can be seen in the figure, following the injury, preferential suppressors are at risk for behavioral dyscontrol. In contrast, reappraisers can still achieve behavioral control in the same ways as they did prior to their injury, assuming that their dorsolateral prefrontal cortex is reasonably intact.

Additionally, prophylactic use of pharmacotherapy has demonstrated some positive effect on mood and rehabilitation when employed early after a CVA (Guang'an, Jinfang, & Lixin, 2004; Niedermaier, Bohrer, Schulte, Schlattmann, & Heuser, 2004; Pomerantz, 2008; Robinson et al., 2008), and has been shown to improve survival rates 9 years later both in patients who were depressed at the time of enrollment and in those who were not (Jorge et al., 2003). What is more, from among patients who receive antidepressant treatment within 3 months after stroke, those who receive treatment earlier show greater improvements in functionality than those who receive treatment later (Narushima & Robinson, 2003).

In addition to depressive symptoms occurring after a large stroke, depression is also associated with vascular disease, especially if accompanied by executive deficits, "silent strokes," and white matter hyperintensities (Kales, Maixner, & Mellow, 2005). Because depression, vascular disease, and executive dysfunction are correlated, the source and causal links among these relationships have increasingly become a target of investigation. In particular, some theoretical accounts suggest that the relationship between vascular disease and depression is bidirectional (Kales et al., 2005) and is in part mediated by premorbid EF weaknesses (Mast, Yochim, MacNeill, & Lichtenberg, 2004). In fact, it has been demonstrated that EF deficits represent a risk factor for depression and/or depression relapse (Alexopoulos et al., 2000; Kales et al., 2005). However, others have suggested that depression precedes executive dysfunction (Cui, Lyness, Tu, King, & Caine, 2007). Lastly, because anxiety is a common comorbidity of depression, it should not be surprising that poststroke anxiety is common among patients with poststroke depression. Interestingly, when poststroke anxiety occurs alone (i.e., without depression), it is more likely to be associated with right frontal, as opposed to left frontal, lesions (Robinson, 1997).

In contrast to secondary depression, poststroke mania is relatively rare, occurring in fewer than 1% of cases (Goyal et al., 2006), and, as mentioned earlier, typically requires family history of mood disorders in order to become expressed (Robinson et al., 1988).

EPILEPSY

There is some evidence that patients with *left frontal* lobectomies for intractable epilepsy are at an increased risk for depression (Suchy & Chelune, 2001), whereas patients with *right temporal* lobectomies are at an increased risk for mania (Carran, Kohler, O'Connor, Bilker, & Sperling, 2003). However, only temporal lobectomy patients were examined in the latter study, leaving the possibility that right frontal lobectomies would also evidence an increased risk.

Additionally, some associations have also been found between interictal depression and left temporal lobe epilepsy (TLE) (Harden, 2002; Hermann, Seidenberg, Haltiner, & Wyler, 1991) and interictal mania and right TLE (Sanders & Mathews, 1994), although other studies on TLE patients have failed to identify such hemispheric differences (Swinkels, van Emde Boas, Kuyk, van Dyck, & Spinhoven, 2006). Lastly, in contrast to interictal and lobectomy findings, *postictal* mania tends to be associated with seizure locus in the *left* frontal or temporal lobes (Nishida et al., 2006). No research has examined postictal depression and seizure locus.

Neuropsychiatric Disorders

Affective dysregulation, whether with respect to poor regulation of internal affective states or overt behavioral displays, is the hallmark of psychopathology. A comprehensive review of neuropsychiatric disorders characterized by affective dysregulation (and frontal lobe dysfunction) is beyond the scope of this chapter. Suffice it to say that the list includes mood disorders, anxiety disorders, trauma-related disorders, substance abuse and addictive disorders, eating disorders, psychotic disorders, and personality disorders—all representing the bread and butter of psychiatry and clinical psychology alike.

Interestingly, there is growing evidence that early weaknesses in the frontal-subcortical circuitry, as well as weaknesses in EF, may represent a vulnerability for the development of psychopathology later in life (Williams et al., 2009). This has been demonstrated with a variety of populations. For example, children who exhibit EF weaknesses early in life are more prone to develop substance abuse (Nigg et al., 2006) and aggressive tendencies in adolescence or adulthood (Giancola, Martin, Tarter, & Pelham, 1996; Giancola, Moss, Martin, Kirisci, & Tarter, 1996). Similarly, early executive dysfunction is associated with features of borderline personality in childhood and adolescence (Coolidge, Segal, Stewart, & Ellett, 2000; Zelkowitz et al., 2004) and even future development of serious mental illness such as schizophrenia (Fish & Kendler, 2005; Mittal & Walker, 2007; Walker, Lewis, Loewy, & Palyo, 1999; Walker, Savoie, & Davis, 1994). Additional topics related to psychopathology in general and major depression in particular, especially as they relate to different affective styles and the impact of a stress response, can be found in Chapters 8 and 10, respectively.

SUMMARY AND CONCLUSIONS

Affective dysregulation secondary to neurological dysfunction or insult typically involves lesions in the frontal lobes and presents as various forms of psychopathology, with symptoms closely resembling those seen in patients with primary forms of psychopathology. Most common forms of dysfunction are secondary depression, secondary anxiety, and secondary psychopathy. Important differences exist between primary and secondary presentations of psychopathy, and these differences may help answer questions about whether the disorder in a given patient was present premorbidly or was acquired due to brain injury. Relatedly, it is important to consider the possibility that differences in adjustment following a brain injury may be a function of different premorbid coping styles, and an interaction of those styles with lesion location. Lastly, poststroke depression is associated with considerable morbidity, and prophylactic pharmacotherapy early in the course of recovery from a stroke may improve both short-term and long-term outcomes.

NOTES

1. Of note, the tendency to ruminate (which can occur in the context of overt emotion suppression) is also associated with *prolonged* amygdalar activation, even following an exposure to stimuli that lead to only brief amygdalar activity in nonruminating individuals (Ray et al., 2005).
2. Although certain types of lesions outside of the left prefrontal cortex, including the medial prefrontal cortex (Drevets, Price, & Furey, 2008) and bilateral basal ganglia (Hama et al., 2007), have also been associated with symptoms that resemble major depression, the underlying deficit in these cases tends to be apathy rather than poor coping.
3. However, note that different subregions of the ventral prefrontal area have been linked to different anxiety disorders. (For a review, see Milad et al., 2007.)

PART III

Emotions, Affective Styles, and Motivation

How Emotions Shape Who We Are and What We Do

INTRODUCTION TO PART III

In Part II of this book, we examined five domains that comprise an emotional response, their neuroanatomic substrates, the syndromes they are associated with, and the implications of each for clinical neuropsychological practice. In Part III, we move beyond the level of discrete domains or even discrete emotional events to examine how the five emotional domains come together in *patterns* of emotional responses, and how such patterns *motivate* behavior. Importantly, the motivating role of emotions is not limited to the phasic seconds or minutes within which a given emotional response plays itself out. Rather, emotions are the fuel behind such tonic phenomena as mood, decision-making styles, and chronic susceptibility to daily stress.

To capture the underlying emotional tone that exists beyond a single emotional experience, Richard Davidson introduced the term *affective style* (Davidson, 1992a, 1992b, 1998a, 1998b). Affective style is a nonunitary construct, encompassing behavioral, cognitive, temperamental, and physiological tendencies (Davidson, 1993; Kagan, 1988). These tendencies are largely biologically determined (Davidson, 2003) and are reflected in various discrete measureable components of emotional response, as discussed in Part II of this book. In particular, affective styles are related to (1) the sensitivity of the emotional trigger mechanism (i.e., the amygdala), as reflected in tonic amygdalar activation (Davidson, Jackson, & Kalin, 2000); (2) multiple measurable features of reflexive emotional responses, including threshold for autonomic reactivity, peak amplitude of an autonomic response, and autonomic recovery time (Davidson, 1998a); (3) experience and communication of emotions (Schaefer, 2007; Sutton & Davidson, 2000); and (4) regulation of affect (Davidson, 2003; Davidson, Jackson, et al., 2000; Dennis, 2007). Consequently, affective styles determine prevail-

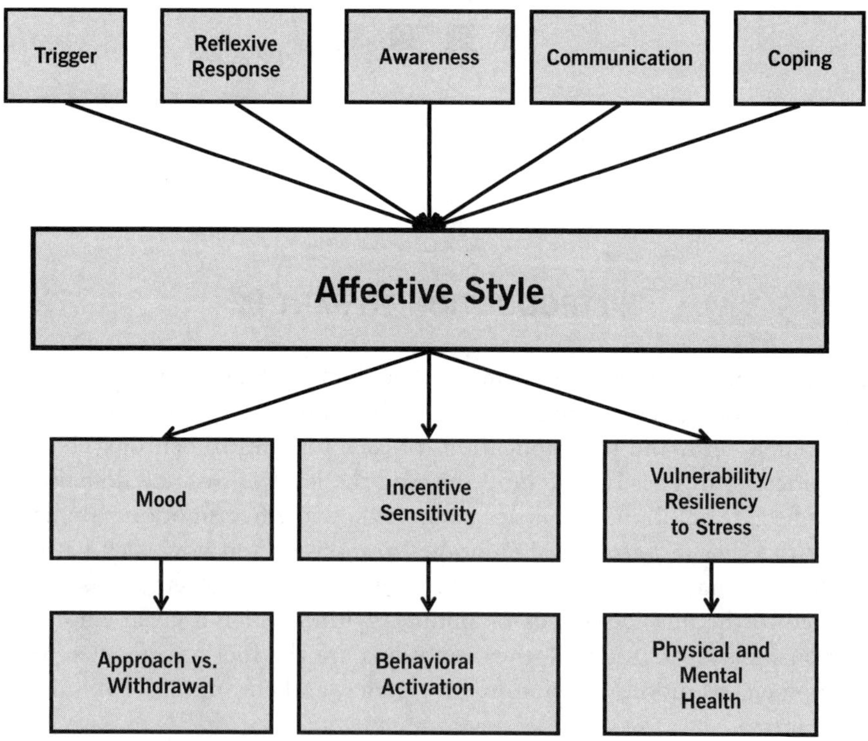

FIGURE III.1. A demonstration of how topics in Part III of the book relate to those examined in Part II. In particular, the five domains of emotional processing determine one's affective style. In turn, affective style translates into prevailing mood tendencies, incentive sensitivities, as well as vulnerabilities to stress. Each of these three "meta-domains" plays a role in motivating behavior in different ways.

ing moods, sensitivity to rewards and punishments, and vulnerability to stress. These tendencies, in turn, motivate behavior in different ways and propel people either away from, or toward, physical and mental health. See Figure III.1.

Readers will notice that the term *motivation* is conceptualized somewhat differently in each chapter, depending on the overarching theoretical framework: In Chapter 8, motivation consists of two opponent systems (approach vs. withdrawal) that ensure behavioral movement in the proper direction; in Chapter 9, motivation refers to a single behavioral activation system that ensures that behavioral output in any form takes place; and in Chapter 10, motivation refers to management of physiological resources that mediate physical and mental health. As was done in Part II, each of the three "outputs" of affective styles is examined from both theoretical and clinical standpoints, highlighting key syndromes, assessment issues, and clinical populations.

CHAPTER 8

Mood and Motivation

Is your glass half full or half empty? You may not ask yourself that question on a daily basis, but, if pressed for an answer, you would likely respond somewhat reflexively—your answer reflecting your basic and stable understanding of who you are. But, from one day to the next, your answer may ring more or less true because from one day to the next, your semantic knowledge of who you are interacts with the apparently inexplicable, but normal, fluctuations in your underlying emotional tone. These fluctuations—what we call *mood*—are a result of a complex collection of hormonal, neurochemical, and metabolic processes that color our thoughts, decisions, and behaviors in ways that we are unable to control or predict. This chapter reviews the emerging understanding of what mood is, where it comes from, and in what ways it motivates human behavior.

THEORETICAL BACKGROUND

Defining the Constructs

Mood

As discussed in Part II of this book, emotions are considered to reflect relatively brief episodes that occur in response to an emotion-evoking stimulus. They are characterized by reflexive physiological and motoric responses, awareness and cognitive elaboration, and down-regulation of affect. In contrast to emotion, personality is characterized by behavioral tendencies that are relatively stable across lifespan. These tendencies are partly determined by the idiosyncrasies of a given person's physiology (i.e., affective reactivity) and partly by past experience (Scherer & Peper, 2001). Thus, personality in part determines the specifics of a given emotional response.

Mood represents a state in between emotional responses, on the one hand, and personality, on the other. It can be conceptualized as the emotional working memory—that is, the substrate for holding important affective information in mind, thereby guiding behavior when immediate salient motivators are no longer present (Davidson, Jackson, et al., 2000). Mood shares processes in common with emotions, such as the sense of "feeling," albeit more long-lasting and somewhat diffused. It also shares processes in common with personality, in that *situation-specific* changes in one's mood occur against the background of mood tendencies that are more prevailing and *person-specific*.

Many of the processes covered earlier in this book contribute to, and interact with, mood. For example, mood tendencies are partly reinforced by amygdalar reactivity (i.e., the emotional trigger mechanism), but they are also known to mediate and moderate amygdalar activation, thereby indirectly influencing reflexive responses such as startle (see Chapter 3). The physiological and behavioral responses that take place following the initial amygdalar activation further influence mood, and, again, are themselves moderated and mediated by mood states (Davidson, Jackson, et al., 2000). See Figure 8.1.

Although one can certainly identify a variety of moods, from happy to excited to sad to angry, this chapter does *not* examine these more discrete mood states individually. Rather, we focus on two overarching mood dimensions known as *positive* and *negative affect* (Tellegen, Tuma, & Maser, 1985).

POSITIVE AND NEGATIVE AFFECT

Positive and negative affect (PA and NA) dimensions have been identified via factor-analytic research on mood and personality, and have been well validated across a variety of methods and populations (Tellegen et al., 1985; Tellegen, Watson, & Clark, 1999). The two dimensions are mutually orthogonal (Steer, Clark, Kumar, & Beck, 2008; Tellegen et al., 1999; Watson, 1988), representing two distinct affective processes. In particular, the PA dimension reflects the amount of positive feelings, ranging from complete absence of pleasure to highly intense pleasurable experience. It is predictive of depressive symptoms, with low PA reflecting anhedonia. In contrast, the NA dimension reflects the amount of negative feelings, again

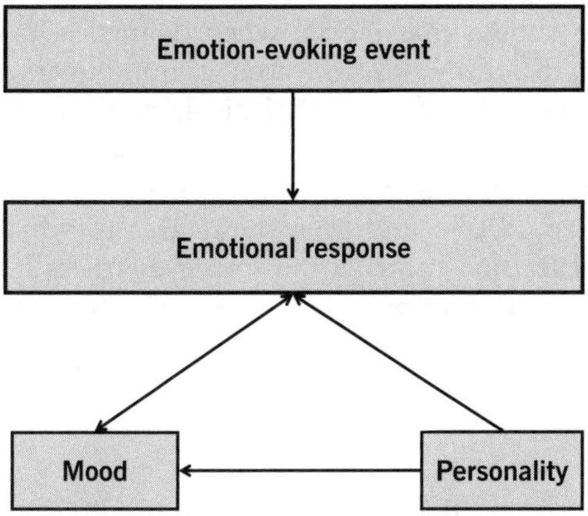

FIGURE 8.1. Mood is partly a function of personality and partly a function of the most recent emotional states. Mood also functions as an emotional working memory, modifying the nature of an emotional response to a subsequent emotion-evoking event.

ranging from complete absence of distress to high levels of intense distress. It is predictive of anxiety, with high NA reflecting unpleasantly high levels of autonomic arousal (Clark, Steer, & Beck, 1994; Clark & Watson, 1991; Kring, Persons, & Thomas, 2007). The amount of negative affect experienced by a given individual is therefore independent of the amount of positive affect that same person experiences. However, please note that due to the common comorbidity of depression and anxiety, the individual with depression is typically marked by both low levels of PA and high levels of NA. The various profiles of NA and PA are described in Table 8.1.

TABLE 8.1. States and Traits Associated with Different PA and NA Profiles

	Positive affect	
Negative affect	High	Low
High	High engagement High arousal Astonishment	Unpleasantness Sadness Distress
Low	Pleasantness Happiness Contentment	Disengagement Sluggishness Anhedonia

Note. For a more detailed description, see Watson and Tellegen (1985).

Research has shown that mood, when defined as PA and NA, influences our actions, including our nonverbal communications (e.g., interpretation and understanding of nonverbal displays of others) (Forgas, 1998; Forgas & East, 2008a, 2008b), affect regulation strategies (Dennis, 2007), conflict resolution strategies (Forgas & Cromer, 2004), the decisions we make (Yuen & Lee, 2003), and even the degree to which we are willing to incorporate misleading information into eyewitness testimony (Forgas, Laham, & Vargas, 2005). In other words, PA and NA appear to play a role in motivating our everyday actions.

Motivation

Motivation is the basic driving force of action. Without motivation, no action is possible. Although a variety of psychoanalytic, spiritual, and moral models of motivation has been proposed, *drive theory* arguably represents the most prominent and scientifically grounded account. According to this theory, behavior is motivated by a desire to reduce drives (Brown, 1961), which include hunger, thirst, sexual needs, and escape from pain (Hull, 1943). However, behavior clearly occurs even when these four drives have been satisfied (or reduced). For example, both animals and humans engage in play, in seeking companionship, or exploring unknown territory as if to satisfy curiosity. To help explain behaviors beyond those motivated by the four basic drives, other modifications of the drive theory have been proposed, such as, for example, the *theory of 16 basic desires* (Reiss, 2000).[1]

Both drive theory and the theory of 16 basic desires are based on the assumption that, ultimately, all behaviors emanate from a *single* common motivation: a movement toward the state of equilibrium, which might be defined as the presence of positive feelings (e.g., satiety) and the absence of negative feelings (e.g., pain, anxiety, or discomfort). Put differently, such equilibrium could be defined as presence of PA and absence of NA.

However, as already discussed earlier, PA and NA are thought to represent not one but *two* separate, mutually orthogonal, affective systems. Thus, if the state of equilibrium is defined as an emotional state characterized by proper balance between PA and NA, and if achievement of such an emotional state represents the fuel behind motivation, then *two separate* overarching motivational systems must exist: one that propels an organism to attain PA (i.e., engaging in *approach* of pleasurable stimuli), and one that propels it to avoid NA (i.e., engaging in *withdrawal* from harmful or unpleasant stimuli).[2]

Which motivational system is engaged in any given moment depends in part on situational factors—that is, on the nature of the emotionally salient stimuli present in the environment—which presumably trigger a predictable emotional response. However, intrinsic (or person-specific) factors also play a role, as individual differences exist not only in emotional processing, but also in the relative strength of each of the two motivational systems. In other words, approach and withdrawal are engaged as a function of not only the external stimulus and the immediate emotional response, but also in relation to an entire array of emotional states and motivational tendencies that fall somewhere between the immediate emotion and the long-standing personality, that is, affective styles.

Neuroanatomic Substrates

Hemispheric Asymmetry of Affective Styles

As mentioned above, *affective style* is related to motivational tendencies of approach and withdrawal. Such tendencies have, in one way or another, been examined by a number of researchers (Gray, van Goozen, Van de Poll, & Sergeant, 1994; Kinsbourne, 1978; Schneirla & Jones, 1959), each proposing somewhat different conceptualizations, but all sharing the notion that withdrawal is subserved by the right cerebral hemisphere, whereas approach is subserved by the left hemisphere. The hemispheric asymmetry of emotional response is nicely in line with the autonomic differences between the two hemispheres (Hugdahl, 1996; Spence et al., 1996; Wittling, 1997; Yoon et al., 1997), such that the left hemisphere plays a role in parasympathetic activation (the very type of activation that is needed during appetitive and approach states), whereas the right hemisphere plays a role in sympathetic activation (the very type of activation that is needed in situations when withdrawal and rapid flight are in order).[3]

In addition to being in line with hemispheric differences in autonomic activation, the approach–withdrawal dichotomy provides a logical parallel to the functional neuroanatomy of relevant behavioral output. In particular, approach behaviors often rely on manual dexterity and complex motor programming, as would be the case when picking berries, participating in mutual grooming activities, or tending to the young. Of course manual dexterity and complex motor programming are well known to be associated with the *left* motor and prefrontal cortices (Haaland, 2006; Harrington & Haaland, 1991; Kawashima et al., 1993; Rushworth, Johansen-Berg, Gobel, & Devlin, 2003; Taylor & Heilman, 1980). In contrast, withdrawal from threats is much less dependent on complex fine motor skills or manual dexterity, and therefore less reliant on the left hemisphere. Rather, withdrawal relies on sustained attention to the external world, clearly a process that is right-hemisphere dominant.

In the contemporary scientific literature, arguably the most comprehensive theoretical and empirical writings in this area have been generated by Richard Davidson and colleagues, with particular focus on neuronal activation asymmetries between the left versus the right anterior temporal and prefrontal cortices (PFC). Davidson and colleagues have used multiple methods in generating an impressive corpus of support for the association between affective style (which, as mentioned above, includes approach and withdrawal tendencies, as well as PA and NA tendencies) and the right versus left PFC (Davidson, 1992a, 1992b). These studies have shown that activation asymmetries in the PFC permeate several levels of emotional phenomenology, including (1) transient shifts in positive versus negative emotions or mood, (2) stable affective tendencies, and (3) psychopathology. The empirical evidence from each of these areas is briefly reviewed below.

TRANSIENT MOOD STATES

Emotional reactions or transient changes in mood are generally studied using a mood induction paradigm. In this paradigm, participants are typically exposed to sad or happy written passages, films, audio-recorded stories, or photographs. Early research has shown that induction of negative affect tends to lead to *relative* increases in the right PFC electrophysiological (as assessed via EEG) activity, whereas positive affect leads to *relative* increases in the left PFC electrophysiological activity (Davidson, Ekman, Saron, Senulis, & Friesen, 1990). Later work using more precise methodology (i.e., positron emission tomography [PET]) revealed that negative and positive mood can be associated with more discrete regions within the prefrontal cortex: The anterior orbital, as well as inferior, middle, and superior frontal gyri of the *right* hemisphere have been implicated in negative mood, whereas the pre- and postcentral gyri of the *left* hemisphere have been implicated in positive mood (Sutton, Davidson, Donzella, & Irwin, 1997).

STABLE AFFECTIVE TENDENCIES

Hemispheric asymmetry also emerges when more pervasive mood tendencies are examined. In a series of studies using a variety of populations, Davison and colleagues have found that there are stable individual differences in the direction and degree of activation asymmetry in the anterior brain regions. In particular, infants and toddlers with greater baseline electrical activity in the right PFC (as compared to the left PFC) exhibit greater tendencies to cry, be shy or inhibited, and generally wary of their surroundings (Davidson & Fox, 1989; Davidson, Rickman, Schmidt, & Schulkin, 1999). Similarly, among adults, the asymmetry in the strength of neuronal activity in the left versus the right PFC was predictive of approach and withdrawal personality styles (Sutton et al., 1997), dispositional mood (Tomarken, Davidson, Wheeler, & Doss, 1992), and reactivity to positive and negative emotional stimuli (Tomarken, Davidson, & Henriques, 1990).

Additionally, individual differences appear to exist with respect to responsiveness to rewards (i.e., an emotional response that reflects approach), and these differences also appear to be related to hemispheric PFC activation asymmetry (Pizzagalli, Sherwood, Henriques, & Davidson, 2005; Sutton & Davidson, 2000).

These stable tendencies have served as the basis for the *diathesis–stress* model of *prefrontal activation asymmetry* proposed by Davidson and colleagues (Davidson, 1998b). According to this model, resting prefrontal activation asymmetries predispose people to respond in certain ways to emotional stimuli, and as such represent a vulnerability for the development of psychopathology under stressful circumstances.

PSYCHOPATHOLOGY

In addition to mood changes in normal populations, research conducted with clinical populations has demonstrated the relationship between hemispheric activation asymmetry and psychopathology. For example, individuals who are currently depressed, as well as those who are in remission but have a history of major depression, exhibit relatively *less left* PFC activity as compared to never-depressed controls; this asymmetry is thought to represent a biomarker for depression (Henriques & Davidson, 1990, 1991). Similarly, individuals suffering from a variety of anxiety disorders have been shown to exhibit relatively *more right* PFC activation when exposed to anxiety-provoking stimuli (Davidson, Lane, & Nadel, 2000). This asymmetry has been found particularly in the right inferior and ventromedial cortices (Rauch et al., 1997), perhaps due to these regions' role in anticipating negative and positive affective consequences (Bechara, Damasio, Damasio, & Anderson, 1994).[4] Together these findings are consistent with the notion of separate systems for positive and negative affectivity (and approach and withdrawal motivations) subserved by the left and the right PFC, respectively.

CRITICAL REVIEW

The approach–withdrawal model of hemispheric asymmetry is seductively elegant. It offers a logical framework for basic organization of behavior that is adaptive and efficient. It forms theoretically solid linkages between physiology, neuroanatomy, cognition, and behavior. It also provides considerable empirical support. However, the model is not without problems. Criticisms or countervailing evidence has emerged in several important domains: conceptual, methodological, and empirical.

The primary *conceptual* problem with this model is that it is sometimes difficult to determine which emotions are associated with approach, and which are associated with withdrawal. For example, running away from threat could also involve running toward home or safety (Blanchard & Blanchard, 1994). Additionally, the distinction between emotional valence (i.e., PA vs. NA), on the one hand, and motivational/action tendencies (i.e., approach vs. withdrawal), on the other, is not always made clear, and the two are sometimes assumed to refer to the same construct. However, there are some clear distinctions between the two. For example, anger is deemed to be a negative emotion, but, if accompanied by aggressive actions, it is also deemed to represent approach. Although this distinction is made clear in some writings (Davidson, Jackson, et al., 2000), the literature, on the whole, is fraught with inconsistencies and confusion. For review, see Murphy and colleagues (2003).

In addition to conceptual limitations, *methodological* questions have plagued the frontal asymmetry model of approach and withdrawal almost from its inception. First, overreliance on EEG has revealed problematic interpretations. For example, one study demonstrated that, depending on the data-analytic approach, EEG activation can be positively, negatively, or not at all correlated with affective reactivity (Hagemann, Naumann, Becker, Maier, & Bartussek, 1998).[5] Additional challenges are inherent in the complexity of the fMRI and PET methodologies, as well as the fact that discrete homologous regions of left and right prefrontal cortices are structurally asymmetric, making activation comparisons difficult (Davidson, Jackson, et al., 2000).

The conceptual and methodological questions are further compounded by inconsistencies in extant *empirical* findings. First, although anterior EEG asymmetry may be related to acute depression, whether it constitutes a *marker* for depression has been questioned (Debener et al., 2000), as some studies have found *no* baseline EEG differences between PA and NA groups (Bell & Fox, 2003; Dawson et al., 1999). Second, contrary to functional imaging research, greater levels of depression have been associated with decreased gray matter volume in the right, but *not left*, prefrontal cortex (Vasic, Walter, Hoese, & Wolf, 2008). Third, relatively greater right prefrontal activation has been found to be related to externalizing, not shy, behaviors in children (Santesso, Reker, Schmidt, & Segalowitz, 2006). Lastly, a recent extensive meta-analysis of fMRI and PET studies found only partial support for the hemispheric specialization in approach and withdrawal. In particular, the study found that whereas approach emotions were associated with greater left than right activation, withdrawal emotions were associated with bilateral activation (Murphy et al., 2003). Incidentally that study found even less support for the hemispheric distinction between emotional valence (i.e., positive vs. negative), as opposed to motivated behavioral output (i.e., approach vs. withdrawal).

EVIDENCE FROM LESION STUDIES

Despite some problems with the studies that use EEG to demonstrate hemispheric asymmetry for affective and motivational styles, lesion research largely supports Davidson's theory. In particular, frontal lobotomy (i.e., bilateral prefrontal disconnection) patients have been characterized by severe apathy (Cohen, Novick, & Ettleson, 1942), consistent with disruption of the two motivational systems presumably subserved by the left and the right PFC. Additionally, as already discussed in Chapter 7, much research has shown that damage to the left frontal lobe tends to be associated with depression (Feinstein et al., 2004; Robinson, 1983; Starkstein & Lischinsky, 2002; Suchy & Chelune, 2001), whereas damage to the right frontal lobe can be associated with mania or disinhibition (Gafoor & O'Keane, 2003; Goyal et al., 2006; Robinson, 1997). However, right prefrontal lesions (particularly orbitofrontal) are also associated with increases in anxiety (Gafoor & O'Keane, 2003; Goyal et al., 2006; Robinson, 1997; Tranel et al., 2002)—a finding that is in direct opposition to the notion that the right PFC supports negative affectivity.

The Anterior Cingulate Cortex: The Motivation–Action Interface

Despite some support for the hemispheric asymmetry of affective style (Davidson, 1992a, 1992b), as well as the role of affective style in motivating the *direction* of a behavioral response (Davidson, 1998a; Davidson, Jackson, et al., 2000), it is important to keep in mind that a *global lack of motivation* is most often associated with lesions in the anterior cingulate cortex and medial prefrontal cortex. This is not surprising, given the role of this brain area in the experience of emotion (see Chapter 5), as well as in autonomic activation (see Chapter 4). In other words, while the left and right PFC may play a role in the generation of mood that facilitates an action in a particular direction, the mood likely cannot be fully experienced and the action cannot be triggered without the involvement of the anterior cingulate cortex. A more extensive discussion of the role of the anterior cingulate cortex in motivation, especially as it relates to responsiveness to rewards and punishments, is presented in Chapter 9.

Interplay with Cognition

The approach and withdrawal dimensions discussed earlier in this chapter are generally described as two motivational systems, that is, systems whose primary purpose is to organize behavioral output in response to emotional experiences. However, the two systems also parallel certain neurocognitive processes that are asymmetrically localized within the left and the right prefrontal cortices. These processes are under the purview of two neurocognitive domains: (1) executive/behavioral control and (2) language.

Executive/Behavioral Control

INITIATION AND INHIBITION

Two executive processes that seem to clearly parallel the notion of approach and withdrawal are *initiation* and *inhibition*. Both processes have been attributed largely to frontal-subcortical circuitry, with much evidence pointing to clearly lateralized networks, with inhibition related to the *right* (Casey, Castellanos, Giedd, & Marsh, 1997; Nielson, Langenecker, & Garavan, 2002; Stuss et al., 2002; Sutton & Davidson, 1997; Vendrell et al., 1995) and initiation to the *left* (Lezak et al., 2004; Stuss et al., 2002) PFC. Given the association between depression and relatively lower activation in the left PFC, it should then not be surprising that depression tends to be associated with initiation deficits and psychomotor retardation (Pier, Hulstijn, & Sabbe, 2004).

SWITCHING

Switching is a core component of executive functioning that has been shown to be lateralized to the left hemisphere. In particular, a number of functional imaging studies have demonstrated substantial *left*-hemisphere activation during task switching (DiGirolamo et al., 2001; Dove, Pollmann, Schubert, Wiggins, & von Cramon, 2000; Dreher & Grafman, 2003; Sylvester et al., 2003); and lesion research has shown that patients with left-hemisphere damage require more time than those with right-hemisphere damage to complete a switch between two tasks (Mecklinger, von Cramon, Springer, & Matthes-von Cramon, 1999; Rogers et al., 1998). Interestingly, consistent with the notion that the *left* prefrontal cortex subserves both cognitive switching and positive affectivity, research has shown that cognitive flexibility improves as positive affect increases (Compton, Wirtz, Pajoumand, Claus, & Heller, 2004; Dreisbach & Goschke, 2004). Lastly, as discussed in Chapter 7, cognitive reappraisal as a coping style is thought to be subserved by the left prefrontal cortex (Ochsner & Gross, 2008), further pointing to an overlap among the substrates for cognitive flexibility, flexible coping, and positive affectivity. For a literature review and a theoretical model of the relationship between PA and improved cognitive flexibility, see Ashby, Isen, and Turken (1999) and Ashby and colleagues (2002).

Language

It is well recognized that expressive and grammatical aspects of speech are subserved by the left frontal networks. Expressive language, of course, can easily be conceptualized as an approach behavior. In fact, carefully articulated verbal discourse is needed if approach toward others is to meet with success; in contrast, inarticulate grunting and growling are sufficient when withdrawal from others is the goal. The hypothesized relationship between language and positive (i.e., approach-oriented) affective style has found some empirical support in Davidson's laboratory. In particular, positive affective style has been found to be associated not only with left frontal activation, but also with better performance on verbal fluency measures (Hoptman & Davidson, 1998). Similarly, affective styles in young children correlate with language skills and predict language abilities 5 years later (Slomkowski, Nelson, Dunn, & Plomin, 1992). Additionally, induction of NA appears to decrease verbal communication in high-conflict situations (Forgas & Cromer, 2004) and impairs verbal associative reasoning (Storbeck & Clore, 2008). Lastly, induced sad mood appears to attenuate the brain activation pattern typically seen during verbal fluency performance (Baker, Frith, & Dolan, 1997), suggesting less effective processing of the task's cognitive demands.

Other Cognitive Domains

Given the presumed association between stronger verbal abilities and PA, one would expect that NA would be related to stronger visual–spatial skills. However, relationships in the expected direction have not been found: In recent studies, participants who were high on negative affectivity exhibited a slight weakness on visual–spatial tasks, as compared to verbal tasks (Bell & Fox, 2003), and induction of PA improved children's visual–spatial task performance (Rader & Hughes, 2005).

INTEGRATING THEORY AND PRACTICE

The presumed relationship between affective styles and hemispheric asymmetry raises a number of questions that have relevance for clinical neuropsychologists. First, if fluctuations in mood impact cognitive performances in experimental settings, perhaps research aimed at better understanding of such fluctuations during clinical assessments may be warranted. Second, if affective styles are associated with stable asymmetries in brain activation and corresponding asymmetries in cognitive strengths and weaknesses, then perhaps they could be controlled for normatively in the same fashion we control for gender, education, or other stable characteristics. Lastly, if affective styles are stable across the lifespan, then perhaps better understanding of the stability, or instability, of such styles in the face of neurological illness may inform diagnostics. The answers to these questions are, to some extent, intuitively obvious to practicing clinicians. However, empirical research on clinical application of these notions is still sorely lacking, and clinicians are left relying on rules of thumb and clinical judgments, rather than empirically driven normative guidelines.

Assessment

Mood and Test Performance

As discussed earlier, there is evidence that increases in positive affect may improve cognitive flexibility (Ashby et al., 1999, 2002), and, in fact, most people can probably relate to being cognitively "stuck" when feeling low, demoralized, or discouraged. However, it is yet unclear whether the experimentally produced effects reported in the literature translate into meaningful fluctuations in performances on neuropsychological measures in clinical situations. Nevertheless, the research reviewed in this chapter supports the typical practice of reassessing patients after difficult life circumstances, such as grieving a loss of a loved one, resolve. Additionally, the research reviewed here serves as a reminder that clinicians need to continue to be vigilant about providing positive, supportive, and encouraging testing environment to patients, so as to minimize undue fluctuations in mood and, potentially, performance.

Psychological Assessment in Dementia

When assessing patients in various stages of dementia, clinicians often wonder to what extent self-reports of mood and personality are valid. With respect to assessment of Axis I disorders, particularly depression and anxiety, patients with cognitive impairment tend to considerably underreport symptoms (Chopra, Sullivan, Feldman, Landes, & Beck, 2008). However, self-reports of positive and negative affectivity as stable personality traits have been shown to be valid and consistent with caregiver reports, at least among patients diagnosed with MCI or mild to moderate Alzheimer's dementia (Rankin, Baldwin, et al., 2005; Ready, Ott, & Grace, 2007). In contrast, patients with frontotemporal degeneration exhibit considerable discrepancies with caregiver reports with respect to a variety of psychiatric symptoms and personality traits (Rankin, Kramer, et al., 2005).

Assessment of Affective and Motivational Styles

The *Positive and Negative Affect Schedule* (PANAS; Watson, Clark, & Tellegen, 1988) is a brief, 20-item scale of PA and NA, consisting of single-word mood descriptors (e.g., *excited, jittery, nervous*) rated on a Likert scale. The PANAS has been shown to have good reliability (*r* values ranging from .84 to .90) (Watson et al., 1988), and a large body of construct validity research has also been conducted. Validity and reliability results have been replicated with Mexican (Robles & Paez, 2003), Chinese (Wang, Li, Liu, & Du, 2007), Italian (Terraciano, McCrae, & Costa, 2003), French Canadian (Gaudreau, Sanchez, & Blondin, 2006), and Dutch (Engelen, De Peuter, Victoir, Van Diest, & Van Den Bergh, 2006) samples, as well as with children (Sandin, 2003) and ethnically diverse rural older adults (Kawata, 2006). Normative and cutting score information can be obtained from Crawford and colleagues (2009). Recently, specific recommendations for additional psychometric improvement of this already psychometrically solid instruments have been made (Tuccitto, Giacobbi, & Leite, 2010), and some suggestions that NA and PA, at least as assessed by this instrument, may not be completely independent have also emerged (Crawford & Henry, 2004; Engelen et al., 2006). Additionally, an International PANAS short form (I-PANAS-SF) has been developed and validated (Thompson, 2007).

Clinical Signs and Syndromes

Major Depression

Major depression is an extreme and pathological instantiation of an affective style characterized by low positive and usually (albeit not always) high negative affect. It ranks among the most common and widespread psychopathologies, affecting about 16% of the population over the lifetime, although only about half of those affected will seek treatment (Kessler et al., 2003). Major depression is associated with an array of cognitive deficits, mostly affecting performances on measures of executive functioning, memory, and speed of processing (McDermott & Ebmeier, 2009). Importantly, the cognitive decrements associated with depression are of clinical significance, with one study reporting that about 50% of patients with depression performed more than two standard deviations below expectations on measures of executive functioning (Veiel, 1997).[6] The same study also found that deficits of similar magnitude could be observed in other cognitive domains (visual and verbal memory, processing speed), albeit with lesser frequency (i.e., about 15% of patients). Such deficits have been reported among depressed individuals of all ages, from childhood and adolescence (Cataldo, Nobile, Lorusso, Battaglia, & Molteni, 2005; Jonsdottir, Bouma, Sergeant, & Scherder, 2006) to young adulthood (Castaneda, Tuulio-Henriksson, Marttunen, Suvisaari, & Loennqvist, 2008) to old age (Sheline et al., 2006).

Notably, a prevailing pattern of left-hemisphere weaknesses, as would be predicted by Davidson's work on the hemispheric asymmetry of affective styles, does not emerge from the literature on the whole. However, it could be argued that most tests of executive functioning, even if not routinely conceptualized as such, rely more heavily on the left, as opposed to the right, prefrontal cortex.[7] From that standpoint, studies that report global executive deficits among patients with depression could be interpreted as actually reflecting a left prefrontal hypoactivity, and, similarly, global executive weaknesses found among patients whose depression is in remission (Paelecke-Habermann, Pohl, & Leplow, 2005) could be viewed as supporting Davidson's hypothesis of left frontal weakness representing a biomarker for depression.[8]

Negative Affect as a Stable Trait

Similar to the association between depression and test performance, even just negative affectivity or dysthymia, in the absence of major depression, appears to relate to cognition and functionality. For example, in a nonclinical sample, individuals who measured high on negative affect reported greater degree of difficulties in the area of executive functioning (Spinella, 2007). In another study, dysthymia was even more strongly associated with poor cognitive flexibility than was depression, perhaps because it reflects a more stable and pervasive cognitive and affective style (Airaksinen, Larsson, Lundberg, & Forsell, 2004). Lastly, older adults who score high on harm avoidance[9] exhibit greater levels of functional disability, irrespective of age, frailty, or cognition (Wilson et al., 2006). Functional disability, in turn, tends to be related to poorer executive functioning (Burton, Strauss, Hultsch, & Hunter, 2006; Cahn-Weiner et al., 2007; Grigsby, Kaye, Baxter, Shetterly, & Hamman, 1998; Royall, Palmer, Chiodo, & Polk, 2005; Suchy, Blint, & Osmon, 1997; Suchy, Kraybill, & Franchow, 2010).

Clinical Populations

As argued throughout this chapter, affective styles represent fairly stable, lifelong, largely biologically determined tendencies of responding to the world. As suggested by Davidson, affective style that is associated with lesser left frontal activation represents a risk factor for psychopathology (Davidson, 1998b). An interesting question for clinical neuropsychology is whether such affective style may also represent a risk factor for cognitive decline in old age.

Neurodegenerative Disorders

DEMENTIAS

There is some evidence that negative affect and recurrent depressive episodes represent a risk factor for cognitive decline or even the development of dementia (Archer et al., 2009; Duchek, Balota, Storandt, & Larsen, 2007; Dux et al., 2008; Wang et al., 2009). For example, among patients with Alzheimer's disease, even mild depressive symptoms lead to considerable declines in functionality (Starkstein, Jorge, Mizrahi, & Robinson, 2005), and patients with a lifelong history of high reactivity to stress exhibit greater memory impairments than their less stressed counterparts (Wilson et al., 2004).[10] This association cannot be explained by increases in depressive symtomatology during prodromal stages of dementia, as at least one very large prospective study found no changes over time in the levels of depression among patients who eventually developed Alzheimer's disease (Wilson, Arnold, Beck, Bienias, & Bennett, 2008). Rather, negative affectivity and depression as risk factors seem to long predate the onset of the disease. These findings point not only to the fact that prodromal dementia does not appear to cause depression, but also to the fact that affective styles appear stable despite the onset of a degenerative disease. In particular, patients in mid to late stages of dementia (mixed sample) exhibit patterns of negative and positive affectivity that are similar to those present premorbidly (Magai, Cohen, Culver, Gomberg, & Malatesta, 1997), and patients with dementia who exhibit behavioral disturbances after dementia onset, in particular with respect to irritability, social withdrawal, and agitation, have a lifelong history of personality styles characterized by negative affectivity (Archer et al., 2007; Gould & Hyer, 2004). In other words, behavioral disturbance in such patients appears to reflect an exacerbation of stable premorbid traits. In contrast, behavioral disturbances observed in patients with frontotemporal-lobar degeneration are often inconsistent with the patients' premorbid traits (Lebert, Pasquier, & Petit, 1995).

Importantly, notice that the above research does not necessarily mean that cognitive decline and behavioral disturbance in old age are related to low positive affectivity or low left frontal activation, as Davidson's diathesis–stress model suggests. Rather, much of the research points to the relationship between cognitive decline and *high negative affect*. Recall that positive affect and negative affect are mutually orthogonal. Thus, it may well be that high negative affect, or a combination of high negative and low positive affect, is the culprit. Additional elaboration of this notion can be found in Chapters 11 and 12.

MULTIPLE SCLEROSIS

Interestingly, similar to dementia, depression and negative affect are predictive of future (i.e., 1 year later) cognitive declines among patients with MS (Christodoulou et al., 2009), as well as future increases in perceived negative impact of the illness on physical and mental functioning (Ytterberg, Johansson, Holmqvist, & von Koch, 2008). Additionally, negative affectivity is related to greater reports of physical and mental fatigue (Bol et al., 2010; Merkelbach, Koenig, & Sittinger, 2003) and may mediate the relationship between slow processing speed and poor cognition among patients with MS (Diamond, Johnson, Kaufman, & Graves, 2008).

Other Neurological Disorders

Pediatric brain injury appears to lead to *decreases in positive affect* and approach behaviors (Landry, Swank, Stuebing, Prasad, & Ewing-Cobbs, 2004). Interestingly, as discussed in Chapter 7, childhood brain injuries involving the orbitofrontal cortex can also be associated with *decreases in anxiety* (i.e., decreases in negative affect) (Vasa et al., 2004). As can be seen in Table 8.1, low levels of both positive and negative affect translate into general disengagement, and may represent a mechanism for other characteristics evidenced in survivors of pediatric TBI; that is, declines in initiation of social behaviors and responsiveness to social interactions (Landry et al., 2004) and increases in antisocial and criminal behaviors (Timonen et al., 2002).

SUMMARY AND CONCLUSIONS

On the whole, research supports the notion that affective styles represent a stable trait that can persist into old age and even beyond the state of dementia (with the exception of frontotemporal degeneration). Low positive and high negative affect among individuals with dementia appears to be associated with poorer executive functioning, or, at least, poor cognitive flexibility, and with a greater tendency to exhibit behavioral problems. When low positive and high negative affect become sufficiently exacerbated to qualify for a diagnosis of major depression, executive weaknesses can translate into clinically significant deficits, and other cognitive abilities begin to suffer, most notably, memory and processing speed. Interestingly, the pattern of cognitive weaknesses associated with low positive and high negative affective style does not appear to follow the expected hemispheric asymmetry for mood (i.e., it is not characterized by left-hemisphere weakness), despite the fact that left frontal lesions among neurological patients represent a reliable risk factor for depression (Chapter 7). Lastly, with respect to pediatric brain injury, research has shown decreases in both positive and negative affect, with increases in social disengagement and possibly criminal behavior.

NOTES

1. According to this theory, although all human beings presumably possess all 16 desires, there are individual differences in the potency of any given desire to motivate behavior, or to prioritize those desires (Reiss, 2004).
2. A related theory of two motivational systems was proposed by Jeffrey Gray (Gray, Gale, & Edwards, 1986). Based on animal research, he proposed that there is a biologically determined behavior activation system (BAS), which propels an animal to approach, and a behavior inhibition system (BIS), which propels an animal to withdraw.
3. These hemispheric differences in autonomic activation were discussed in more detail in Chapter 4.
4. This latter line of research is addressed further in Chapter 9.
5. Davidson offered extensive explanations of methodological challenges, stating that most studies fail to examine condition (or group) by hemispheric interactions, which he views as crucial step in this line of research (Davidson & Irwin, 1999).
6. The findings of this study are based on a meta-analysis.
7. The most common clinical measures of executive functioning, including the Trail Making Test Part B, the Stroop test, and verbal fluency (Ravnkilde, Videbech, Rosenberg, Gjedde, & Gade, 2002; Zakzanis, Mraz, & Graham, 2005), have all been linked to *left* prefrontal activation or damage. Figural (design) fluency has been shown to rely on the *bilateral* prefrontal cortex (Kramer et al., 2007; Suchy, Sands, & Chelune, 2003).
8. However, other viable interpretations exist, including simply general (not left) prefrontal weakness (see Chapter 11), as well as the deleterious effects of stress (see Chapter 10). Nevertheless, research conducted with a variety of neurological patients with acquired left-hemisphere damage provides strong evidence of lateralization of mood and depression. Please see Chapter 7, particularly the sections on secondary depression.
9. *Harm avoidance* reflects a motivational style characterized by withdrawal, rather than approach, and as such is related to negative affectivity.
10. For additional mechanisms of cognitive decline, as they relate to stress, see Chapter 10.

CHAPTER 9

Motivation and Sensitivity to Incentives

Imagine the world, just as it is, except no rewards, no punishments. A world like that would also mean no purpose, no goals, no action. Plants could still exist, passively receiving nutrients and energy from the air, water, and sun. So could perhaps some bacteria, or plankton, or maybe even algae. But certainly no species that relies on *active* pursuit of food or shelter or procreation could survive, or, in fact, even evolve. In other words, sensitivity to rewards and punishments is absolutely crucial not only for generation of adaptive behavior, but for the very survival of all but the simplest organisms.

THEORETICAL BACKGROUND

Defining the Constructs

Rewards and Punishments

Rewards and *punishments* refer to experiential *outcomes* that are pleasurable or aversive, respectively, and therefore desirable to pursue or avoid, respectively. As such, rewards and punishments serve the purpose of teaching us about how to interact with the world around us. Some rewards and punishments can be inherent to a given organism, such as sweet versus bitter taste, satiety versus hunger, comfort versus pain, as well as social acceptance versus shunning by other members of one's social group (Berridge & Kringelbach, 2008; Schulkin, 2004). Additionally, stimuli that are inherently neutral can acquire rewarding or punishing properties via direct or social learning. Such secondary rewards and punishments can come from many categories, including monetary, artistic, or even altruistic (Berridge & Kringelbach, 2008).

Because of the clear role of rewards and punishments in learning, these constructs invoke behavioristic theory. However, unlike behaviorism, the neuropsychology of rewards and punishments focuses less on the externally observable behavioral outcomes and more on what happens *inside* what the behaviorists would refer to as the "black box."[1] This chapter focuses on those brain mechanisms that comprise the *reward* and *punishment systems*.

As is implied in the term *system*, the processing of rewards and punishments is multifaceted, relying on at least three separate modules that serve three separate purposes: (1) experiencing the pleasurable or aversive characteristics of a *sensation*, (2) *learning* which behaviors lead to pleasurable and aversive outcomes, and (3) *being motivated* to engage in such learned behaviors. Within the reward system, these three components have also been described in the literature as *liking, learning*, and *wanting*, respectively (Berridge & Kringelbach, 2008). We examine these in turn below.

SENSATIONS

As Berridge and Kringelbach (2008) put it, *liking* is the "hedonic gloss [painted] onto mere sensations" (p. 464). Similarly, then, one could describe aversion as perhaps the "noxious patina" of sensations. But beyond these metaphors, the constructs of hedonic gloss and noxious patina are difficult to operationalize: For one thing, the act of pursuing or avoiding a stimulus cannot serve as an operationalization of sensations, as the motivation to pursue or avoid, on the one hand, and the experience of pleasure or displeasure, on the other, represent two processes that are distinct from one another. In fact, increases in reinforced behaviors can occur *in the absence* of pleasurable feelings (Wyvell & Berridge, 2000), and the act of avoiding a stimulus does not necessarily correspond to the magnitude of aversion (Seligman & Maier, 1967).

Autonomic activation, too, is inadequate as an index of liking and aversion because physiological reactions to pleasurable stimuli are fairly minimal (Rousmans, Robin, Dittmar, & Vernet-Maury, 2000) and appear relatively unrelated to the magnitude of the subjective hedonic experience (Leterme, Brun, Dittmar, & Robin, 2008). If anything, physiological responses associated with hedonic experience simply prepare the organism for the bodily demands that are linked with such an experience: For example, a sweet taste leads to activation of the hepatic branch of the vagus nerve, presumably in preparation for digestion (Niijima, 1991). With respect to aversion, research tells us that autonomic changes do occur in response to punishing outcomes such as pain (Aslaksen, Myrbakk, Hoifodt, & Flaten, 2007), fear (Dembiec, LeDoux, Shiromani, Keane, & LeDoux, 2009), embarrassment (Keltner & Buswell, 1997), shame (McClendon & Kadis, 1994), and even unpleasant taste (Rousmans et al., 2000). However, the specific profiles of such autonomic changes vary with different punishments, and, once again, it is yet unclear whether the intensity of the aversive experience corresponds with the strength or pattern of the physiological response.

Thus, it appears that reflexive autonomic and behavioral changes that are a central part of an emotional response (Chapter 4) and that contribute importantly to the subjective awareness of emotions (Chapter 5) do *not* seem to be sufficient to explain, or measure, the sensation of pleasure and aversion. Other processes, likely involving biochemical changes in the brain, must play a role. However, until reliable and valid measurements of such changes become available, researchers will be left to assessing sensations via self-report, or relying on clearly imperfect inferences based on behavioral and autonomic responses.

Aside from the difficulty with operationalization, and therefore the study, of sensations, it is not clear if conscious sensations serve a purpose, or whether they are mere epiphenomena generated by the reward and punishment systems. In fact, activation of the sensation circuitry at levels that are too low to be consciously detected are sufficient for motivation and behavior to occur (Fischman & Foltin, 1992; Fischman, Sudakov, Ganten, & Nikolov, 1989; Lamb, Preston, Schindler, & Meisch, 1991), suggesting that the actual experience of pleasure or pain may not serve a purpose. Although, as we'll see later, it is possible that sensations play a role in emotional decision making, such that they may help rank potential outcomes and prioritize behaviors, the degree to which conscious awareness is needed for this process is not clear.

LEARNING

In Chapter 3, we discussed the role the amygdala–hippocampus complex plays in learning associations between initially neutral stimuli and emotionally relevant outcomes, such as a gun signaling danger. However, in order to maximize pleasure and minimize aversion, it is not enough to learn that certain stimuli are associated with certain properties, nor is it sufficient to engage in reflexive emotional responses. Rather, one must learn the link between the pleasurable or aversive properties of various stimuli and the *behaviors* that achieve pleasurable or avoid aversive outcomes. The following example is offered to illustrate this distinction:

You are at home, sleeping in your bed, but suddenly are awakened by the piercing sound of a smoke detector. The screeching sound "trips" your emotional trigger (Chapter 3), causing a reflexive startle and a cascade of autonomic changes (Chapter 4). Next, you will likely become aware of your distress (Chapter 5) and communicate it to other family members (Chapter 6). Lastly, you will employ emotion regulation strategies (Chapter 7) that will facilitate your taking care of the problem, in this case perhaps a smoking pot that had been mistakenly left on the stove with the heat still turned on.

Now consider the following: After you have identified the source of the smoke, picked up the pot with a heavy oven mitt, taken it gingerly out into the yard and left it there under the cool stream from a garden hose, there you are, back in the house, still being pounded by the piercing, punishing sound of the alarm. In contrast to the initially reflexive and mindless emotional cascade that took over your body when the smoke alarm first woke you up, you are now experiencing a single-minded, goal-directed motivation to *eliminate* the deafening sound. Having been exposed to this aversive stimulus before, you know exactly what to do: You grab a broom from the broom closet and swing it against the ceiling, knocking the smoke alarm open and dislodging the battery that has been fueling the noxious screeching.

Importantly, having once learned this response is not enough, as rewarding and punishing contingencies may change. For example, if you replace your battery-operated smoke alarm with one that is hardwired, your previously learned broom trick will no longer work. In other words, new learning must be able to override old learning, so as to facilitate actions that are most relevant and adaptive at any given time.

So, to recap, whereas the role of the emotional system (described in Chapters 3 through 7) is to generate, and subsequently down-regulate, reflexive physiological and behavioral responses that will maximize our chances for survival, the role of the reward and punishment systems is to continuously teach us *new adaptive behaviors*—behaviors that, too, in the long run, will maximize our chances for survival.

However, just because learning has taken place doesn't necessarily mean that an action will follow. In other words, one needs to be *motivated* to engage in a given behavior. This aspect of the reward system is explored next.

MOTIVATION

As already discussed in Chapter 8, motivation is the driving force behind action. This statement, however, begs the question, what is the driving force *behind motivation*?

If we were to make a guess, we might propose that we are likely driven and motivated by the pleasurable and aversive experiences that our actions generate. This would be a very reasonable and intuitively appealing guess—and one that would in fact be in line with the long-held beliefs about reinforcement and learning. However, there are two problems with this notion. First, it is undeniably circular. In other words, it states that we want the things that we like because we like the things that we want. The second problem is that, as already alluded to in the section "Sensations," the motivation for action is separable from the pleasurable or aversive sensations of an outcome. For example, electrical stimulation in the substrates presumed to subserve motivation to achieve rewards leads to reward-seeking actions but *not* to concomitant pleasurable feelings (Wyvell & Berridge, 2000). Similarly, it is possible to experience an increased desire for a drug, even if the amounts initially administered are too small to be noticed, let alone experienced as pleasure (Fischman & Foltin, 1992; Fischman et al., 1989; Lamb et al., 1991). By the same token, impairments in motivation are *not* always necessarily accompanied by decreases in pleasurable or aversive experiences (Berridge & Kringelbach, 2008). Rather, once a particular behavior becomes accompanied by activation within the motivation module (whether it be via pleasurable experiences or pharmacological manipulation), the motivation to engage in that behavior is present even in the absence of additional pleasurable or aversive feelings.

Consider, for example, a Thanksgiving dinner. You had your first helping of turkey, mashed potatoes, and string bean casserole, and enjoyed it tremendously. Now, you ponder your empty plate and the still tall, albeit disheveled, piles of food on platters and in bowls in the center of the table in front of you. You are no longer hungry. In fact, you are beginning to feel somewhat stuffed. Yet, you are aware of a persistent nagging feeling that you must go back for seconds. And so you do: more turkey, more mashed potatoes, more string bean casserole. You finish your second helping, now feeling quite uncomfortably stuffed with food. You reflect on your behavior and think to yourself: *Why did I finish that second plate? It didn't even taste good to me anymore . . .*

In other words, the pleasure of eating was gone, but the motivation to engage in the behavior nevertheless persisted. In fact, even after you have finished your second plate, you may, at some point, reach for a piece of meat or a spoonful of mashed potatoes, not fully understanding why you are doing that, but giving in to that nagging motivation nonetheless. Clearly, then, once the association between eating turkey and pleasurable feeling has been made, the act of eating the turkey alone becomes self-motivating, and very little reinforcement of that behavior is needed in order for it to be maintained.

And so, the driving force behind motivation is . . . well, there is no driving force behind motivation. Rather, motivation is an entity in its own right, sometimes described as *psychomotor* or *incentive sensitization* (Robinson & Berridge, 2000), other times as *behavioral activation* (Salamone, Correa, Farrar, & Mingote, 2007; Salamone, Cousins, & Snyder, 1997), and other times simply as *wanting* (Berridge & Kringelbach, 2008). The differences among these terms are largely semantic. Ultimately, all the terms refer to a neural circuit that mobilizes action, in general. Once mobilized, behavioral output is generated from among the available repertoire of actions that have been previously learned and that fit the extant contextual cues. The purpose of this behavioral activation is thought to be twofold: On the one hand, it increases the likelihood that a given behavioral response, perhaps one that is important for survival, will actually take place. On the other hand, it also produces behaviors *repeatedly*, thus allowing implicit calculation of the odds of positive versus negative outcomes. Consequently, high levels of motivation are often experienced when contingencies are uncertain, such as during gambling. In the absence of viable contextual cues (i.e., when no cues are available to help select a given action from the available repertoire), such behavioral activation becomes agitation and can be seen, for example, among addicts in inpatient settings where the cues for specific drug-seeking behaviors are removed. Alternatively, agitation can also result from the presence of too many *competing* cues, requiring that a decision to engage in one behavior over another be made.

DECISION MAKING AND SENSITIVITY TO REWARDS AND PUNISHMENTS

Multiple stimuli that signal rewards and punishments are present everywhere around us, often all at once, requiring us to select from among many previously reinforced actions. To complicate the matters further, some stimuli can be sometimes rewarding and other times punishing. It seems that at any given moment, prior to any given action, one is faced with an array of questions: Is it better to pursue a reward or to avoid punishment? Which reward, or which punishment, is the most relevant for survival? And which reward, which punishment, is the most relevant—not yesterday, not tomorrow, but *right now*?

As mentioned earlier, awareness of sensations may aid with this process. To better understand how a potentially limited range of sensations can aid in making complex choices, one needs to consider the following: No external action the world imposes upon an individual, no matter how salubrious or horrific it may seem to an external observer, can have rewarding or punishing properties unless the brain processes it as such. Research tells us that the brain has the capacity to generate experiences of pleasure or distress in a dynamic fashion, such that current moods (Davidson, Jackson, et al., 2000), individual and situational differences (Delahunty et al., 2007; Giardino et al., 2008; Pizzagalli et al., 2005), and even developmental stages (van Duijvenvoorde, Zanolie, Rombouts, Raijmakers, & Crone, 2008) and the amount of circulating hormones (Li, Huang, Lin, & Sun, 2007; van Honk et al., 2004) can influence how something is experienced. It is these various contexts that elevate some of the pleasant or noxious experiences above others, thereby aiding us in the process of sorting through the excess of various rewarding and punishing signals. This finely graded sensitivity to rewards and punishments is the basis for an exquisitely fine-tuned process known as emotional decision making.

Neuroanatomic Substrates

For many years, it was believed that the mesolimbic dopaminergic system—the neuronal system that delivers dopamine from the ventral tegmental area via the medial forebrain bundle to the nucleus accumbens—is the be-all and end-all of the reinforcement circuitry (Fibiger & Phillips, 1988). This belief was based on empirical evidence consisting of literally millions upon millions of bar presses generated by scores of rats and other rodents that tirelessly sought the delivery of voltage, dopamine, amphetamines, and other stimulants into various components of this circuit. This relentless bar pressing was taken as evidence that the mesolimbic dopaminergic system in general, and the release of dopamine in the nucleus accumbens in particular, subserved learning of new behaviors as well as the maintenance of basic behaviors needed for survival, including eating, drinking, and sexual activity. This powerful influence over behavior was believed to be driven by the experience of intense pleasure, presumably associated with the release of dopamine in the nucleus accumbens, and led to the dubbing of this structure "the pleasure center" of the brain (Puccetti, 1969).[2]

However, in recent years, these interpretations have been questioned. First, the mesolimbic circuit appears to play a role in behavioral outputs that are motivated not only by pleasurable, but also by aversive, stimuli (Reynolds & Berridge, 2002), demonstrating that, in the very least, the nucleus accumbens does not "specialize" in pleasure alone. Second, with respect to pleasure, research has shown that (a) the mesolimbic dopamine system does *not* become activated in response to pleasurable sensation or pleasurable properties of reinforcing stimuli, (b) the intensity of pleasure does *not* appear to be related to the intensity of stimulation within the system, and (c) pleasurable experiences are *not* abolished by interfering with the mesolimbic dopamine (Berridge, 1996; Berridge & Robinson, 1998; Salamone et al., 1997). In other words, whatever it was that led the rats to engage in bar pressing, it apparently was not the experience of pleasure. And lastly, with respect to learning, evidence has emerged that the mesolimbic dopamine system does *not* appear to be necessary for making associations between neutral stimuli and pleasurable outcomes (Robinson, Sandstrom, Denenberg, & Palmiter, 2005).

Taken together, these findings demonstrate that the mesolimbic dopamine system is neither the "pleasure center" that it was once held out to be (Puccetti, 1969) nor the substrate for learning. Yet, the millions upon millions of bar presses are difficult to ignore. So what, then, is the role of this system? We address this question next.

Motivation

When the learning and the sensation components of reinforcing situations are teased apart, activation within the mesolimbic dopamine system and the release of dopamine in the nucleus accumbens correlate with the *anticipation* of rewards (and punishments), *calculation* of the probabilities that a particular outcome will occur, and the amount of behavioral effort and behavioral *activation* exerted in pursuit of rewards or avoidance of punishments (Faure et al., 2008; Fuchs, Ramirez, & Bell, 2008; Knutson, Adams, Fong, & Hommer, 2001; Mingote et al., 2008; Pessoa, 2009; Robbins & Everitt, 2007; Salamone et al., 2007). These findings have led to a *re*interpretation of the role of the mesolimbic dopamine, attributing motivational properties to it, outside of the context of liking and learning.

Beyond the nucleus accumbens, motivation to act is further elaborated in the anterior cingulate gyrus, which receives projections from the nucleus accumbens (Pessoa, 2009). Importantly, at least some studies have found that both the nucleus accumbens and the anterior cingulate gyrus become activated during incentive (reward or punishment) anticipation, but not incentive consumption (Dillon et al., 2008; Knutson, Fong, Adams, Varner, & Hommer, 2001), further supporting the dissociation between "wanting" and "liking." Additionally, the anterior cingulate gyrus also receives information from "hotspots" responsible for the generation of strong liking and aversion feelings (Petrovic et al., 2008). These hotspots are discussed next.

Sensation

LIKING

The neuroanatomic substrates of liking have been referred to as the "hedonic hotspots." These *hotspots* have been localized in the rostral dorsal quadrant of the nucleus accumbens, the posterior half of the ventral pallidum, and the parabrachial nucleus in the pons (Mahler, Smith, & Berridge, 2007; Smith & Berridge, 2007), although other yet-to-be identified hotspots likely exist within the limbic system and the brainstem. The hedonic hotspots are approximately 1 cubic centimeter large, and, when stimulated with opioids or other related neurochemicals, they considerably enhance liking reactions (Pecina & Berridge, 2005).

The study of the *hedonic hotspots* has generally relied on two paradigms: (1) electrical or biochemical stimulation of the presumed hotspots, with the expectation of enhanced subjective liking sensations, and (2) biochemical or surgical disruption of the hotspots, with the expectation of decreased liking sensations. These two lines of research have together demonstrated that some, but not all, hotspots are *sufficient*, and some, but not all, *necessary*, for pleasure generation. In other words, while stimulation of a given hotspot may enhance pleasurable experience during, say, the act of eating, disruption of the same circuit may *not* abolish the ability to enjoy food (Berridge & Kringelbach, 2008). These findings point to the considerable redundancy within the sensation module of the reward system, pointing to the evolutionary importance of hedonic pleasure, whether processed consciously or not.

AVERSION

Less is known about possible "hotspots" for aversion, although some aversion-sensitive areas do appear to exist in close proximity to those identified for pleasure. For example, the nucleus accumbens, particularly its more caudal areas, responds to aversive stimuli (Reynolds & Berridge, 2002), although it is thought that the discrimination between pleasurable versus aversive sensations may be more related to the patterns of neurochemical activity than to specific location within this structure (Roitman, Wheeler, Wightman, & Carelli, 2008).

Learning

There is general consensus that the orbitofrontal cortex represents the brain region most involved in coding the associations between reinforcing qualities (i.e., pleasurable or aversive sensations) and stimuli from all five sensory modalities (Rolls, 2004). It is also generally agreed that the orbitofrontal cortex has the ability not only to code such associations, but to update them rapidly. Thus, when contingencies change, new learning overrides old learning. This rapid updating takes place not only when contingencies reverse—that is, when something that was once pleasurable subsequently becomes punishing—but also when the hedonic value of stimuli decreases, such as after becoming satiated. Lastly, the orbitofrontal cortex also codes information about the *probability* of negative versus positive outcomes, which is gathered by repeated behavioral output motivated by the mesolimbic dopamine system.

However, with respect to the functions of individual subregions of the orbitofrontal cortex, the theoretical accounts and the empirical findings are far from clear. In general, the literature has considered functional differences between lateral versus medial orbitofrontal cortex, and it can be divided into three theoretical accounts: (1) the steadiness hypothesis, (2) the valence hypothesis, and (3) the somatic marker hypothesis. For a review, see Rolls (2004) and Windmann and colleagues (2006).

THE STEADINESS HYPOTHESIS

The notion that there is a neuroanatomic dissociation in the orbitofrontal cortex between responsiveness to steady versus changing contingencies was first proposed by Elliott and colleagues (Elliott, Dolan, & Frith, 2000). Evidence for this segregation comes primarily from functional imaging research that has shown that the lateral aspects of the orbitofrontal cortex respond to rewards that are uncertain or changing, requiring that previously reinforced responses be suppressed, whereas the medial aspect of the orbitofrontal cortex is activated when rewards are steady and predictable. Thus, for example, during the performance of the Wisconsin Card Sorting Test (WCST; Heaton, Chelune, Talley, Kay, & Curtiss, 1993), responses would initially rely more on the lateral aspects of the orbitofrontal cortex, because it is not yet clear which responses will be reinforced. Once the first sorting principle is identified, responses would begin to rely on the medial orbitofrontal cortex, maintaining the same, previously reinforced set. But as the initial sorting principle changes, the lateral aspects of the orbitofrontal cortex would once again need to be engaged, and so on and so forth. This is an elegant and theoretically appealing explanation of two opponent processors, that is, essentially, set maintenance and set switching. However, alternative explanation of essentially the same data is offered by the valence hypothesis.

THE VALENCE HYPOTHESIS

The valence hypothesis suggests that whereas the medial orbitofrontal cortex responds to rewards, the lateral orbitofrontal cortex responds to punishments. Support for a segregation of substrates that mediate learning based on rewards versus punishments is provided by functional imaging studies, which have found greater medial activation in response to rewards, and greater lateral activation in response to punishments (Grabenhorst, Rolls, Margot, da Silva, & Velazco, 2007; Markowitsch, Vandekerckhove, Lanfermann, & Russ, 2003; Rolls, 2004; Rolls, Kringelbach, & de Araujo, 2003; Rolls, O'Doherty, et al., 2003; Ursu & Carter, 2005).

Interestingly, individuals with greater capacity for experiencing pleasure exhibit stronger activation in the medial orbitofrontal cortex in response to pleasureable stimuli (Harvey, Pruessner, Czechowska, & Lepage, 2007), a result that provides support for the notion that the medial orbitofrontal cortex responds to pleasure rather than to "steadiness." In contrast, at least one study found equal medial orbitofrontal activation during delivery of both rewards and punishments (Dillon et al., 2008). However, it is not clear whether activation during incentive delivery necessarily translates into learning.

Regardless, the same hypothetical pattern of activation during WCST performance, described under the steadiness hypothesis, could apply to the valence hypothesis as well. In other words, since the medial orbitofrontal cortex would be activated during the steadily reinforced portions of the test, one could simply describe these portions of the test as being rewarding. In contrast, those portions of the test that are characterized by uncertainty and, presumably, reliance on the lateral prefrontal cortex, can also be conceptualized as simply being associated with punishment. This conceptually difficult distinction between the two theoretical accounts highlights how little we understand not only about the substrates, but also about the constructs of set switching and set maintenance.

THE SOMATIC MARKER HYPOTHESIS

Similar to the valence hypothesis, the somatic marker hypothesis, proposed and elaborated by Antonio Damasio and colleagues in the 1990s, also suggests segregated systems for learning about rewards and punishments. Unlike the valence hypothesis, however, the somatic marker hypothesis proposes that the substrate for learning from punishments is located in the ventromedial[3] prefrontal cortex.

According to this hypothesis, the brain has the ability to store associations between behavioral responses and markers of "somatic states." In other words, if a particular behavior leads to an intense physiological change, future initiation of a similar behavior will lead to reactivation of a similar physiological change, causing one to abort such behavior before it has a chance to trigger a full-blown negative outcome. What is more, such physiological changes can occur on a purely unconscious level, allowing for a highly economic guidance of behavior based on "gut feelings" rather than lengthy deliberation[4] (Bechara & Damasio, 2005).

Much of the research on the somatic marker hypothesis has utilized the Iowa Gambling Task (IGT; Bechara, Damasio, Tranel, & Damasio, 1997). In this task, examinees are presented with four decks of cards, turned face down, and asked to take cards from the decks with the goal of maximizing their winnings in the course of 100 trials. Two of the four decks are "bad," containing cards that provide very large winnings but, occasionally, even larger losses (for the overall loss by the end of the 100 trials), whereas the other two decks are "good," containing cards that provide small winnings, but even smaller losses (for the overall gain by the end of the 100 trials). Consistent with the somatic marker hypothesis (Bechara & Damasio, 2005), healthy normal examinees initially sample all four decks but fairly quickly, and without conscious awareness, begin to favor the good decks. What is more, these individuals also exhibit an increase in autonomic arousal as they begin to reach for the bad decks, which is believed to represent the "gut feeling" that guides their behavior away from the bad decks. In contrast, individuals with certain types of brain lesions seek out the larger winnings of the bad decks, while *not* being dissuaded by the larger losses. In other words, these individuals exhibit greater sensitivity to rewards than to punishments. What is more, such individuals fail to exhibit the anticipatory autonomic arousal (i.e., the presumed somatic markers) when they begin to reach for the bad decks.

According to the original somatic marker hypothesis, the somatic markers were thought to be stored in the ventromedial prefrontal cortex. In fact, behavioral and autonomic deficits on the IGT have been demonstrated among patients with ventromedial, but not other cortical, damage (Bechara et al., 1994; Bechara, Damasio, Tranel, & Damasio, 2005; Bechara, Tranel, & Damasio, 2000). Subsequent research has led to an elaboration of the original hypothesis, suggesting that the ventromedial prefrontal cortex damage in the right, but not the left, hemisphere alone is sufficient for such deficits (Bechara, 2004; Clark, Manes, Antoun, Sahakian, & Robbins, 2003; Tranel et al., 2002).[5]

Despite its elegance, the somatic marker hypothesis has been criticized on several grounds (Dunn, Dalgleish, & Lawrence, 2006; Maia & McClelland, 2005). First, individuals with bilateral amygdalar damage exhibit deficient IGT performance (Brand, Grabenhorst, Starcke, Vandekerckhove, & Markowitsch, 2007; Weller, 2007). Thus, perhaps any disruption of the connections between the amygdala and the substrate for the somatic markers would also lead to impairment. Second, research from other laboratories has shown that lesions elsewhere within the prefrontal cortex, including dorsolateral or dorsomedial prefrontal convexities (Fellows & Farah, 2005; MacPherson, Phillips, Della Sala, & Cantagallo, 2008; Manes et al., 2002), disrupt normal IGT performance. Lastly, there is some evidence that other cognitive functions, such as attention (Loesel & Schmucker, 2004) and memory (Premkumar et al., 2008), may mediate impairment on the IGT, at least for some populations. Thus, although the somatic marker hypothesis provides an elegant theoretical explanation for the mechanism behind "gut decisions," the neuroanatomic underpinnings of somatic markers have yet to be definitively identified.[6]

Summary

In summary, it appears clear that the orbitofrontal cortex (both the lateral and the medial portions thereof) plays a role in learning and updating based on emotionally salient incentives. However, the exact mechanisms of this learning process, and the degree to which the circuitry for such learning can be simply dichomized based on valence, steadiness, or any other simple characteristic, is not clear. Likely, much more complex mechanisms are at play.

Interplay with Cognition

The impact of dysfunctional reward and punishment systems on neurocognitive functioning is twofold. First, effective learning clearly cannot take place if this system is dysfunctional. But, perhaps even more importantly, a number of processes that fall under the umbrella of executive functions clearly must also be impaired. These include decision making, judgment, cognitive flexibility, and motivation. Cognitive flexibility, in particular, deserves further attention.

Cognitive flexibility (sometimes referred to as "switching") is the ability to stop a given cognitive or behavioral response and to initiate a new and different response. Ample evidence suggests that switching from one task to another, in the absence of tangible rewards and punishments, is related primarily to the dorsolateral prefrontal cortex (Demakis, 2003). However, when rewards and punishments are involved, the associations between rewards, punishments, and stimuli relies on the integrity of the orbitofrontal cortex. (For a review, see Clark, Cools, & Robbins, 2004.) In other words, simply informing an examinee about the need to switch appears to rely on different neuroanatomic substrate than when the cue to switch reflects a reward or punishment. This notion is supported by evidence that certain populations, such as criminal psychopaths, exhibit perseverative responding only when concrete rewards and punishments are administered (R. J. R. Blair et al., 2004; Newman, Patterson, Howland, & Nichols, 1990). For the clinical implications of the distinction between cognitive and emotional decision making, see the section "Assessment" later in this chapter.

INTEGRATING THEORY AND PRACTICE

Clinical Signs and Syndromes

Disorders of Diminished Motivation

APATHY, ABULIA, AND AKINETIC MUTISM

According to the diagnostic guidelines put forth by the American Congress of Rehabilitation Medicine (1995), disorders of diminished motivation are characterized by (1) diminished emotional reactivity to goal-related events or stimuli, (2) diminished goal-oriented cognitions, and (3) diminished goal-related behavioral output. These decreases should occur in the context of normal levels of consciousness, attention, language, and sensorimotor capacity, as well as normal eye tracking. *Apathy, abulia*, and *akinetic mutism* represent three examples of syndromes characterized by diminished motivation and are sometimes thought of as discrete entities. However, in reality, diminished motivation occurs along a continuum (see Figure 9.1.), with akinetic mutism representing the most severe form of motivational impairment, and apathy, the least severe or debilitating form. Abulia is typically considered to be somewhere in between the two levels of severity, with the boundaries distinguishing it from the other two disorders being somewhat arbitrary (American Congress of Rehabilitation Medicine, 1995).

Often, these disorders result from damage to the mesololimbic dopamine system (i.e., the ventral tegmental area and the nucleus accumbens) or to structures that receive mesolimbic dopaminergic projections—that is, the anterior cingulate gyrus and the ventral pallidum (American Congress of Rehabilitation Medicine, 1995; Marin & Wilkosz, 2005; Pessoa, 2009). Disorders of diminished motivation have been observed in a wide range of neurological conditions, including neurodegenerative disorders (particularly frontotemporal degeneration, progressive supranuclear palsy, and Hunting-

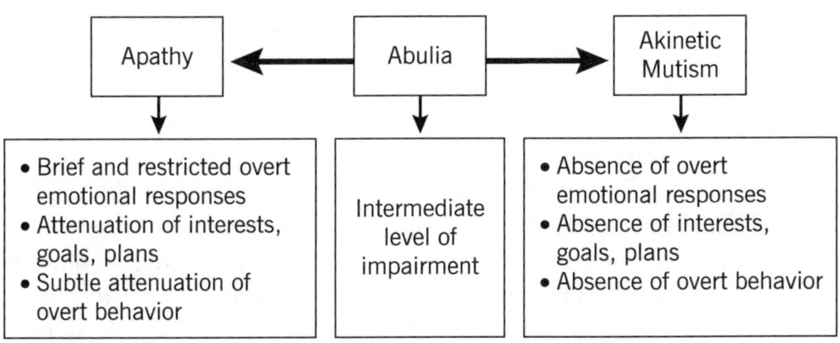

FIGURE 9.1. The relationship among apathy, abulia, and akinetic mutism, and the classic symptoms that define each.

ton's and Parkinson's diseases), cerebral vascular accidents (particularly thalamic, anterior cerebral artery, and right middle cerebral artery), white matter disease, TBI, brain tumor, and anoxia (Marin, Chakravorty, Silver, McAllister, & Yudofsky, 2004). Lastly, diminished motivation is also commonly associated with a variety of neuropsychiatric disorders, including major depression (Marin, Firinciogullari, & Biedrzycki, 1994) and schizophrenia (Roth, Flashman, Saykin, McAllister, & Vidaver, 2004).[7]

ANHEDONIA

Anhedonia is generally conceptualized as a diminished capacity to experience pleasure, although several lines of recent research have demonstrated that perhaps even more prominent feature is the lack of motivation to pursue rewards (Treadway, Buckholtz, Schwartzman, Lambert, & Zald, 2009). Some research even suggests that individuals with anhedonia report normal experience of pleasure in response to pleasurable stimuli (Germans & Kring, 2000). Interestingly, reward anticipation (which has been conceptualized as the motivation component of the reward circuitry) is associated with increases in self-reported happiness (Knutson, Adams, et al., 2001), suggesting a mutually reciprocal link between a lack of motivation and depressed mood.

Anhedonia is generally thought to be related to abnormalities within the mesolimbic dopaminergic system (i.e., the motivation component of the reward system), specifically a diminished dopamine release in the nucleus accumbens and medial prefrontal cortex (Di Chiara & Tanda, 1997; Putnam, Pizzagalli, Gooding, Kalin, & Davidson, 2008; Sarchiapone et al., 2006; Willner, Lappas, Cheeta, & Muscat, 1994). Neuroanatomically, trait anhedonia is associated with smaller volume in the basal ganglia (primarily the anterior caudate and ventral striatum, including the nucleus accumbens) (Harvey et al., 2007; Wacker, Dillon, & Pizzagalli, 2009). These findings are consistent with the suggestions that anhedonia is a disorder of motivation.

Anhedonia is a common comorbidity of depression, although it has been shown to represent a distinct construct (Loas, Noisette, Legrand, & Boyer, 2000). As a stable trait, it appears to be a risk factor for the development of schizophrenia (Docherty & Sponheim, 2008), and as an acute state it differentiates among subtypes of depression (Fawcett, Clark, Scheftner, & Hedeker, 1983) and predicts depression treatment outcomes (Clark, Fawcett, Salazar-Grueso, & Fawcett, 1984). Additionally, anhedonia is common among individuals with alyxithymia (Warnes, 1986). Importantly, anhedonia is seen among patients with neurodegenerative disorders, such as Parkinson's disease (Costa et al., 2007), vascular dementia (Lavretsky et al., 2008), and dementia with Lewy bodies and Alzheimer's disease (Rockwell, Choure, Galasko, Olichney, & Jeste, 2000).

CONCLUDING THOUGHTS

According to the reviewed literature, both anhedonia and the apathy–akinetic mutism spectrum appear to rely on the same circuitry, and appear to be associated with similar motivational problems. Although there seems to be a different connotation for the words *anhedonia* and *apathy*, with one focusing more on the experience of pleasure and the other on behavioral output, it may be that this distinction is largely arbitrary, or that the two phenomena represent two symptom groups that are a part of the same neuropsychiatric syndrome. However, research examining this question is still quite limited, and much past research has relied on animal models, making interpretation difficult.

Disorders of Abnormal Sensitivity to Rewards and Punishments

Although the ability to respond to both rewards and punishments needs to be present for survival of an organism, considerable individual differences exist with respect to the *relative* sensitivity to rewards versus punishments. These differences appear to be a function of genetic predispositions (Schmitz et al., 2009), hormonal factors (Li et al., 2007; van Honk et al., 2004), and environmental influences (Dadds & Salmon, 2003). This variability is normal and accounts for an array of individual traits, including decision-making styles (Franken & Muris, 2005a), personality characteristics (Mitchell et al., 2007), and even food craving and body mass index (Franken & Muris, 2005b).

However, as imbalances between the sensitivity to positive versus negative outcomes increase, so do maladaptive behavioral biases, such as pathological anxiety centered around avoidance of potential threats (Mueller, Nguyen, Ray, & Borkovec, 2010), or impulsive and indiscriminate responding to rewards accompanied by failures to respond to punishments (Martin & Potts, 2009). The latter form of imbalance is particularly troublesome, leading individuals to make apparently impulsive or illogical choices that are in contrast to their stated, and perhaps genuinely desired, goals. Thus, not surprisingly, the majority of the research in this area has focused on various forms of psychopathology characterized by impaired impulse control and propensity for making maladaptive decisions.

This line of research has shown that children with attention-deficit disorder (Holroyd, Baker, Kerns, & Mueller, 2008; Masunami, Okazaki, & Maekawa, 2009; Wang, Zhu, Wang, & Wang, 2008), as well as conduct disorder, oppositional defiant disorder, and externalizing behavior (Fairchild et al., 2009; Matthys, Van Goozen, Snoek, & Van Engeland, 2004; Yechiam et al., 2006) are characterized either by greater sensitivity to rewards, or lesser sensitivity to punishments, or both. Similar profiles are seen among adults with psychopathy (Blair, Morton, Leonard, & Blair, 2006), addicts (Genovese & Wallace, 2007), and individuals exhibiting Cluster B personality disorders[8] (Voelm et al., 2007).

CONSIDERING THE COMPONENTS OF THE REWARD AND PUNISHMENT SYSTEMS

As discussed earlier, the reward and punishment systems each consists of at least three components: sensation, learning, and motivation. Thus, at least theoretically, imbalance between sensitivity to rewards or punishments could occur in all or just some of the three components. For example, learned helplessness is clearly associated with low motivation to pursue rewards and escape punishments, although the ability to experience and learn from rewarding and punishing outcomes may very well be normal. Unfortunately, research that has examined such imbalances among different clinical populations has not always clearly distinguished among the three processes. Nevertheless, based on available research, one can postulate theoretical models of how imbalances in the three components of the reward and punishment systems would affect behavior. See Table 9.1.

Assessment

Sensitivity to Rewards and Punishments in Neuropsychological Evaluations

One clinical measure that is clearly relevant for the discussion of rewards and punishments is the Wisconsin Card Sorting Test (WCST; Heaton et

TABLE 9.1. Hypothesized Imbalances between Rewards and Punishments for Select Clinical Syndromes

	Components of the reward and punishment systems		
Clinical syndromes	Sensation	Learning	Motivation
Anhedonia	Low sensitivity to rewards	Normal	Low sensitivity to rewards
Addiction, psychopathy, and ADHD	Normal	High sensitivity to rewards and low sensitivity to punishments	High sensitivity to rewards and low sensitivity to punishments
Anxiety	High sensitivity to punishments	High sensitivity to punishments	High sensitivity to punishments
Learned helplessness	Normal	Normal	Low sensitivity to rewards and punishments

al., 1993). It is generally assumed that performance of this test relies on highly *cognitive* processes, such as reasoning and problem solving, cognitive flexibility, and set maintenance, with the dorsolateral prefrontal cortex representing the primary substrate (Demakis, 2003). In addition, in order to perform the test properly, the examinees need to have the capacity to properly process the feedback they receive about their performance. However, test feedback may have very different meaning to different examinees. In other words, whereas one person may process such feedback as factual information, another person may experience it as rewarding or punishing. Consequently, then, the test may tax primarily the dorsolateral prefrontal cortex (i.e., processing of the factual information so as to accomplish a switch) for some individuals, whereas for others (i.e., for those for whom the test is more emotional) it may tax primarily the orbitofrontal cortex. See Figure 9.2, Panel A.

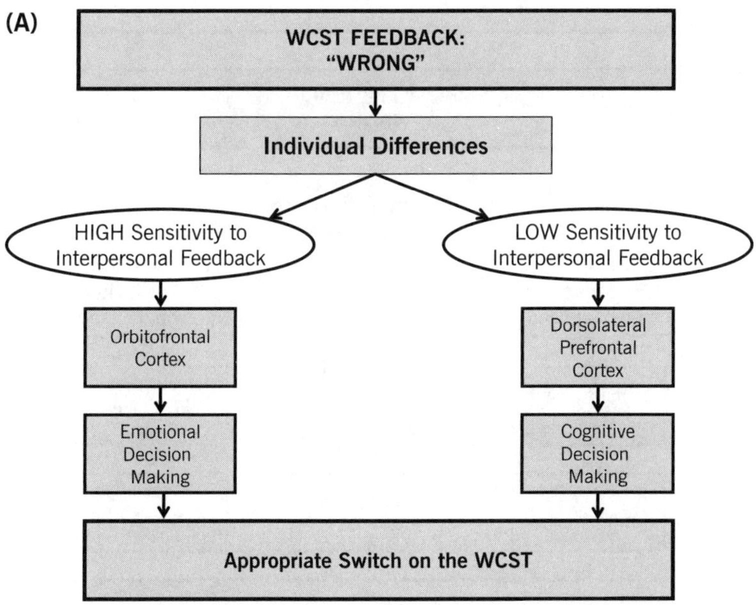

FIGURE 9.2. Irrespective of one's interpersonal style, the Wisconsin Card Sorting Test (WCST) can be performed well, albeit by relying on different regions of the prefrontal cortex (Panel A). However, damage to either the orbitofrontal (Panel B) or the dorsolateral (Panel C) prefrontal cortex could have very different effects on performance, depending on individual differences in sensitivity to interpersonal feedback.

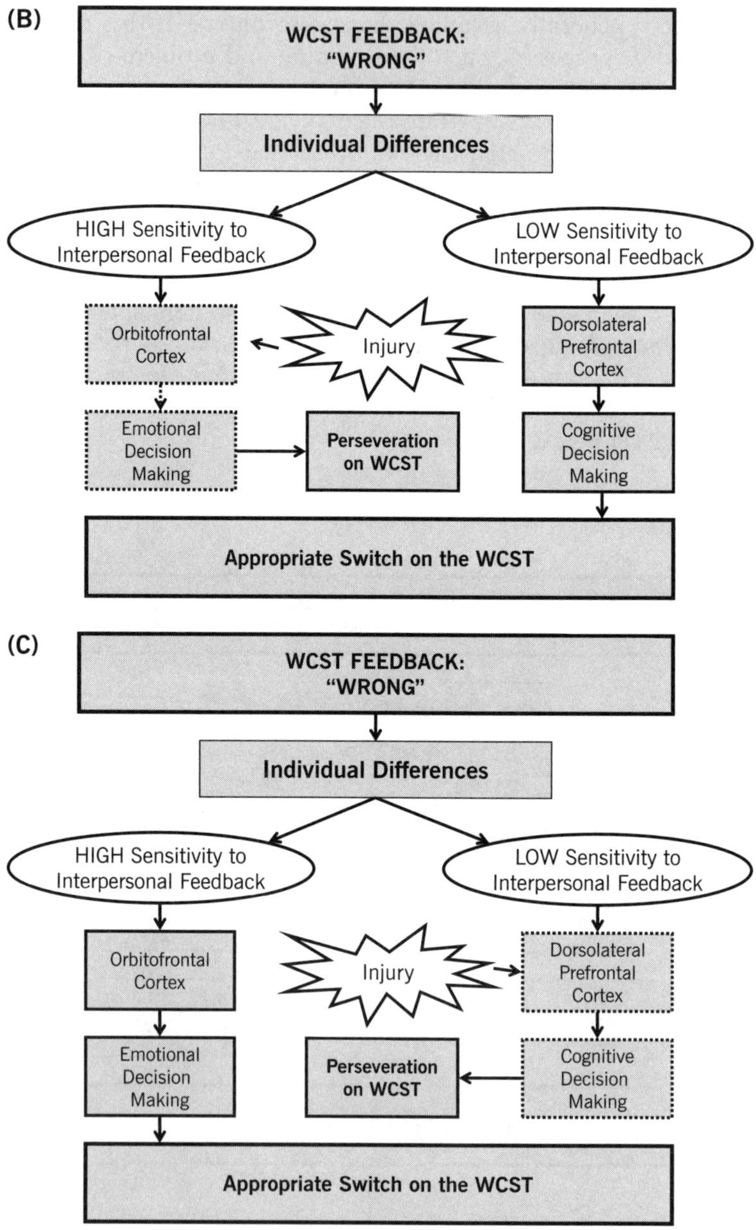

FIGURE 9.2. *(cont.)*

Of course, in a healthy brain, this distinction may well be irrelevant, as either cortical area should be equally capable of managing the challenges presented by the test demands. However, individuals with weaknesses or lesions in different areas of the prefrontal cortex may differentially succeed or fail, depending on their idiosyncratic experience of the feedback. In other words, those individuals for whom the feedback is primarily perceived as rewards and punishments may exhibit deficits after lesions to the orbitofrontal cortex, whereas individuals who perceive the feedback more factually may be more impaired after lesions to the dorsolateral prefrontal cortex (see Figure 9.2, Panels B and C).[9]

Some empirical support for this notion exists, as simply just decreasing the rewarding and punishing quality of the feedback is sufficient to improve or worsen performances in some populations. For example, children with autism exhibit deficits on the WCST when it is administered by a person, but *not* when it is administered by a computer (Ozonoff, 1995), and criminals with psychopathy exhibit deficits when provided with tangible rewards, but *not* during typical administration (Howland & Newman, 1993). These patterns of performance are suggestive of an orbitofrontal dysfunction in both these populations. Utilizing other assessment procedures, dissociation between emotional and cognitive decision making has also been demonstrated in people with schizophrenia (Y. Lee et al., 2007).

Importantly, performances on other tests that do not involve direct administration of rewards and punishments may also be deleteriously affected by dysfunctional reward and punishment systems, as assessment procedures rely on a patient being motivated to, in the very least, engage in the sort of socially appropriate collaborative discourse that a testing situation requires.

Assessment of Emotional Decision Making

The Iowa Gambling Task (IGT; Bechara et al., 1997), described in more detail earlier in the section on "Somatic Marker Hypothesis," has enjoyed a prolific career as a research measure of choice for assessment of emotional decision making. Much research has demonstrated that IGT performance is impaired in a variety of clinical populations, including those with substance abuse, pathological gambling, and criminal offenses (Buelow & Suhr, 2009). Additionally, as already outlined in the section on neuroanatomy, the involvement of the frontal lobes in successful performance of the IGT has been demonstrated with lesion and neuroimaging studies, although the specific substrates *within* the frontal lobes continue to be a source of controversy (Buelow & Suhr, 2009).

Recently, the IGT has become available as a clinical tool (Bechara, 2007). Despite its conceptual richness and theoretical contributions, the

IGT as a clinical tool has some limitations. An excellent recent review (Buelow & Suhr, 2009) has outlined these limitations in considerable detail, and they will be only briefly summarized here. First, no reliability studies have been conducted with the IGT or listed in the manual. Second, with respect to correlations with other measures of similar constructs, the findings are mixed. Lastly, depressed mood and impulsive or sensation-seeking personality traits can have deleterious effects on performance even in the absence of neurological or psychiatric dysfunction. Consequently, although the IGT may contribute to the characterization of a given patient's level of functioning and decision-making style, its contribution to differential diagnosis remains questionable.

Assessment of Diminished Motivation

As discussed earlier, deficient reward and punishment systems can result in diminished motivation, a common correlate of many neurological and neuropsychiatric disorders. The instrument of choice for assessment of diminished motivation is the *Apathy Evaluation Scale* (AES; Marin, Biedrzycki, & Firinciogullari, 1991), an 18-item scale that has self-rated, informant-rated, and clinician-rated versions. Although apathy and depression share some features and can often be comorbid, the AES has been shown to measure a construct that is separate from depression (Marin, Firinciogullari, & Biedrzycki, 1993). Recent extensive review of the literature confirms that the AES has high internal consistency, test–retest reliability, and interrater reliability, and shows good discriminant, convergent, and criterion validities (Clarke, van Reekum, Patel, et al., 2007). The AES has been extensively validated for clinical use in a number of populations, including those with dementia (Clarke, van Reekum, Simard, et al., 2007), TBI (Andersson & Bergedalen, 2002; Lane-Brown & Tate, 2009), and schizophrenia (Faerden et al., 2008). A German version of the AES has been validated with a mixed clinical sample (Lueken et al., 2006), and a short version of the AES for use in nursing homes has also been developed (Lueken et al., 2007).

Assessment of Anhedonia

Several scales for assessment of anhedonia currently exist. The *Snaith–Hamilton Pleasure Scale* (SHAPS; Snaith, Hamilton, Morley, & Humayan, 1995) is a brief measure that has good internal consistency and test–retest reliabilities, as well as good convergent and discriminant validities. It has been validated both with nonclinical and clinical populations (Franken, Rassin, & Muris, 2007). The *Chapman Physical Anhedonia Scale* (CPAS; Chapman, Chapman, & Raulin, 1976) also has good psychometric properties, but has been criticized for obsolete item content. This scale is more suitable for assessment of anhedonia as a stable trait, given that it asks questions about lifelong anhedonia characteristics. As such, it has shown considerable stability over time in clinical populations (Horan, Reise, Subotnik, Ventura, & Nuechterlein, 2008). Lastly, the *Fawcett–Clark Pleasure Scale* (FCPS; Fawcett, Clark, Scheftner, & Gibbons, 1983) also has good psychometric properties and has been extensively validated with normal and clinical populations, demonstrating good ability to discriminate among different patient groups (Loas & Boyer, 1993; Loas, Boyer, Fremaux, & Gayant, 1995; Loas et al., 2000; Loas, Perot, Hardy, & Jouvent, 1994). Factor-analytic research has shown that hedonic capacity is most strongly related to the SHAPS, and, to a lesser extent, the FCPS (Leventhal, Chasson, Tapia, Miller, & Pettit, 2006). See Table 9.2 for a summary of scale characteristics.

Assessment of Sensitivity to Rewards and Punishments

The behavior activation system (BAS) and the behavior inhibition system (BIS) represent two opponent motivational processors proposed by Jeffrey Gray in his work with animals (Gray et al., 1986). These theoretical constructs are thought to reflect relative sensitivity to rewards and punishments.

TABLE 9.2. Comparison of Three Scales Used for Anhedonia Assessment

	SHAPS	FCPS	CPAS
Number of items	14	36	61
Scale type	4-point Likert	5-point Likert	True–false
Responses reflect	Last few days	Current state	Throughout lifetime
Domains	Sensory experience Social interaction Interest/pastime Food/drink	Sensory experience Social interaction Sense of mastery	Sensory experience Social interaction Interest in activities Pastime Food/drink
Reliabilities	Cronbach α = .91–94 Test–retest = .70	Cronbach α = .94–.96	Cronbach α = .72–.85
Validations with clinical populations	Depression, schizophrenia, substance abuse	Depression, schizophrenia, substance abuse	Depression, schizophrenia

Note. SHAPS, Snaith–Hamilton Pleasure Scale; FCPS, Fawcett–Clark Pleasure Capacity Scale; CPAS, Revised Chapman Physical Anhedonia Scale; MADRS, Montgomery–Asberg Depression Rating Scale.

The *BIS/BAS Scale* (Carver & White, 1994) was developed to provide a way of operationalizing the BIS and the BAS constructs in work with humans. It consists of 24 statements to which examinees respond on a 4-point Likert scale. The items load on one BIS factor and three BAS factors[10] (Carver & White, 1994; Knyazev, Slobodskaya, & Wilson, 2004), although some inconsistencies in the factor structure have been reported (Gomez, Cooper, & Gomez, 2005; Heubeck, Wilkinson, & Cologon, 1998; Heym, Ferguson, & Lawrence, 2008; Poythress et al., 2008), and simple two-factor (BIS vs. BAS) solutions have also been proposed (Caci, Deschaux, & Bayle, 2007; Knyazev et al., 2004; Strobel, Beauducel, Debener, & Brocke, 2001). The two-factor solutions tend to have better reliabilities (in the .7–.9 range) than the four-factor solutions (Beck, Smits, Claes, Vandereycken, & Bijttebier, 2009; Franken, Muris, & Rassin, 2005). The scale has been validated with a number of populations, including school children (Blair, 2003), adolescents (Cooper, Gomez, & Aucote, 2007), and college students (Voigt et al., 2009), patients with bipolar disorder (Meyer, Barton, Baur, & Jordan, 2010), anxiety disorder (Campbell-Sills, Liverant, & Brown, 2004; Vervoort et al., 2010), eating disorders (Beck et al., 2009), and offenders with psychopathy (Poythress et al., 2008), as well as in Polish (Mueller & Wytykowska, 2005), German (Strobel et al., 2001), French (Caci et al., 2007), Chinese (Li et al., 2008), Italian (Leone, Pierro, & Mannetti, 2002), Norwegian (Bjornebekk, 2009), and Dutch (Franken et al., 2005) samples. Normative data across the adult lifespan can be found in Jorm and colleagues (1999).

Clinical Populations

Neurodegenerative Disorders

FRONTOTEMPORAL-LOBAR DEGENERATION

A recent review of the literature confirmed a strong association between disorders of diminished motivation and FTD (Mendez, Lauterbach, & Sampson, 2008), with about 70% of patients displaying apathy (Engelborghs et al., 2005). This association appears to be strongest among patients with late-onset FTD (Shinagawa et al., 2008). However, unexpectedly, apathy in this population seems unrelated to atrophy in the ventral striatum, that is, the reward system substrate (Links et al., 2009). Rather, apathy in FTD is most strongly related to atrophy in the dorsolateral prefrontal cortex[11] and anterior cingulate gyrus; in contrast, impulsivity in this population *is* associated with atrophy in the nucleus accumbens and medial orbitofrontal cortex, as well as superior temporal sulcus and mediotemporal limbic structures (Massimo et al., 2009; Zamboni, Huey, Krueger, Nichelli, & Grafman, 2008). These findings suggest that whereas apathy in this population may not be caused principally by a disruption of the reward system, impulsivity may be related to an imbalance between sensitivity to rewards and punishments. Importantly, apathy symptoms appear to be separate from symptoms of depression (Blass & Rabins, 2009). Last but not least, apathy and disinhibition represent the most burdensome symptoms reported by caregivers of FTD patients (Massimo et al., 2009).

ALZHEIMER'S DISEASE

Reports of apathy among patients with AD range from 10 to 76% (Starkstein, Jorge, & Mizrahi, 2006). This discrepancy may be due to the comorbidity of apathy with depression, although apathy appears to be more common in this patient population than depression (Tatsch et al., 2006). In contrast to the findings with patients who have FTD, apathy among patients with AD does appear to be related to decreased metabolism in the anterior cingulate gyrus and medial orbitofrontal cortex (Marshall et al., 2007), suggesting an involvement of the reward system. Apathy among patients with mild cognitive impairment (MCI) appears to be a risk factor for a rapid decline in functionality (Lechowski et al., 2009), as well as conversion to AD within 3 years (Robert et al., 2008). Lastly, about 37% of patients with autopsy-confirmed AD have been reported to exhibit symptoms of anhedonia (Rockwell et al., 2000).

DEMENTIA WITH LEWY BODIES

Apathy and anhedonia represent an extremely common neurobehavioral presentation of dementia with Lewy bodies (DLB) (Borroni et al., 2008; Simard, van Reekum, & Cohen, 2000), with apathy identified in 50% of DLB cases (Martinez et al., 2008) and anhedonia identified in as many as 76% of autopsy-confirmed DLB cases (Rockwell et al., 2000). At least one study found that progressively growing apathy is more common among patients with DLB as compared to those with AD, and may in fact help with differential diagnosis (Galvin, Malcom, Johnson, & Morris, 2007). Recall from earlier discussion of the topic that the distinction between apathy and anhedonia is not clear. The fact that both apathy and anhedonia are extremely common among patients with DLB reinforces the notion that both syndromes may share a common underlying cause.

PARKINSON'S DISEASE

Given the role of dopamine in the motivational aspect of the reward and punishment systems, it is not surprising that patients with PD exhibit decreased responsiveness to rewards, in particular with respect to reward anticipation, leading to impairments in reinforcement-based learning (Mattox, Valle-Inclan, & Hackley, 2006). Relatedly, anhedonia and/or apathy is a common comorbidity of PD, occurring in about 70% of patients at some point in the course of the illness (Pedersen, Alves, Aarsland, & Larsen, 2009). Anhedonia/apathy often occurs in conjunction with depression (Bahroo & Appleby, 2009), but can also occur in the absence of other depressive symptoms (Kirsch-Darrow et al., 2006). Additionally, patients with PD exhibit greater frequency of anhedonia/apathy than patients with other, similarly disabling conditions, providing additional support for the notion that these symptoms are a function of the disease itself, rather than a psychological reaction to it (Pluck & Brown, 2002).

Other Neurological Disorders

The most common cause of abnormally functioning reward and punishment systems is damage to the ventral aspects of the prefrontal cortex. This, of course, occurs most commonly among patients with TBI. These patients are sometimes characterized by abnormal processing of rewards (Larson, Kelly, Stigge-Kaufman, Schmalfuss, & Perlstein, 2007), with diminished capacity to utilize rewards toward improvements in performance (Konrad, Gauggel, Manz, & Schoell, 2000; McCauley, McDaniel, Pedroza, Chapman, & Levin, 2009). Consequently, emotional decision making is also often impaired (Bonatti et al., 2008; Fujiwara, Schwartz, Gao, Black, & Levine, 2008). Additionally, apathy/anhedonia are seen relatively commonly following a TBI (Lane-Brown & Tate, 2009; Rao, Spiro, Schretlen, & Cascella, 2007).

Neuropsychiatric Disorders

ADDICTION

Individuals who are addicted to a variety of substances, including alcohol, cocaine, opioids, and cannabis, as well as pathological gamblers, exhibit impaired emotional decision making, evidenced not only by their maladaptive lifestyles, but also by poor performances on the IGT (Buelow & Suhr, 2009). This abnormality is also associated with abnormally strong responses to rewards, as well as abnormal patterns of prefrontal activation in response to rewards (Goldstein, Alia-Klein, et al., 2007; Goldstein, Tomasi, et al., 2007).

ANTISOCIAL BEHAVIOR AND PSYCHOPATHY

There is increasing evidence that antisocial behavior is genetically based, with approximately 50% of variance accounted for by genes (Moffitt,

2005). At least seven different genes have been associated with antisocial behavior, with the monoamine oxidase A (*MAOA*) gene showing perhaps the strongest association with antisocial behavior and aggression (Abrahamson, Baker, & Caspi, 2002; Buckholtz & Meyer-Lindenberg, 2008; Caspi et al., 2002; Moffitt, 2005; Viding, Blair, Moffitt, & Plomin, 2005). Interestingly, this gene has also been implicated in volume reduction in the amygdala and the orbitofrontal cortex (Meyer-Lindenberg et al., 2006), leading to impairments in emotional processing in general, and in emotional learning and decision making in particular. It should therefore not be surprising that individuals with psychopathic tendencies are more sensitive to rewards than to punishments (Arnett, Smith, & Newman, 1997; Newman et al., 1990; Newman & Schmitt, 1998). Because psychopathy is characterized by a failure to attain adult lifestyles, goals, or plans (Cleckley, 1976), the notion that psychopaths are particularly sensitive to rewards is in line with research showing that children, up until about the age of 11 years, also respond better to rewards than to punishments (van Duijvenvoorde et al., 2008). Additionally, given the association between relatively higher levels of testosterone and criminal aggression, it is interesting that higher levels of testosterone are also associated with greater sensitivity to rewards than punishments (Li et al., 2007; van Honk et al., 2004).

SUMMARY AND CONCLUSIONS

The primary problems associated with dysfunctional reward and punishment systems involve (1) deficits in motivation and (2) an imbalance between the sensitivity to rewards and punishments. Disorders of diminished motivation are generally related to lesions that disrupt the motivation component of the reward system, subserved by mesolimbic dopamine and its targets, primarily the nucleus accumbens and anterior cingulate gyrus. Disorders of diminished motivation are associated with a variety of neurological conditions that affect these structures, including neurodegenerative disorders and acquired brain injuries. Clinical presentations can range from severe absence of motivation (i.e., akinetic mutism) to less debilitating forms (i.e., apathy). Anhedonia, contrary to popular belief, also appears to be a disorder of diminished motivation, and may in fact be indistinguishable from apathy. In contrast to disorders of diminished motivation, disorders characterized by an imbalance between sensitivity to rewards and punishments tend to be associated with orbitofrontal lesions, as well as with a number of neurodevelopmental disorders that are characterized by impulsivity as a result of excessive sensitivity to reward and diminished sensitivity to punishments.

NOTES

1. In behaviorist terminology, (1) positive reinforcement refers to a rewarding stimulus that, when presented, increases the frequency of given behavior; (2) negative reinforcement refers to a punishing stimulus that, when removed, increases the frequency of a given behavior; and (3) punishment refers to a punishing stimulus that, when added, results in a decrease in the frequency of a given behavior.
2. The release of dopamine in the nucleus accumbens has also been implicated in the development of drug addiction, drug craving, and drug abuse relapse (Balfour, 2001; Fibiger & Phillips, 1988; Self, 1998; Shippenberg et al., 1992; van Furth & van Ree, 1996; West & Michael, 1990).
3. In the somatic marker hypothesis literature, the term *ventromedial* is consistently used. For that reason, the same term is used in this section. Although there is some disagreement as to the exact boundaries of this area, the term *medial orbitofrontal* refers to the same *general* brain region and is therefore often used interchangeably.
4. This conceptualization also invokes the construct of "embodied emotions" discussed in more detail in Chapter 6.
5. This elaboration is also consistent with the theoretical view of the right hemisphere playing a role in withdrawal actions (Davidson & Irwin, 1999), as described in Chapter 8.
6. Functional imaging research has implicated additional regions above and beyond the ventromedial prefrontal cortex. In particular, decision making during ambiguous contingencies (as is the case in the IGT) also activated the medial frontal gyrus and the insula, and the learning aspect of decision making relied on the lateral orbitofrontal cortex and the presupplementary motor area (Lawrence, Jollant, O'Daly, Zelaya, & Phillips, 2009). Yet another study implicated similar regions, but found different associations between regions and specific aspects of test performance (Lin, Chiu, Cheng, & Hsieh, 2008). In particular, this study found that it was the basal ganglia and the insula that responded during the anticipation phase of test performance, whereas the medial prefrontal cortex was activated during the high punishment contingencies. Additionally, the inferior parietal lobule was activated during the outcome phase. These inconsistencies point to the potentially confounding influence of even subtle conceptual or methodological differences among functional imaging paradigms.
7. Symptoms resembling impairments in motivation can also be seen in patients suffering from autonomic hypoarousal due to damage to the networks controlling the sympathetic nervous system, including the right hemisphere (Chapter 4).
8. Cluster B includes histrionic, narcissistic, antisocial, and borderline personality disorders.

9. Such individual differences may account for reports of normal WCST performance despite dorsolateral prefrontal damage (Heck & Bryer, 1986).
10. The three BAS factors are (1) drive, (2) fun seeking, and (3) reward responsiveness.
11. Recall that apathy was also a prominent feature of people with frontal lobotomies (Cohen et al., 1942).

CHAPTER 10

Stress and Motivation

Richard Lazarus, the prominent psychologist and theorist in the field of emotion research, bemoans in his book *Stress and Emotion* (1999, p. 35) that the literature on stress and the literature on emotions have been largely evolving along separate paths, as if stress and emotion were not at all related. He refers to the separation between the two constructs as "absurdity." Interestingly, a similar schism appears to prevail between the research on stress and the writings on the neuropsychology of emotion. This chapter attempts to integrate the research on stress and emotion, focusing on the theoretical, neuroanatomic, and clinical constructs that are of relevance to clinical neuropsychology.

THEORETICAL BACKGROUND

Defining the Constructs

Stress and Stress Response

STRESS

Stress is typically defined as a mental, emotional, or physical strain that often occurs in response to perceived or real threat to one's physical or psychological integrity. As such, stress reflects an internal state rather than an environmental context. Stress that is relatively mild, occurs acutely and briefly, and is perceived as controllable is often referred to as "good stress" and is considered to be good for one's well-being. In particular, brief doses of stress lead to adaptive responses in the body, such as appropriate increases in autonomic activation and temporary improvements in attention and concentration (Ohmura et al., 2009). Importantly, brief doses of stress early in life appear to have an "inoculation" effect, leading to attenuated stress responses in later years (Parker et al., 2006). In contrast to mild, phasic stress, stress that is severe, chronic, or long-lasting, as well as unpredictable and uncontrollable, has been termed "bad stress" and has been empirically shown to have deleterious effects on physical, mental, and neurocognitive health (van Heck et al., 2008).

The extent to which a stressful situation results in bad stress varies from one person to the next. This variability is a function of two factors: (1) affective style, such that individuals with higher levels of negative affectivity have been shown to have stronger and longer-lasting reactions to minor stressors than their more positively affected counterparts[1] (Kirschbaum, Pruessner, Stone, & Federenko, 1995), and (2) individual differences in the effectiveness and the health of a complex hormonal cascade known as the stress response.

THE STRESS RESPONSE

The stress response consists of two principal processes: (1) *sympathetic adrenomedullary (SAM)* system activation (already covered in Chapter 4 under autonomic and endocrine responses), which results from a release of adrenaline into the bloodstream and is controlled directly via sympathetic innervations of the core (also known as the medulla) of the adrenal gland; and (2) *HPA* (*hypothalamic–pituitary–adrenocortical*) *axis activation* (described in more detail under "Neuroanatomic Substrates" below), which ultimately serves to contain the stress response. The HPA axis interacts reciprocally with a variety of other hormonal and neurotransmitter systems, including dopaminergic, serotonergic, and norepinergic. Activation of the HPA axis leads to, among other things, a release of glucocorticoids into the bloodstream. As is explained later in this chapter, proper management of glucocorticoid levels in the bloodstream has serious implications for physical and mental health, including neurocognitive health, which makes this aspect of emotional processing particularly relevant for clinical neuropsychology. See Figure 10.1.

Stress and Motivation

Stress motivates behavior in two primary ways. The first relies on the reward and punishment systems described in Chapter 9, and the second is a

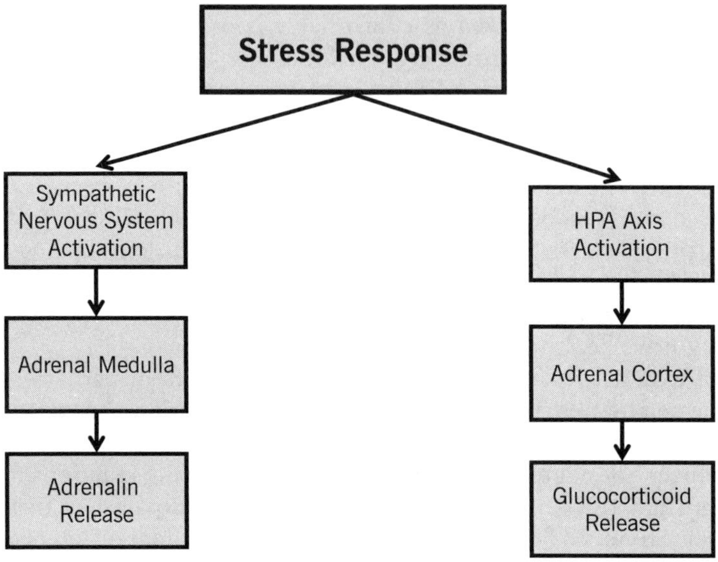

FIGURE 10.1. The stress response consists of two reactions. The first is activation of the sympathetic adrenomedullary (SAM) system, which occurs via direct sympathetic innervations of the adrenal medulla and subsequent release of adrenaline. The second is the hypothalamus–pituitary–adrenocortical (HPA) axis activation, which consists of a hormonal cascade involving the hypothalamus, the pituitary gland, and the adrenal cortex, and ultimately leads to a release of glucocorticoids.

function of biochemical changes in the body that signal threats to homeostasis and are preprogrammed to facilitate certain behaviors.

First, as mentioned earlier, "good" stress can have salubrious effects on one's physical and mental health. Additionally, good stress is also experienced as pleasant, exciting, and rewarding. Thus, assuming a healthy reward system (Chapter 9), people tend to actively seek out behaviors and situations associated with good stress, such as competitions, games, and sports activities. "Bad" stress, on the other hand, is experienced as unpleasant or punishing. Typical examples of bad stress include inescapable financial hardship or a terminal illness in a loved one. But even less serious situations, such as public speaking, can be associated with bad stress. Because bad stress tends to be experienced as unpleasant or punishing, behaviors or situations associated with bad stress are likely to be avoided. Thus, for example, individuals who suffer from social anxiety exhibit high levels of stress when forced to interact with others, and these same individuals tend to engage in socially avoidant behaviors (Cavigelli et al., 2007; Roelofs et al., 2009).

Interestingly, it appears that the subjectively experienced noxious quality of bad stress is related to the presence of stress hormones. This is suggested by the fact that unpleasant stressful situations motivate behaviors that have been shown to dampen the release of stress hormones. Among these are seeking close social interaction (Kirschbaum, Klauer, Filipp, & Hellhammer, 1995; Wittig et al., 2008) and ingestion of sweet and fatty foods (Gibson, 2006).[2]

Importantly, chronic elevations in stress hormones tend to lead to passivity by altering the biochemistry of the reward system (Chapter 9). Thus, when chronic stress is unavoidable or uncontrollable, such as financial hardship, illness, or abuse, biochemical changes in the body occur that lead to a *decrease* in reward-related motivation, as may be seen, for example, among individuals with anhedonic depression (Kleen, Sitomer, Killeen, & Conrad, 2006). However, somewhat counterintuitively, extremely *low* levels of stress hormones tend to be associated with aggression and antisocial tendencies (J. J. Kim et al., 2007; Putman, Hermans, & van Honk, 2007).

Neuroanatomic Substrates

The HPA Axis

The HPA axis represents the physical substrate of the self-regulatory portion of the stress response. The HPA axis accomplishes self-regulation via a negative feedback loop that can be divided into two steps: initiation and containment. We consider these two stages separately.

INITIATION

Recall from Chapter 4 that the hypothalamus contains receptors for a variety of stress signals, including neuronal projections from the amygdala, hormones signaling hunger and thirst, as well as serotonin, epinephrine, and norepinephrine signaling autonomic arousal. In response to these signals of physiological, physical, or mental distress, as well as specific modulating effects of norepinephrine and serotonin, the paraventricular nucleus of the hypothalamus produces corticotropin-releasing hormone (CRH) and vasopressin. These neurochemicals in turn stimulate the anterior pituitary gland into releasing adrenocorticotropic hormone (ACTH). The ACTH then travels via the bloodstream, reaching the cortex of the adrenal glands located above the kidneys, which then release adrenal steroids, most notably glucocorticoids.

Glucocorticoids (also known as *cortisol* in humans and *corticosterone* in rodents) travel via the bloodstream and bind to receptors in various tissues of the body, serving four primary purposes. First, in conjunction with adrenaline, they enhance the readiness of the body for stress by facilitating conversion of proteins and lipids into glycogen, which then can be used as fuel by the muscles. Second, glucocorticoids suppress immune responses to trauma and injury, such as inflammations and fever. Third, glucocorticoids motivate behavior, particularly food-seeking (so as to provide fuel to the body that is in distress) and aggressive (so as to defend against threats) behavior. Lastly, glucocorticoids curb what would otherwise become a positive feedback loop of the stress response (McEwen, 2005; McEwen & Lasley, 2003). As Marius Tausk, an influential endocrinologist, put it, glucocorticoids "limit the water damage caused by the fire brigade" (de Kloet & Oitzl, 2006, p. 15). This process is discussed next.

CONTAINMENT

Recall again that the hypothalamus responds to signals of stress, including the presence of epinephrine (i.e., adrenaline). Thus, once a stress response is initiated, it could theoretically continue ad infinitum, simply because the presence of adrenaline itself would continue to stimulate additional activation of the sympathetic nervous system. To contain this positive feedback loop, a negative feedback loop is built into the system that relies heavily on glucocorticoid receptors in the hippocampus (also known as the Type II receptors). Activation of these receptors interferes with production of CRH and vasopressin by the paraventricular nucleus of the hypothalamus, thereby interfering with the release of the ACTH, with the final outcome of curbing additional release of glucocorticoids by the adrenal gland (McEwen, Angulo, Cameron, & Chao, 1992).

In addition to this direct containment, glucocorticoids contain the stress response indirectly by dampening metabolic processes in the cortex, as well as interfering with the synthesis of catecholamines, most notably epinephrine (Noble, 1968; Pacak et al., 1992). This entire process takes approximately 5 minutes, such that heart rate, used as an index of sympathetic activation, returns to baseline within approximately 5 minutes following a single episode of acute stress (Jamieson, Flood, & Lavoie, 1994). See Figure 10.2.

HABITUATION

However, many stressful situations take longer than 5 minutes to resolve, requiring a more prolonged stress response. In such situations, in order to avoid repeated shutting down of the very response that the body needs, the HPA axis temporarily *habituates*, leading to a *temporary decrease* in the release of glucocorticoids (McEwen, Magarinos, & Gorman, 2004; Yehuda & McEwen, 2004), thereby allowing more prolonged circulation of adren-

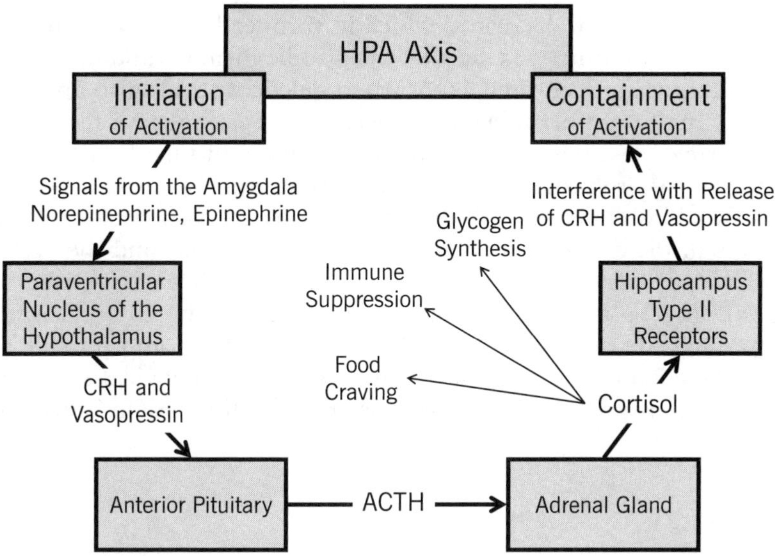

FIGURE 10.2. The principal steps of the initiation and containment stages of the HPA (hypothalamus, pituitary, adrenal) axis activation. In response to signals from the amygdalae, as well as in response to the presence of certain neurotransmitters and hormones, the hypothalamus releases CRH (corticotropin-releasing hormone) and vasopressin, which stimulate the anterior pituitary to release ACTH (adrenocorticotropic hormone). ACTH travels via the bloodstream to the cortex of the adrenal gland, which then releases cortisol (glucocorticoid) into the bloodstream. Cortisol has multiple effects on the body and also binds on the Type II receptors in the hippocampus. Activation of Type II receptors interferes with further release of CRH and vasopressin by the hypothalamus, thereby containing further HPA activation.

aline in the bloodstream (Schommer, Hellhammer, & Kirschbaum, 2003). However, if stress is chronic, the opposite of habituation occurs: The HPA axis becomes sensitized, leading to hyperactivity and chronic elevations of cortisol, which in turn lead to temporary or even permanent atrophy of neurons in the hippocampus and the cerebral cortex. The mechanism behind this process is described in more detail in the section "Clinical Signs and Syndromes" later in this chapter.

Interplay with Cognition

Hyperactivity of the HPA axis may represent one of the primary mechanisms for the cognitive difficulties associated with stress. Much research has now demonstrated that chronic or severe stress leads to atrophy of hippocampal and cortical dendrites, which in turn leads to declines in attention and executive functions, as well as episodic memory and memory for contexts. In addition, chronic exposure to glucocorticoids also appears to lead to lasting (if not permanent) decreases in dopamine levels in the prefrontal cortex.[3] Decreases in prefrontal dopamine in turn lead to further exacerbation of problems in attention, concentration, and executive functioning (Robbins & Arnsten, 2009). If the exposure to cortisol is relatively time-limited, the deleterious effects on the hippocampus and the prefrontal cortex are reversible; consequently, cognitive declines associated with stress can also be reversed (Liston, McEwen, & Casey, 2009). Together, these findings are consistent with clinical observations and provide support for the common practice of repeating neuropsychological evaluations after patients' psychiatric symptoms or stressful life circumstances have resolved.

Stress and Aging

However, during prolonged chronic stress, dendritic atrophy leads to permanent loss of neurons, leading to permanent cognitive deficits. It has been hypothesized that the neuronal loss associated with cumulative effects of chronic stress over the lifespan is responsible for brain atrophy and cognitive changes associated with aging (Finch, Seeman, Bengtson, & Schaie, 1999; Lupien, Meaney, Wang, & Snyder, 1998; Maggi, Tavola, & Gala, 1996). This so-called glucocorticoid cascade hypothesis of aging is based on animal (Dellu, Mayo, Vallee, Maccari, & Piazza, 1996; Montaron et al., 2006) and human (Keller, Buckley, Schatzberg, Roose, & Sackeim, 2004; Nichols, Zieba, & Bye, 2001; O'Dwyer & Orrell, 1994; Pruessner et al., 2004; Sackeim & Roose, 2004) studies that have shown greater dysregulation of the HPA axis, greater hippocampal atrophy, as well as greater memory impairment among elderly individuals who have experienced unusually high levels of stress in their life. These deleterious effects of stress appear to be particularly prominent among individuals who carry a particular variant of the serotonin transporter gene (O'Hara et al., 2007; S. E. Taylor et al., 2006; W. D. Taylor et al., 2005).

Stress and Early Development

Because chronic glucocorticoid exposure interferes with neurogenesis, stress early in life has deleterious effects on normal brain development and cognition. For example, children who are chronically exposed to stress due to poor economic conditions, abusive or neglectful home environment, or chronic illness tend to exhibit developmental delays (Cahill, Kaminer, &

Johnson, 1999; Dukewich, Borkowski, & Whitman, 1999), hippocampal atrophy evident in adulthood (Bremner, Randall, Vermetten, & Staib, 1997), and smaller cerebral volume (De Bellis, Hooper, & Sapia, 2005). Additionally, prenatal stress appears to lead to HPA hyperactivity, predisposing the unborn child not only to cognitive decrements (particularly deficits in learning and attention), but also increased vulnerability for psychopathology (Kapoor, Kostaki, Janus, & Matthews, 2009; Kinney, Munir, Crowley, & Miller, 2008; Lee, Brady, Shapiro, Dorsa, & Koenig, 2007; Lucassen et al., 2009; Rieger et al., 2004; Yaka, Salomon, Matzner, & Weinstock, 2007).

INTEGRATING THEORY AND PRACTICE

Clinical Signs and Syndromes

As discussed earlier in this chapter, healthy functioning of the HPA axis is crucial for physical, mental, and neurocognitive health. A dysfunction of the HPA axis can emerge over time via a gradual process of prolonged exposure to stress, or, more acutely, via brain injury. Additionally, abnormal levels of cortisol can be a result of a neuroendocrine disease, or can emerge as a side effect of certain pharmacotherapies. These mechanisms are reviewed in turn below.

Sensitization of the HPA Axis

When stress becomes chronic and prolonged, *sensitization* of the HPA axis occurs, leading to *chronic elevations* in the levels of glucocorticoids (McEwen et al., 2004; Yehuda & McEwen, 2004). Such chronic elevations lead to structural and functional changes in the brain that cumulatively can result in considerable impact on neurocognitive health. First, chronic elevations in cortisol interfere with neurogenesis in the hippocampus (Malberg & Duman, 2003), as well as lead to atrophy of the pyramidal cell dendrites in the hippocampus (McEwen, 1999) and the prefrontal cortex (Liston et al., 2006, 2009; Radley et al., 2006), leading to predictable concomitant cognitive declines. Second, these structural changes also include a decrease in the functionality of the Type II receptors in the hippocampus (i.e., the receptors become resistant to cortisol), leading to a breakdown in the HPA containment mechanism; consequently, the release of glucocorticoids, and their deleterious effects, go unchecked. Third, this resistance to cortisol appears to be true also for receptors elsewhere in the body, including the receptors that play a role in suppression of the immune system; consequently, the immune system becomes overactive, leading to the presence of excessive inflammatory markers in the bloodstream, as well as exacerbation of inflammatory illnesses such as rheumatoid arthritis and multiple sclerosis (Chrousos, Kino, Judd, & Sternberg, 2009; Kendall-Tackett, 2007). Lastly, these effects are further exacerbated by the fact that chronically elevated levels of glucocorticoids also lead to *hyper*trophy in the amygdala (Vyas, Mitra, Rao, & Chattarji, 2002), which in turn leads to excessive sensitivity to emotional stimuli (Chapter 3) and thus greater opportunity for the HPA axis to become activated.

While these various effects are reversible over the course of weeks or months (Heine, Maslam, Zareno, Joels, & Lucassen, 2004), severe or prolonged chronic stress that continues unchecked for months or years can lead to neuronal death and permanent structural and functional changes in the brain (Bremner et al., 1997; Hoeschl & Hajek, 2001; Uno, Ross, Else, Suleman, & Sapolsky, 1989).

Cushing Syndrome

Cushing syndrome (CS) is a disorder caused by a chronic exposure to extremely high levels of cortisol. Individuals with CS are characterized by a heavy upper body with relatively thin limbs, round face and thick neck, and fragile skin prone to bruising. Women also sometimes exhibit facial hair. Additional symptoms include fatigue and muscle weakness, hypertension, high blood glucose, and increased thirst and urination. Psychiatric symptoms commonly include depression, mania, irritability, anxiety, sleep disturbance (Sonino & Fava, 2001; Starkman, Wolkowitz, & Rothschild, 2003), and even psychosis (Myhill, Sillars, Starkstein, Annus, & Yeap, 2008). The majority of cases of CS are iatrogenic, caused by prolonged treatment of asthma, rheumatoid arthritis, or other inflammatory disorders with steroidal anti-inflammatory drugs such as prednisone. The remaining cases are usually a result of various forms of both benign and malignant tumors affecting either the central nervous system (e.g., pituitary adenoma) or other parts of the body (e.g., pancreatic cancer).

Given what is known about the effects of cortisol on the brain, it should not be a surprise that CS sufferers exhibit structural and functional changes in the hippocampus and the amygdala (Bourdeau et al., 2005; Maheu et al., 2008), generalized brain volume loss (Bourdeau et al., 2005), and premature cognitive aging characterized primarily by memory and learning weaknesses (Michaud, Forget, & Cohen, 2009). These effects seem to correlate with cortisol levels (Starkman, Giordani, Berent, Schork, & Schteingart, 2001) and are at least partly reversible with treatment (Hook et al., 2007). For a comprehensive review of the literature, see Bourdeau and colleagues (2005).

Adrenal Insufficiency

Adrenal insufficiency is a syndrome characterized by low levels of adrenocortical hormones, particularly costisol and aldosterone. *Primary* adrenal insufficiency, also known as *Addison disease*, refers to a dysfunction of the adrenal cortex, rendering it unable to produce cortisol and other hormones. Primary adrenal insufficiency is typically caused by an autoimmune disease, although other causes, such as infections, tumors, or genetic abnormalities, can also occur. *Secondary* adrenal insufficiency, which is much more common than Addison disease, refers to an insufficient production of ACTH by the pituitary gland. Such failure can be caused by a tumor or an infection, pituitary ischemia, pituitary necrosis secondary to radiation, or surgical removal of the hypothalamus or the pituitary gland.

Regardless of the etiology, adrenal insufficiency is typically accompanied by fatigue and muscle weakness, loss of appetite and weight loss, as well as an array of other symptoms such as nausea, hypotension, excessive sweating, headaches, and hypoglycemia. In women, irregular or absent periods are common. Psychiatric symptoms include irritability, depression, lack of motivation, and, rarely, psychosis. Because onset is insidious, it is not uncommon for adrenal insufficiency to be misdiagnosed as a psychiatric condition or perimenopausal complications. The severe worsening of symptoms, called *Addisonian* or *adrenal* crisis, is characterized by abdominal pain, back pain, dehydration, diarrhea and vomiting, severe drops in blood pressure, and eventually loss of consciousness and death. For additional information, see Munver and Volfson (2007) and Williams and Dluhy (2008).

Low levels of cortisol have been shown to lead to memory deficits in animal studies (Vaher, Luine, Gould, & McEwen, 1994), and mental status changes in patients with Addison disease have also been reported (Anglin, Rosebush, & Mazurek, 2006), but on the whole the literature on the neurocognitive sequelae of this disorder is sorely lacking.

Posttraumatic Hypopituitarism

It has now been almost 100 years since the first case of pituitary dysfunction following a head trauma was reported (described in Benvenga, 2003). Reports of similar cases have since emerged occasionally in the literature, and the syndrome of dysfunctional pituitary following TBI has come to be known as *posttraumatic hypopituitarism* (PTHP) (Horn, 1988). However, only recently has PTHP been systematically studied, with prevalence rates reported anywhere between 15 and 68% following moderate to severe TBI (Behan, Phillips, Thompson, & Agha, 2008; Rothman, Arciniegas, Filley, & Wierman, 2007). Despite this high prevalence, it appears that most cases of PTHP remain undiagnosed and untreated (Benvenga, 2003). For these reasons, an international panel of endocrinologists has recently produced consensus guidelines for assessment of PTHP among patients with TBI (Ghigo et al., 2005).

PTHP can lead to a variety of hormonal abnormalities, including sexual dysfunction, hypothyroidism, hypoadrenalism, and growth hormone deficiencies. Although a dysfunction of the HPA axis is not officially on the list of PTHP symptoms, recent studies have reported that between 2 and 13% of patients who have suffered moderate to severe TBI are characterized by HPA axis dysfunction; this dysfunction presents as a deficiency in cortisol levels and often persists into the chronic phase of recovery. For a review, see Schneider, Kreitschmann-Andermahr, Ghigo, Agha, and Stalla (2007).

Clinical Populations

Neuropsychiatric Disorders

Because hyperactivity of the HPA axis is commonly associated with various forms of psychopathology, most notably depression, posttraumatic stress disorder (PTSD), and psychosis, it is likely that elevations of cortisol are partly responsible for some of the cognitive deficits seen in these populations.

MAJOR DEPRESSION

A large body of evidence supports the notion that depression is associated with HPA axis sensitization or hyperactivity. First and foremost, patients with depression have higher levels of cortisol in their system and exhibit enlarged and overactive pituitary and adrenal glands (Claes, Nemeroff, Corveleyn, Luyten, & Blatt, 2005). Additionally, these patients exhibit a breakdown in the HPA containment system, such that their HPA activity is not suppressed by injections of the synthetic glucocorticoid, dexamethasone. In other words, the Type II receptors in the hippocampus are resistant to cortisol (Pariante & Lightman, 2008). As mentioned before, resistance to cortisol also leads to overactivity of the immune system, explaining why depression is associated with exacerbation of autoimmune disorders such as rheumatoid arthritis and multiple sclerosis (Chrousos et al., 2009; Kendall-Tackett, 2007). Interestingly, treatment with antidepressants appears to reverse this resistance of the cortisol receptors, both in the brain and in the periphery. For a review, see Pariante (2006).

Based on the above findings, it was originally believed that the HPA axis hyperactivity and the concomitant inflammatory response are simple epiphenomena of the chronic stress associated with depressed mood. However, in recent years, this notion has begun to yield to a new reconceptualization of the relationship between depression and the HPA axis, in which HPA hyperactivity is thought to represent a risk factor for, rather than an outcome of, depression. This risk is believed to be conferred by HPA axis changes stemming from early life experiences (Gillespie & Nemeroff, 2007; Pariante & Lightman, 2008) as well as genetic predisposition (O'Hara et al., 2007; Taylor et al., 2006). In particular, research with rodents and nonhuman primates has shown that prolonged maternal separation early in life is associated with HPA changes that persist into adulthood (Sanchez, Ladd, & Plotsky, 2001), and men and women who experienced abuse or trauma in childhood exhibit a hyperactive HPA axis in adulthood (Heim, Mletzko, Purselle, Nemeroff, & Musselman, 2008; Heim, Newport, Mletzko, Nemeroff, & Miller, 2008). Given the deleterious effects of chronic cortisol exposure on brain structure and function, it should then not be surprising that a recent, large, meta-analysis found that major depression is associated with lower hippocampal volume (Campbell, Marriott, Nahmias, & MacQueen, 2004), and a large-scale study examining over 8,000 patients found that memory functions decline in direct proportion to the length of previous depressive history (Gorwood, Corruble, Falissard, & Goodwin, 2008). Relatedly, cortisol levels explain memory and executive deficits among patients with depression, above and beyond psychiatric symptom load (Egeland et al., 2005).

POSTTRAUMATIC STRESS DISORDER

About 8% of individuals exposed to extreme, uncontrollable stress develops PTSD (Kessler, Sonnega, Bromet, & Hughes, 1995). It has been well established that PTSD is associated with hyperactivity of the HPA axis (Bremner, Vythilingam, Vermetten, Khan, et al., 2003), as well as increased amygdalar volume or activation, decreased hippocampal volume (Bremner et al., 1997; Bremner, Vythilingam, Vermetten, McGlashan, et al., 2003; Geuze et al., 2005), and decreased memory functions (Bremner, Vermetten, Afzal, & Vythilingam, 2004; Bremner, Vythilingam, Vermetten, Charney, & Vaccarino, 2004). However, given that exposure to severe stress or trauma in childhood predisposes individuals both to hippocampal atrophy and to the development of PTSD later in life, it is not clear whether smaller hippocampi among sufferers of PTSD are truly a result of PTSD or a premorbid risk factor accrued during early life.

Importantly, recall from Chapter 3 that the hippocampus plays a role in modulating the activity of the amygdala by providing information about the context in which a given emotion-evoking stimulus is encountered. Thus, the same stimulus may lead to a large, or a small, amygdalar response, depending on how the hippocampus interprets the contextual cues. However, hippocampal atrophy is thought to lead to declines in memory for contexts, thereby precluding it from effectively influencing amygdalar activity. Consequently, individuals with PTSD have difficulty effectively distinguishing between threatening and nonthreatening situations, therefore reacting emotionally to any potentially threatening stimulus, regardless of whether contextual cues suggest otherwise (McEwen & Lasley, 2003). The result is a chronic flooding with glucocorticoids and continued damage to the stress response substrates.

SCHIZOPHRENIA

It has been suggested that inherent hyperactivity of the HPA axis may represent an underlying neurodevelopmental mechanism in the development of psychosis (Corcoran et al., 2003; Walker, Mittal, & Tessner, 2008). This hypothesis has been supported by numerous studies that have found enlarged pituitary glands in patients with schizophrenia or schizophrenia spectrum disorders, and even in unaffected relatives (Mondelli et al., 2008; Takahashi et al., 2009), as well as higher ACTH levels in first-episode drug-naive patients with schizophrenia (Ryan, Sharifi, Condren, & Thakore, 2004). Consistent with other disorders characterized by a hyperactive HPA axis, schizophrenia is also associated with smaller hippocampal volume (Phillips et al., 2006; Yuii et al., 2007).

Aging and Dementia

Among older adults HPA axis dysregulation appears to be relatively common (O'Dwyer & Orrell, 1994), placing the aging brain at an increased risk for developing cortisol-related structural and functional abnormalities. In fact, this increased vulnerability may be the very mechanism behind "pseudodementia" among older adults (Mitchell, 1995).

However, it should be noted that structural and functional abnormalities associated with depression among older adults may have two fully independent etiologies. On the one hand, there are elderly individuals with depression who have a lifelong history of the disorder; on the other hand, there are those with late-onset depression. In a recent study, both groups exhibited hippocampal atrophy, as compared to healthy older adults, but the patterns of atrophy appeared to be different for the two groups. In particular, individuals with late-onset depression exhibited prominent changes in the CA1 area of the hippocampus and the subiculum, a pattern of atrophy that is typical of mild cognitive impairment and/or early Alzheimer's disease, suggesting that among these patients depression may have been a reaction to subtle, preclinical signs of dementia. In contrast, lifelong history of depression was associated with more widespread hippocampal atrophy, also involving areas CA2 and CA3, which are thought to play a role in the HPA axis containment (Ballmaier et al., 2008). However, a combination of the two etiologies is also likely to play a role, given that dementia appears to progress faster when associated with cortisol elevations (Csernansky et al., 2006). Lastly, higher levels of cortisol have been found in patients with Alzheimer's disease and vascular dementia (Spada et al., 2001), nursing home residents with dementia of various etiologies (Woods et al., 2008), and individuals suffering from delirium (Robertsson et al., 2001).

Other Neurological Disorders

MULTIPLE SCLEROSIS

MS and other autoimmune disorders are known to become exacerbated by stress. It has been suggested that these exacerbations are related to stress-related sensitization, or hyperactivity, of the HPA axis, or, put differently, a resistance of glucocorticoid receptors (Mohr & Pelletier, 2006). As mentioned earlier, glucocorticoids bind not only to receptors in the hippocampus, but also to receptors in other tissues in the body, playing a role, among others, in suppression of the immune system. When glucocorticoid receptors develop resistance to cortisol, the normal suppression of the immune system does not occur. Thus, somewhat counterintuitively, although patients with MS exhibit elevations of plasma cortisol (Ysrraelit, Gaitan, Lopez, & Correale, 2008), which, under normal circumstances, should suppress autoimmune flare-ups, these increased levels of cortisol lead to an overactivity of the immune system and, consequently, to an MS relapse. Additionally, higher levels of cortisol have been shown to correlate with indicators of cerebral inflammation as well as depressive symptomatology in this population (Fassbender et al., 1998).

TRAUMATIC BRAIN INJURY

As mentioned earlier, moderate to severe TBI has been shown to be associated with between 15 and 68% prevalence rates of PTHP (Behan et al., 2008; Rothman et al., 2007) and with between 2 and 13% of patients exhibiting HPA axis dysfunction (Schneider et al., 2007). This dysfunction presents as a deficiency in cortisol levels and often persists into the chronic phase of recovery (for review, see Schneider et al., 2007). Although severely low levels of cortisol can be life-threatening, in less severe cases they generally lead to low energy levels and weight loss (Schneider et al., 2007). Importantly, among survivors of TBI, low levels of cortisol have been found to correlate with reported fatigue 1 year postinjury (Bushnik, Englander, & Katznelson, 2007), as well as dysfunctional sleep patterns that resemble those associated with major depression (Frieboes et al., 1999).

To date, only one study has examined the effect of *mild* TBI on cortisol levels (Sojka, Stalnacke, Bjornstig, & Karlsson, 2006), demonstrating a pattern of dysregulation that is different from that seen in moderate to severe TBI cases. In particular, this study found that among patients with mild TBI, cortisol was *elevated upon admission* to the hospital, but generally began to *decrease* by 7 hours *postinjury*. This decrease, however, was not ubiquitous, as some patients continued to exhibit elevated cortisol over the long term. These persistent (i.e., still present after 7 hours) cortisol elevations were predictive of posttraumatic stress symptoms 1 year postinjury, providing a viable explanation for why a minority of patients with mild TBI continue to experience distress beyond the typical period of recovery. Additional support for differential endocrine response to mild versus moderate to severe TBI was also provided by a recent animal study, in which rats that underwent mild TBI showed greater reactivity to stress (i.e., greater cortisol release) than both those with moderate to severe injuries and noninjured controls. Importantly, this effect persisted for more than 2 months after the injury (Taylor et al., 2008).

TUMORS

Corticotropic pituitary adenomas are small benign brain tumors that produce ACTH,[4] causing the adrenal gland to produce excessive amounts of cortisol. They account for the majority (about 70%) of noniatrogenic cases of Cushing's syndrome. When Cushing's syndrome is caused by a pituitary adenoma, it is typically referred to as Cushing's disease. It is about five times more common among women than among men. Although pituitary adenomas are relatively common, accounting for about 15% of all intracranial neoplasms, only a small proportion of these are corticotropic. Pituitary adenomas also can be associated with visual disturbance due to pressure on the optic chiasm. For additional information, see Ezzat and colleagues (2004).

In addition to pituitary adenomas, other types of tumors, both benign and malignant, have been shown to lead to increases in ACTH and cortisol levels, including some lung, pancreatic, and medullary cancers. When Cushing's syndrome is caused by such tumors, it is referred to as *ectopic ACTH syndrome*.

SUMMARY AND CONCLUSIONS

As the literature reviewed above suggests, HPA axis abnormalities and concomitant neurobiological changes likely account for at least some of the neurocognitive abnormalities seen among neuropsychiatric populations.

This is particularly true for depression and PTSD. Additionally, breakdown in the HPA axis is commonly seen among older adults, and has been suggested as a potential mechanism for brain changes associated with aging. Lastly, certain poorly understood manifestations among neurological populations are beginning to be understood in the context of HPA axis breakdown, including stress-related exacerbations of autoimmune disorders and some counterintuitive sequelae of mild versus moderate to severe TBI. In particular, whereas moderate to severe TBI is associated with abnormally low levels of cortisol, some patients with mild TBI exhibit lasting posttraumatic *elevations* in cortisol levels, offering a viable explanation for persistent postconcussive syndrome in a subset of patients with mild TBI. Considering stress as a source of potentially permanent brain injury or even as a progressive neurodegenerative process represents a considerable paradigm shift for clinical neuropsychology, but one that promises to offer exciting new discoveries as well as improvements in clinical care.

NOTES

1. See Chapter 8 for a discussion of positive and negative affectivity.
2. However, an alternative explanation for why stress hormones lead to food craving is that they facilitate replacement of energy stores expended during stress (McEwen, 2005; McEwen & Lasley, 2003).
3. In animals, these changes have been shown to last for several weeks following the removal of chronic stress (Biggio, Dazzi, Serra, & Smith, 2004; Mizoguchi, Shoji, Ikeda, Tanaka, & Tabira, 2008).
4. Not all pituitary adenomas produce ACTH. Other hormones produced by these types of tumors are growth hormone, thyroid stimulating hormone, and prolactine, among others.

PART IV

A Glimpse at Tomorrow from an Interdisciplinary Perspective

INTRODUCTION TO PART IV

Whereas Part I of this book focused primarily on whence neuropsychology of emotion came and Parts II and III reviewed where neuropsychology of emotion is today, Part IV examines the *future* of this growing area. The future, like the past, will undoubtedly be interdisciplinary, with reciprocal benefits for clinical neuropsychology and for other allied disciplines. In this interdisciplinary spirit, Part IV of this book offers guest contributions from a health psychologist, Paula G. Williams, who specializes in studying the interface between personality, health, and executive functioning. Additionally, Part IV offers thoughts on specific scientific and clinical endeavors that would further facilitate integration of the neuropsychology of emotion into everyday clinical practice, "sneaking a peek" at what *clinical* neuropsychology of emotion might look like in years to come.

CHAPTER 11

Temperament, Personality, and Heritability of Individual Differences in Executive Functioning

with Paula G. Williams

In clinical neuropsychology, temperament and personality are often considered only as they relate to psychopathology, and often only if such psychopathology is meaningfully linked to the referral question, test performance and interpretation, or treatment recommendations. Rarely do neuropsychologists consider the normal variability in personality and temperament that occurs among psychologically healthy individuals. However, in recent years, personality researchers have begun to explore the neurobiological underpinnings of personality traits and, consequently, the relationship between personality and cognition. Subtle individual differences in executive functioning (EF), in particular, have emerged as correlates of personality, and the mechanisms underlying these associations, as well as those underlying the normal variability in EF, are the topics of this chapter.

DEFINING THE CONSTRUCTS

Temperament

Temperament refers to individual differences in emotional, motor, and attentional reactivity, and is often characterized as the initial state from

Paula G. Williams, PhD, is Associate Professor in the Department of Psychology at the University of Utah.

which personality develops in interaction with experience (Rothbart, 2007). Importantly, temperament is considered to be biologically based, and identification of the underlying neural networks has become a focus of research (e.g., Posner, Rothbart, & Sheese, 2007). Although there has been a variety of temperament taxonomies, Rothbart and colleagues (e.g., Rothbart & Sheese, 2007) have provided support for three higher-order temperament factors: (1) negative emotionality, (2) positive emotionality, and (3) effortful control.

As already reviewed in Chapter 8, positive and negative emotionality, or affective styles, have been linked to hemispheric asymmetry in frontal metabolism and relate to approach-versus-withdrawal behavioral tendencies as well as to sensitivity to rewards versus punishments, respectively. Importantly, recent research suggests that positive emotionality is heterogeneous; in addition to reflecting approach/reward tendencies, positive emotionality can also be related to interpersonal bonds (sometimes called *affiliation*) (e.g., Kochanska, Aksan, Penney, & Doobay, 2007). Effortful control, on the other hand, is characterized as the ability to override dominant emotional tendencies (i.e., negative or positive affectivity) to successfully engage in goal-directed behavior and, therefore, is thought to be central to self-regulation, generally, and to emotion regulation, specifically (Rothbart & Sheese, 2007). Recall from Chapter 7 that emotion regulation is related to various aspects of EF, and, depending on the strategy used, also relates to different frontal networks. These relationships are revisited later in this chapter.

Personality

Broadly defined, *personality* refers to characteristic patterns of thinking, feeling, and behaving. Personality research in the lexical tradition (i.e., factor-analytic examination of descriptive adjectives) has consistently yielded five broad personality factors. The five-factor model (FFM) (or "Big Five") is a widely accepted personality trait taxonomy (Digman, 1990) with well-validated measures (e.g., NEO Personality Inventory—Revised [NEO PI-R]; Costa & McCrae, 1992). In this chapter, the primary labels used to designate the major personality traits correspond to the factor labels of the NEO PI-R (Costa & McCrae, 1992), a frequently utilized measure of the FFM. These are *neuroticism*, *extraversion*, *openness to experience*, *agreeableness*, and *conscientiousness* (see Table 11.1).

Neuroticism, sometimes termed *trait negative affectivity*, *trait anxiety*, or *emotional (in)stability*, is characterized by the propensity to experience emotional distress (i.e., anxiety, anger, depression) and vulnerability to adverse stress responses. Extraversion (also termed *trait positive affectivity*) is the propensity to prefer intense and frequent social interactions and

TABLE 11.1. Elements of the Five-Factor Model of Personality

Trait	Opposite pole	Facets
Neuroticism	Emotional Stability	Anxiety, Angry Hostility, Depression, Self-Consciousness, Impulsiveness, Vulnerability
Extraversion	Introversion	Warmth, Gregariousness, Assertiveness, Activity, Excitement Seeking, Positive Emotion
Openness	Closed Mindedness	Fantasy, Aesthetics, Feelings, Actions, Ideas, Values
Agreeableness	Antagonism	Trust, Straightforwardness, Altruism, Compliance, Modesty, Tender-Mindedness
Conscientiousness	Unreliability	Competence, Order, Dutifulness, Achievement Striving, Self-Discipline, Deliberation

Note. From Williams, Smith, Gunn, and Uchino (in press; adapted from Costa & McCrae, 1992). Reprinted with permission from Springer Publishing Co.

to be energized and optimistic. Openness to experience (sometimes called *intellect* or *culture*) refers to cognitive and behavioral inquisitiveness, as reflected in active imagination, aesthetic sensitivity, attentiveness to inner feelings (both positive and negative), preference for variety, intellectual curiosity, and independence of judgment. Agreeableness (vs. antagonism) is the tendency to regard others with sympathy and to act unselfishly and cooperatively with others. Conscientiousness reflects the propensity to control behavior in the service of goals. Individual differences in organization and orderliness, persistence, dutifulness, self-discipline, deliberateness/impulse control, and perceived competence are all aspects of conscientiousness (sometimes termed *constraint*).

The FFM of personality has been characterized with respect to the underlying temperament dimensions (Rothbart, 2007; Shiner & Caspi, 2003) reviewed above (i.e., positive emotionality, negative emotionality, and effortful control). The relationships between these temperamental dimensions and the five personality factors are summarized in Table 11.2. Specifically, neuroticism has been associated with negative emotionality and the behavioral inhibition system (BIS),[1] involving enhanced sensitivity to punishment cues (Gray, 1982, 1987), as well as a moderate (negative) association with effortful control (Evans & Rothbart, 2007). The temperament precursor to extraversion is positive emotionality (sometimes called

TABLE 11.2. Relationships between Personality Factors and Temperament Factors

Personality factors	Temperament factors: Negative emotionality	Positive emotionality	Effortful control
Neuroticism	High	N/A	Moderately low
Extraversion	N/A	High (approach)	Moderately low
Conscientiousness	N/A	N/A	High
Agreeableness	N/A	High (affiliation)	High

surgency) and reflects high-intensity pleasure, activity level, and impulsivity (Rothbart, Ahadi, Hersehy, & Fisher, 2001). Sensitivity to reward cues (i.e., behavioral activation system [BAS][1]) (Gray, 1970) is a proposed temperament substrate of extraversion. Positive emotionality in the context of reward cues (i.e., "approach") is negatively associated with effortful control (Kochanska et al., 2007). There is evidence that the temperament factor of effortful control is the developmental precursor to conscientiousness (Rothbart, Ahadi, & Evans, 2000). Agreeableness also appears to be developmentally linked to temperamental effortful control (Ahadi & Rothbart, 1994). For example, children who are rated as more agreeable by their peers perform better on tasks requiring effortful behavioral regulation (Cumberland-Li et al., 2004). Importantly, Kochanska and colleagues (2007) demonstrated that positive emotionality expressed during mother–child interactions, interpreted as reflecting high affiliation, was positively associated with behavioral indices of effortful control.

Heritability of Individual Differences in EF

Subtle individual differences in EF among normal (i.e., non-brain-injured, nonpsychiatric) individuals are central to understanding temperament and personality. Although such individual differences partly reflect environmental influences, there is also considerable evidence of genetic determinants. This evidence is reviewed below.

One line of evidence pointing to the heritability of EF comes from twin studies. Such studies have found significant heritability in executive attentional control as assessed with the Attention Network Test (ANT)[2] (Fan, Wu, Fossella, & Posner, 2001) and the Continuous Performance Test (CPT) among normal (i.e., non-ADHD) participants (Cornblatt et al., 1988), and some twin studies have found significant heritability in performance on the Wisconsin Card Sorting Test (WCST; Anokhin, Heath, & Ralano, 2003).[3] Notably, a recent twin study, using a composite score of "inhibition," "set switching," and "updating of working memory," yielded high heritability estimates, indicating that EF may be among the most heritable of psychological traits (Friedman et al., 2008).

Another line of research has focused on identifying candidate genes that can be linked to various indices of EF. Because some aspects of the dopamine system (primarily the mesocortical system) have been implicated in EF (e.g., Lumme, Aalto, Ilonen, Nagren, & Hietala, 2007), the search for candidate genes that underlie individual differences in EF has focused largely on those that influence dopaminergic communication. This search has yielded significant associations between various indices of EF and the genes controlling various aspects of the dopamine system. The summary of this literature can be found in Table 11.3.

In addition to the dopamine system, the serotonin system may also play a role in executive attention and cognitive control (Canli et al., 2005; Reuter, Ott, Vaitl, & Hennig, 2007), particularly in the context of emotion regulation. The short allele of the serotonin transporter gene (*5-HTTLPR*) is associated with anxiety-related temperament traits (Schinka, Busch, & Robichaux-Keene, 2004; Sen, Burmeister, & Ghosh, 2004), depression, and enhanced amygdalar activity during processing of emotional information (Hariri et al., 2002, 2005). This allele has also been associated with activity in the circuit linking the amygdala and the anterior cingulate cortex during processing of fearful stimuli (Heinz & Smolka, 2006; Pezawas et al., 2005). Additionally, the gene associated with the tryptophan hydroxylase enzyme, which constrains serotonin production, is implicated in anger expression and aggression, indicative of poor emotion regulation and difficulty modulating interpersonal behavior and, thus, suggesting associations with EF (Manuck et al., 1999).

In summary, twin studies, examination of EF–polymorphism association, and imaging genomic research support the notion that there are identifiable individual differences in EF that show relatively high heritability. Multiple genes, primarily those involved in dopamine metabolism, have associations with various indices of EF, including performance on EF measures and brain activation during EF task performance.

COGNITIVE AND NEUROANATOMIC SUBSTRATES FOR PERSONALITY

Given that individual differences in EF are inherited, at least in part, and given that such differences manifest in characteristic ways of thinking and behaving, it is important to examine associations between EF and established individual differences in temperament and personality. In this section, relations between individual differences in temperament/personality and EF are examined.

TABLE 11.3. The Association between the Genetic Underpinnings of the Dopamine System and Performance on Measures of Executive Functioning

Gene	Function	Index of EF	References
DRD2	D2 receptor protein synthesis	Wisconsin Card Sorting Test	Rodriguez-Jimenez et al. (2006)
		fMRI ACC activation during performance of the ANT task	Fan, Fossella, Sommer, Wu, & Posner (2003)
DRD4	D4 receptor protein synthesis	Executive attention	Fossella, Posner, Fan, Swanson, & Pfaff (2002)
		fMRI ACC activation during performance of the ANT task	Fan et al. (2003)
		ADHD susceptibility	Gornick et al. (2007)
MAOA	Synthesis of MAOA, responsible for degradation of monoamines	Executive attention	Fossella et al. (2002)
		fMRI ACC activation during performance of the ANT task	Fan et al. (2003)
COMT	Synthesis of COMT, responsible for degradation of dopamine	Conflict resolution; performance on clinical EF measures	Bishop, Cohen, Fossella, Casey, & Farah (2006); Gallinat et al. (2003); Blasi et al. (2005); Diamond, Briand, Fossella, & Gehbach (2004); de Frias et al. (2005)
		Processing efficiency[a] in PFC and ACC during a WM and attentional control tasks, respectively	Heinz & Smolka (2006)

Note. MAOA, monoamine oxidase A; COMT, catechol-O-methyltransferase; ACC, anterior cingulate cortex; PFC, prefrontal cortex; fMRI, functional magentic resonance imaging; ANT, Attentional Network Test; EF, executive functioning; WM, working memory; ADHD, attention-deficit/hyperactivity disorder.

[a]"Processing efficiency" refers to better performance in the context of lesser fMRI activation.

Neuroticism

As explained earlier, neuroticism is associated with a tendency toward negative affectivity and sensitivity to punishment. Thus, neuroticism can also be conceptualized in EF terms as reflecting enhanced conflict monitoring. This notion is supported by findings that neuroticism is associated with anterior cingulate gyrus activation during processing of negative emotional[4] information (Haas, Omura, Constable, & Canli, 2007), as well as *non*emotional conflict tasks (Luu, Collins, & Tucker, 2000). Similarly, individuals scoring high on a self-report measure of the BIS (Carver & White, 1994), which, as mentioned earlier, is considered to be a temperament underpinning of neuroticism, evidence greater ERPs in conflict trials of the go/no-go task (Amodio, Master, Yee, & Taylor, 2008), reflecting greater anterior cingulate activity (Botvinick, Braver, Barch, Carter, & Cohen, 2001; Yeung, Cohen, & Botvinick, 2004).

Importantly, moderately enhanced conflict monitoring evidenced among individuals with high neuroticism may facilitate the development of EF, as it relies on the recruitment of higher-order cognitive control mechanisms. In other words, somewhat counterintuitively, the development of EF is, to some extent, dependent on signals from neural pathways that are associated with neuroticism, as evidenced in developmental studies that indicate that negative emotionality/fearfulness in childhood may be important in the development of self-regulatory abilities (see Rothbart, Ellis, & Posner, 2004, for review).[5] However, neuroticism is also associated with enhanced activity in the amygdala in response to negative emotional stimuli (Haas et al., 2007). Thus, at very high levels, neuroticism may be associated with chronic stress, which, as reviewed in Chapter 10, may lead to an eventual decline in EF. Indeed, Denburg and colleagues (2009) found that neuroticism is related to poorer performance on a decision-making task, but only in older adults, pointing to the cumulative deleterious effect of stress over time as a potential mechanism for this association. Taken together, these findings suggest a possible curvilinear, dynamic association between neuroticism and EF that awaits definitive empirical demonstration.

Extraversion

Unlike neuroticism, which is associated with sensitivity to punishment, extraversion is associated with greater sensitivity to reward cues (i.e., BAS) (Gray, 1970). As already suggested by the review of the literature in Chapter 9, a number of clinical populations characterized by weaknesses in EF, such as children with attention-deficit disorder (Holroyd et al., 2008; Masunami et al., 2009; Wang et al., 2008) and adults with psychopathy (Blair et al., 2006) or addictions (Genovese & Wallace, 2007), also exhibit greater sensitivity to reward. High sensitivity to reward has been demonstrated to disrupt higher-order executive processes (MacCoon et al., 2004; Suchy & Kosson, 2006; though see Lieberman & Rosenthal, 2001, for contradictory findings). Consistent with this notion, in studies of children, high BAS is associated with poorer EF (Blair, Peters, & Granger, 2004), and high positive emotionality in reward/approach tasks, as opposed to that expressed in interpersonal interaction, is associated with poorer performance on behavioral effortful control tasks (Kochanska et al., 2007).

Extraversion has also been the focus of studies examining attentional bias toward positive emotional/reward information. For example, extraversion is associated with increased anterior cingulate activation in response to positive compared to neutral words in the emotional Stroop task[6] (Haas, Omura, Amin, Constable, & Canli, 2006). Additionally, extraversion is positively associated with the thrill-seeking factor of impulsivity (Flory et al., 2006) and negatively associated with inhibitory control among adults (Evans & Rothbart, 2007) as well as children and adolescents (Abe, 2005). Consequently, it should not be surprising that extraversion (particularly the sensation-seeking aspect thereof) is associated with an increased incidence of TBI (O'Jile, Ryan, Parks-Levy, Betz, & Gouvier, 2004) and substance abuse, which may lead to additional EF declines (Blume & Marlatt, 2009), thus further strengthening the association between extraversion and poorer EF in adulthood.

Lastly, associations with dopamine-related genetic polymorphisms with known links to EF are also relevant. For example, sensation or thrill seeking, which is an aspect of extraversion, has been associated with the *DRD4* allele (Swanson et al., 2000), and individual differences in dopamine transmission figure prominently in neurobiological models of extraversion (Depue & Collins, 1999).

Taken together, the literature suggests that temperamental (nonaffiliative) positive emotionality and reward sensitivity may interfere with the development of EF in childhood, as well as phasically disrupt EF in highly rewarding situations. Such chronic and phasic weaknesses may be further exacerbated by injuries to the brain and the frontal lobes as a consequence of lapses in behavioral control.

Openness to Experience

Openness to experience reflects one's desire and ability to seek new experiences (Hughes, Case, Stuempfle, & Evans, 2003). Of course, new experiences inherently require that one be flexible in thought and action and capable of generating solutions to novel problems. Thus, it should not be surprising that openness to experience is associated with several indices of EF, including critical thinking skills (Clifford, Boufal, & Kurtz, 2004;

Ennis, 1987), goal maintenance and achievement (Farsides & Woodfield, 2003), cognitive flexibility (McCrae, 1987), and the ability to consider different vantage points (McElroy & Dowd, 2007). Importantly, openness is associated with performance on experimental cognitive tasks presumably associated with dorsolateral prefrontal cortex functioning (DeYoung, Peterson, & Higgins, 2005)—that is, a neural region associated with EF, as well as with performance on neuropsychological tests of EF in older adults (Williams et al., 2010).

Additionally, researchers have linked higher levels of openness to an enhanced ability to attend to internal and external environmental cues (Baer, Smith, & Allen, 2004; Wise, Mann, & Shay, 1992) as well as greater auditory P3 ERP amplitude (Gurrera, O'Donnell, Nestor, Gainski, & McCarley, 2001), which is associated with attending to stimuli and transferring information into consciousness (Polich & Kok, 1995). These findings suggest that higher levels of openness may be related to greater attention to environmental information, which may result in greater awareness and more in-depth processing of stimuli (Ford, Pfefferbaum, Tinklenberg, & Kopell, 1982). These abilities, in turn, represent essential precursors for effective self-regulation (Stegg, Terwogt, & Gross, 2007; Tangney et al., 2004). Consequently, higher openness to experience may be associated not only with better reasoning and problem solving, but also with better emotion regulation.

Agreeableness

Agreeableness reflects the ability to inhibit disagreeable tendencies, particularly emotional expressions that may affect relationship quality, in favor of socially appropriate responses (Tobin, Graziano, Vanman, & Tassinary, 2000). In support of this notion, the behavioral disinhibition factor of impulsivity is most strongly (negatively) related to agreeableness (Flory et al., 2006). Thus, to the extent that agreeableness reflects the ability to inhibit negative tendencies in the service of interpersonal harmony, EF appears to be involved.

The associations between agreeableness and EF-related constructs have been less studied than other FFM constructs, and, to our knowledge, only one study thus far has directly examined the relationship between EF (a composite of four traditional EF measures) and agreeableness assessed with the NEO PI-R (Williams et al., 2010). This study found a significant positive association between agreeableness and EF.

Some support exists for the association between low or even clinically deficient EF and low agreeableness, as manifested in social inappropriateness (von Hippel, 2007). For example, lesions to EF-associated brain circuits are often manifest in dysregulated and interpersonally inappropriate behavior (Boccardi, Della Sala, Motto, & Spinnler, 2002; Harlow, 1868; Mathiesen, Farster, & Svendsen, 2004; Starkstein & Robinson, 1997). Executive functioning deficits are also associated with "off-target verbosity" (i.e., talking excessively about topics irrelevant to the stream of conversation) among older adults (Pushkar et al., 2000). Older individuals are also more likely than younger individuals to discuss socially embarrassing information in public settings, and this difference is explained by performance on tasks of response inhibition (von Hippel & Dunlop. 2005). Moreover, individual differences in inhibitory ability among young adults (i.e., Stroop performance) also predict social inappropriateness under socially challenging circumstances (von Hippel & Gonsalkorale, 2005).

In summary, agreeableness is an adaptive trait that allows one to negotiate everyday social situations toward better achievement of interpersonal goals. Although evidence suggests a positive association between agreeableness and EF, the majority of the findings thus far only imply this association by demonstrating poor EF among individuals who are socially inappropriate. Only one study has demonstrated high agreeableness in the context of above-average EF skills.

Conscientiousness

Conscientiousness refers to the ability to reliably and adaptively engage in planning, organization, and completion of tasks while overriding distracting or competing emotional states or stimuli—in other words, the ability to engage in goal-directed behavior. From that descriptive standpoint, individual differences in conscientiousness are virtually analogous to individual differences in EF. Thus, it should not be a surprise that the putative developmental precursor of conscientiousness is the temperamental tendency known as effortful control, which, as mentioned earlier, is itself related to emotion regulation and EF. It is also noteworthy that conscientiousness increases in young adulthood (Robins, Fraley, Roberts, & Trzesniewksi, 2001), corresponding to the completion of myelination of the prefrontal cortex and related circuits that subserve EF (Stuss, 1992; Welsh, Pennington, & Groisser, 1991). Lastly, low conscientiousness is a well-established personality correlate of attention-deficit disorder (Nigg et al., 2002), which is, in turn, well known to be associated with EF weaknesses (Seidman, 2006).

Although limited in scope, research linking these constructs to performance on cognitive tasks has supported the notion that conscientiousness/effortful control reflects underlying differences in EF. For example, in young children, parent-reported temperament marked by effortful control is associated with better performance on EF tasks (Gerardi-Caulton, 2000; Rothbart, Ellis, Rueda, & Posner, 2003). Among adults, extreme self-reported difficulties in effortful control associated with borderline personality disorder have also been linked with poorer response selection as measured by the ANT (Posner et al., 2002). Impulse control, considered to be a facet of conscientiousness (Roberts et al., 2005), has been associated with performance on cognitive tasks assessing the inhibitive aspects of EF (Keilp, Sackeim, & Mann, 2005; Pietrzak et al., 2008; though for contradictory findings, see Cheung, Mitsis, & Halperin, 2004; Reynolds, Ortengran, Richards, & de Wit, 2006).[7]

Taken together, these results generally support the intuitively apparent association between conscientiousness and EF. However, it is important to consider that strength in EF alone is insufficient for greater conscientiousness behavior, as the desire to utilize one's EF strengths toward adaptive goals is also likely needed. In contrast, a deficient EF system is likely sufficient for precluding sustained conscientious actions.

SUMMARY AND CONCLUSIONS

Outside of neuropsychology, there has been an increasing interest in identifying neurobiological substrates of temperament and personality, with heritable variability in EF representing one of a number of studied mechanisms. In this chapter, we reviewed the theoretical underpinnings for the hypothesized relationships between personality, temperament, and EF, as well as the available empirical support. The theoretical and empirical accounts reviewed in this chapter suggest that (1) neuroticism may have a curvilinear relationship with EF, such that intermediate levels of neuroticism are associated with optimal EF; (2) aspects of extraversion, especially sensation seeking, are associated with lower EF; and (3) openness to experience, agreeableness, and conscientiousness are generally associated with higher EF. However, much research is needed to further clarify these relationships.

NOTES

1. BIS and BAS systems are typically assessed using the BIS/BAS Scale (Carver & White, 1994) reviewed in Chapter 9. Also see Chapter 8 for a discussion of the approach–withdrawal motivational systems more generally.
2. The ANT is a computerized reaction time flanker task assessing the ability to inhibit a prepotent response.
3. However, some studies have failed to find genetically linked variability on the WCST performance (Kremen, Eisen, Tsuang, & Lyons, 2007), likely due to the test's limited score range among normal individuals.

4. Particularly sad (but not fearful or happy) faces.
5. The importance of emotional input for normal behavioral and executive control is also supported by the literature on emotional decision making, reviewed in Chapter 9.
6. The emotional Stroop task requires that participants name the color of ink in which emotionally loaded words, such as *death* or *tragedy*, are printed.
7. Note that impulsivity has been demonstrated to be a multidimensional construct, with facets that include thrill seeking, nonplanning impulsivity, and disinhibited behavior (Flory et al., 2006). Flory and colleagues (2006) have shown that conscientiousness is most strongly (negatively) associated with nonplanning impulsivity (which also has a modest positive association with neuroticism). The other aspects of impulsivity are more strongly associated with extraversion/behavioral approach and agreeableness.

CHAPTER 12

Stress Regulation, Executive Functioning, and Physical and Mental Health

with Paula G. Williams

As already covered in Chapter 10, chronic stress is associated with deleterious structural and functional brain changes that are of considerable relevance to clinical neuropsychology. Stress also figures prominently in biopsychosocial models of the maintenance of health and the development of illness. Indeed, understanding individual differences in stress risk and resilience has been a cornerstone of health psychology and behavioral medicine. Individuals vary greatly in the extent to which they are "exposed" to stress, the magnitude of their physiological and emotional responses to potentially stressful events, the length of time it takes to recover from stressful events, and the extent to which there is adequate restoration during or following times of stress. As suggested in Chapters 7 and 11, this variability is moderated, at least in part, by individual differences in EF. In this chapter, we review how EF moderates each of the stress processes (exposure, reactivity, recovery, and restoration), thereby also moderating susceptibility to physical and mental illness.

DEFINING THE CONSTRUCTS

Stress Regulation

Stress regulation is a broad term that refers to cognitive, behavioral, and physiological processes that serve to alter, foster adaptation to, or transform psychological stress.[1] Stress, however, is not a unitary construct. Rather, it consists of a several component processes, including stress exposure, stress reactivity, stress recovery, and restoration. These processes are central to recent theoretical frameworks for understanding the mechanisms by which stress affects health (Hawkley & Cacioppo, 2004; Uchino et al., 2007). Thus, stress regulation can be thought of in relation to the occurrence of stressful events, aspects of a person that increase or decrease the probability of experiencing adverse circumstances, as well as responses to those events.

Importantly, stress regulation should be distinguished from emotion regulation discussed in Chapter 7. Both *stress* and *emotion* can be considered in the superordinate category *affect*, which also includes mood and impulses (Gross & Thompson, 2007). Whereas both *stress* and *emotion* refer to whole-body responses to events, stress usually refers to a negative affective state in the context of taxing circumstances; emotions, on the other hand, can be negative or positive in valence. Because *emotion regulation* refers to a process whereby one decreases, enhances, or alters an internal emotional experience and an external emotional display, it plays an important role in stress regulation processes. For example, any given emotion regulation strategy may serve to increase or decrease stress exposure, reactivity, recovery, and restoration. See Table 12.1 for examples of ways in which emotion regulation may affect stress regulation processes.[2]

Stress Exposure

Stress exposure generally refers to the frequency and severity of adverse events (i.e., "stressors") that an individual experiences in daily life. Stressors may take the form of major life events (e.g., divorce, loss of job) or daily hassles (e.g., an argument with a coworker, getting a traffic ticket). Stressful circumstances may be either acute (i.e., time limited), such as difficulty finding a parking space, or may be chronic, such as serving as a caregiver for a family member with Alzheimer's disease. Stress exposure may also include cognitive processes such as anticipation of a stressor (worry) and mentally reimagined stressors (rumination). That is, stress exposure can occur in the absence of an external stimulus to the extent that an individual is distressed by the possibility of a future stressor or engages in thought processes that involve "reliving" a past stressor.

TABLE 12.1. Hypothesized Effects of Emotion Regulation Strategies on Stress Regulation

Emotion regulation strategy	Hypothesized effect on stress regulation
Proactive	Avoids stressful situations. Modifies stressful situations by self-assertion. Prevents prolonged emotional reactions to stressful situations by self-distraction.
Reactive reappraisal	Decreases perception of situations as stressful by reinterpretation or distancing.
Reactive suppression	Produces emotional displays that may reduce the likelihood of escalation of stressful situations. May prolong stress recovery.

Note. Emotion regulation strategies outlined in this table are based on models proposed by Gross et al. (2006) and Ochsner and Gross (2008).

Stress Reactivity

The term *stress reactivity* describes the immediate response to a potentially stressful event and involves one's perception of the event (i.e., appraisal; Lazarus & Folkman, 1984), subjective distress, and physiological arousal (e.g., increased heart rate, increased blood pressure, release of stress hormones such as cortisol). As briefly reviewed in Chapter 10, the sympathetic adrenomedullary (SAM) system and the HPA axis are central to the body's characteristic responses to stress. Studies of stress reactivity, therefore, often focus on cortisol, the stress hormone indicative of HPA axis activation, and systolic and diastolic blood pressure (SBP, DBP) and heart rate (HR), indicative of SAM-mediated cardiovascular activation. More recently, the variability in HR that corresponds to changes in respiration, often referred to as heart rate variability, has been studied. Phasic change in high-frequency heart rate variability (HF-HRV), also called respiratory sinus arrhythmia (RSA), is an index of parasympathetic activation.[3] Recall from Chapter 4 that parasympathetic activation can be conceptualized as a "brake" that periodically suppresses sympathetic activation (Porges, 2007). Additionally, there is a variety of anatomic links between the nervous and immune systems, including immune receptors for neurotransmitters and hormones that are either produced or regulated by the nervous system (Ader, Felton, & Cohen, 2001); thus, physiological responses to stress also include immune system responses (Segerstom & Miller, 2004).[4]

In addition to these psychophysiological indicators, stress reactivity can also be conceptualized as the subjective distress experienced in response to a stressful event, which can occur even in the absence of enhanced physiological reactivity. Furthermore, the strength or duration of neurophysiological responses to stressful events, assessed via brain imaging, may also be considered "reactivity." For example, enhanced amygdalar activation during the processing of negative emotional stimuli may indicate the breakdown of down-regulation of the emotional trigger mechanism by the prefrontal cortex or by the hippocampus (also see Chapters 3, 7, and 10).

Stress Recovery

In the context of the stress response, *recovery* typically refers to levels of emotional or physiological arousal that persist after termination of the stressor. Stress recovery is often operationalized as the time required for the individual to return to baseline levels after termination of the stressor. Central to cardiovascular stress recovery is the activity of the parasympathetic nervous system. Of particular relevance to the current chapter, parasympathetic activation, as indexed by HF-HRV (or RSA), is associated with prefrontal cortex (PFC) activity (Lane, Reiman, Ahern, & Thayer, 2001). Specifically, this region supports stress-dampening self-regulatory activity through connections to the heart via the vagus nerve. Furthermore, as described above, researchers have noted that physiological responses to stress occur during worry (i.e., in anticipation of a stressor) and rumination about stressful events (which may occur even years after an event), leading to a proposal to expand the construct of recovery to include *prolonged cardiovascular activation* (Pieper & Brosschot, 2005).

Restoration

During and after the experience of stress, restorative processes operate to "refresh, buttress, and repair various forms of cellular damage" and to return an individual to baseline levels (Cacioppo & Berntson, 2007, p. 73). Sleep, wound healing, and humoral immunity (i.e., mediated by secreted antibodies) are examples of restorative processes. Related concepts are allostasis and allostatic load. *Allostasis* refers to the active process by which stability or homeostasis is maintained via mediators such as stress hormones. *Allostatic load* refers to the disruption of homeostatic mechanisms (e.g., stress hormones do not "turn off" when stress is over) related to either repeated stress or poor management of systems that promote allostasis (McEwen, 2007). It is hypothesized that inadequate restoration may lead to allostatic load, which in turn may further disrupt restorative processes, such as sleep (e.g., development of insomnia). Finally, although it might alternatively be characterized as "illness behavior," the capacity to retreat from daily stress to recuperate following a time of increased stress and/or illness can also be considered restoration and may, in fact, be adaptive.

COGNITIVE AND NEUROANATOMIC SUBSTRATES OF STRESS REGULATION

There is much evidence that effective stress regulation relies on intact EF, or, alternatively, on neuroanatomic substrates that overlap with those known to control EF. Initial evidence for the role of EF in stress regulation comes from documented associations between EF and psychopathologies that involve impaired emotion regulation and are known to be associated with high levels of stress. For example, individuals with borderline personality disorder, a psychopathology characterized by poor emotion and stress regulation, evidence deficits in some aspects of EF (Fertuck, Lenzenweger, & Clarkin, 2005; Posner et al., 2002). Executive functioning deficits have also been implicated in anxiety disorders, depression, and bipolar disorder (Gruber, Rathgeber, Braunig, & Gauggel, 2007; Olley, Malhi, & Sachdev, 2007; Paeleck-Habermann et al., 2005; Rubinsztein, Michael, Paykel, & Sahakian, 2000), as well as in substance abuse and addiction disorders, eating disorders, aggression, and criminal behavior (Blume & Marlatt, 2009; Brand, Franke-Sievert, et al., 2007; Stevens, Kaplan, & Hesselbrock, 2003), all of which are associated with high levels of stress. Finally, ADHD, considered to be a disorder of EF (Seidman, 2006), is highly comorbid with substance abuse, mood, and anxiety disorders (Biederman et al., 1993). A growing body of research suggests that the disinhibitory problems associated with ADHD may develop in parallel with emotion regulation difficulties (Mullin & Hinshaw, 2007), and it has even been suggested that ADHD is better explained by deficient emotion regulation than by deficient EF (Martel, 2009).

Similarly, brain injuries that affect EF circuitry also have deleterious effects on stress regulation. For example, as already discussed in Chapter 7, patients with TBI often exhibit behavioral disinhibition and social inappropriateness, as well as a difficulty modulating emotional responses. Because many patients with such injuries exhibit minimal decline in IQ, language abilities, or perceptual and motor skills, they at first blush appear unaffected by their injury. However, when faced with the complexities and demands of everyday life (i.e., "daily hassles" or interpersonal challenges), the victims of TBI appear unable to cope (Marschark, Richtsmeier, Richardson, Crovitz, & Henry, 2000), the final result being high levels of stress in their daily lives. Such changes in stress regulation are often attributed to an injury-induced "personality change" or to the so-called "postconcussive syndrome." The latter syndrome, in particular, tends to be associated with a variety of psychiatric, cognitive, and somatic complaints, including depression, anxiety, irritability, difficulty concentrating, fatigue, sleep dysregulation, headaches, dizziness, and many others (Eslinger et al., 1996). In other words, relatively minor declines in EF can lead to a breakdown in emotion regulation, which in turn leads to a breakdown in stress regulation and declines in both mental and physical health. Given emerging theoretical perspectives on stress regulation, described above, associations between EF and stress exposure, reactivity, recovery, and restoration are now considered.

EF and Stress Exposure

Individual differences in EF may influence stress exposure in a variety of ways. There is considerable evidence that individuals interact reciprocally with their environments to enhance or diminish the probability of experiencing stressful events. One behavior–genetic mechanism by which this can occur is the environment–gene correlation; in other words, genetically influenced factors, such as EF (see Chapter 11), enhance or diminish the probability of exposure to stressors (Jang, Wolfe, & Larston, 2006). For example, individuals with poor EF and poor emotion regulation abilities have difficulty overriding dominant emotional tendencies, staying on task, organizing and planning, and making decisions, all of which will place them in a position of increased stress exposure. Individuals with poor EF may struggle with substance use and addiction and may engage in a variety of impulsive and risk-taking behaviors, all of which also have the potential to be stress generating. Importantly, EF influences self-regulation in interpersonal contexts. Thus, individual differences in EF may determine, in part, the extent to which individuals are vulnerable to interpersonal difficulties—which represents a primary source of stress—and a breakdown in social support networks—which represents a potential buffer against the adverse effects of stress.

EF and Stress Reactivity

Although the relationship between stress exposure and EF is driven largely by externally observable behaviors, stress reactivity may be moderated by individual differences in EF due to an overlap or proximity of underlying neuroanatomic networks. In particular, as already reviewed in Chapter 4, activity of the dorsal anterior cingulate gyrus (along with coactivation of the insula region of the temporal lobe) is associated with sympathetic responses to emotive stimuli or threat (see Critchley, 2005, for review), suggesting that individual differences in anterior cingulate function will predict sympathetic responses to perceived stress. Additionally, individual differences in response inhibition (i.e., Stroop interference) are associated with greater systolic and diastolic blood pressure reactivity, at least among middle-age and older adults (Waldstein & Katzel, 2005).

PFC functioning also figures prominently in recent models of self-regulation, including the neurovisceral integration model (Thayer & Lane,

2007; Thayer, Hansen, Saus-Rose, & Johnsen, 2009) and polyvagal theory (Porges, 2007). As previously described, the PFC has rich connections to the heart via the vagus nerve. Porges (2007) has likened resting or tonic vagal activation (i.e., resting HF-HRV or RSA) to a "brake" that actively suppresses sympathetic nervous system activity. Release of the brake (i.e., vagal withdrawal or decreased HF-HRV) allows rapid engagement of sympathetically driven "fight-or-flight" stress responses. Low resting HRV also predicts cortisol reactivity and recovery during performance of cognitive tasks (Thayer et al., 2009). Taken together, these findings suggest that individual differences in EF are reflected in physiological indices of autonomic balance (i.e., high sympathetic reactivity and low parasympathetic tone), which will manifest in both stress reactivity and recovery.

It is also the case that, as already reviewed in Chapter 7, some aspects of EF may serve to alter appraisal processes that will influence both physiological reactivity and subjective distress in response to adverse events. For example, cognitive flexibility and comfort with novelty may moderate the interpretation of events that others' may view as potentially threatening.

EF and Stress Recovery

As described above, in addition to associations with stress reactivity, PFC functioning is hypothesized to predict prolonged activation to stress. Furthermore, the extent to which individual differences in EF influence propensity to worry or ruminate may be a related mechanism for associations with poor stress recovery and prolonged cardiovascular activation to stress. In particular, research has identified EF deficits among individuals prone to rumination, such that rumination is associated with deficits in inhibiting prior mental sets on the WCST (Davis & Nolen-Hoeksema, 2000) and a switching task (Whitmer & Banich, 2007). Other research has demonstrated that the act of rumination itself may tax cognitive resources, leading to deterioration of cognitive flexibility (Watkins & Brown, 2002). Thus, there appears to be a reciprocal association between ruminative tendencies and EF: Individual differences in the cognitive flexibility aspects of EF are associated with propensity to ruminate, which in turn leads to further decrements in EF.

EF and Restoration

Individual differences in EF may act reciprocally with restorative processes over time. Most notably, as described above, weaknesses in EF are associated with prolonged activation in response to stressors, which in turn is associated with high presleep cognitive and physiological arousal—a strong predictor of sleep disruption and chronic sleep difficulties (Bastien,

St.-Jean, Morin, Turcotte, & Carrier, 2008). Poor sleep quality, in turn, negatively affects EF (Nilsson et al., 2005; Van Dongen, Maislin, Mullington, & Dinges, 2003). Relatedly, sleep disruption affects the neuroanatomic circuitry underlying emotion regulation. For example, sleep-deprived individuals exhibit greatly enhanced amygdalar activity in response to emotional imagery, but decreased activity of the medial prefrontal cortex, suggesting a disruption of the emotional modulation circuitry (Yoo et al., 2007).

Lastly, to the extent that individual differences in EF influence educational attainment, socioeconomic status, and career success, there may be indirect influences of EF weaknesses on restoration. For example, individuals of low SES often may need to retain multiple low-paying jobs, with minimal flexibility; thus, their life circumstances may preclude the conditions necessary for adequate restoration (e.g., resulting in sleep loss, inability to take sick days) (Cacioppo & Berntson, 2007).

EXECUTIVE FUNCTIONING AND STRESS REGULATION: PATHWAYS TO PHYSICAL AND MENTAL HEALTH

Individual differences in EF appear to represent an important source of risk and resilience to both stress exposure and to the negative effects of stress. As shown in Figure 12.1, individual differences reflective of EF can be identified at multiple levels, including genetic, neuroanatomic, cognitive, and temperamental/personality (also see Chapter 11). Environmental factors, particularly early stress exposure, influence EF and stress regulation. As described below, each stress regulation process may have particular pathways to poor mental and physical health outcomes. Although it is beyond the scope of this chapter to thoroughly explicate the mechanisms by which stress affects all mental and physical health outcomes, primary hypothesized pathways are outlined and several key examples are highlighted.

Current evidence suggests a reciprocal relationship between EF and stress; individual differences in EF confer vulnerability to adverse stress responses, which in turn contribute to further decrements in EF. That is, environmental forces shape genotypic expression of EF. Stress, particularly chronic traumatic stress, appears to negatively influence EF via a variety of pathways, including cortisol effects on the brain. Animal research suggests that chronic stress leads to glucocorticoid receptor down-regulation in the PFC, contributing to decreased dopaminergic transmission and associated cognitive deficits (Mizoguchi et al., 2004). Moreover, extreme stress in young animals is associated with reduced basal activity in the medial prefrontal cortex in adulthood (Stevenson, Marsden, & Mason, 2008),

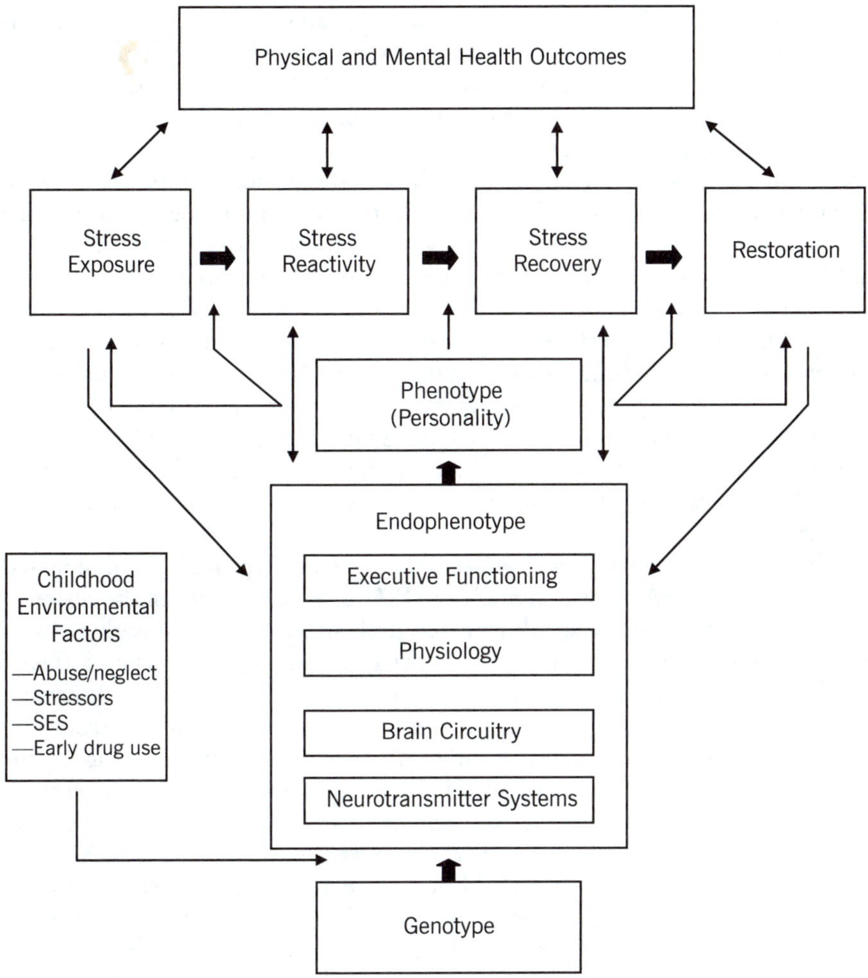

FIGURE 12.1. Schematic representing levels of individual differences related to executive functioning and hypothesized theoretical relations to stress processes. From Williams, Suchy, and Rau (2009). Reprinted with permission from Springer Science+Business Media. SES, socioeconomic status.

suggesting stress effects on the neural substrates of EF. Although cortisol associations with hippocampal-mediated memory problems in humans have been consistently reported (Lupien et al., 2005), research has also found associations with EF in older adults (B. K. Lee et al., 2007).

The stress processes described above—exposure, reactivity, recovery, and restoration—evidence both cascading and reciprocal associations with each other, as well as with EF; these putative associations can inform our understanding of mechanisms linking stress to adverse mental and physical health outcomes. For example, a principle mechanism by which stress exposure may lead to poor mental and physical health is via stress reactivity, which in turn may influence recovery, which may then affect restorative processes in a cascading fashion, with each component process having its own set of pathways to illness. Stress exposure may also have a negative effect on health via changes in health behavior, such as exercise and alcohol consumption (Ng & Jeffrey, 2003); alterations in health behavior, in turn, may affect stress responses, such as when increased substance use disrupts restorative sleep.

With respect to pathways between stress reactivity and health, repeated activation of the SAM system and the HPA axis may influence the onset or progression of disease. Indeed prior research suggests that individuals who evidence enhanced cardiovascular reactivity (i.e., blood pressure, heart rate) to stressors are at increased risk for the development of cardiovascular disease (see Treiber et al., 2003, for review). This so-called "reactivity hypothesis" for stress–cardiovascular disease associations highlights the role of endothelial injury (both mechanical, e.g., "shearing," and chemical, e.g., catacholamines) in the development of disease (Krantz & Manuck, 1984). Research has also focused on the inflammatory processes that may follow endothelial injury as an additional mechanism for stress reactivity–disease associations (e.g., Libby, 2002). Furthermore, subjective distress in response to a stressor, particularly if communicated in social interactions, may serve to increase exposure to interpersonal conflict or to prolong stress responses. Thus, a mechanism by which emotional reactions to stress may influence health is via reciprocal relations to other stress processes.

In the case of cardiovascular recovery, it has been hypothesized that the duration of stress-related cardiovascular responses may be as important as the magnitude of initial reactivity in the development of cardiovascular diseases (Brosschot, Gerin, & Thayer, 2006; A. R. Schwartz et al., 2003). Indeed, poor cardiovascular recovery has been associated with increases in blood pressure over several years (Mosely & Linden, 2006; Stewart, Janicki, & Kamarck, 2006). Furthermore, prolonged activation, particularly as manifest in presleep arousal, is associated with poor sleep quality (Bastien et al., 2008). Prolonged activation in relation to stressful events is inherent in several forms of psychopathology, most notably clinical depression (rumination) and generalized anxiety disorder (worry).

With respect to restoration, poor sleep, especially sleep deprivation, is related to impaired immune functioning (Lange, Perras, Fehm, & Born, 2003) and predicts all-cause mortality (Dew et al., 2003). Recent research suggests that even modest reductions in restorative sleep are associated with increased susceptibility to illness (Cohen et al., 2009) and coronary artery calcification (King et al., 2008) in otherwise healthy individuals. Importantly, there is accumulating evidence that sleep disturbance precedes the onset of depression (Johnson, Roth, & Breslau, 2006; Ohayon & Roth, 2003) and is not merely a symptom of depression. Although more specific mechanisms linking poor sleep to adverse mental and physical health outcomes have not been well studied, increasing evidence suggests that sleep-mediated changes in inflammatory processes may be important (e.g., Irwin, 2002).

SUMMARY AND CONCLUSIONS

In this chapter, we have provided evidence that individual differences in EF play a central role in stress regulation. Over time, individuals with poorer EF are vulnerable to enhanced stress exposure (e.g., interpersonal conflict). Individuals with poor EF also appear to have enhanced physiological reactivity to stress and prolonged activation to stress, which may cascade into insufficient restorative process, particularly sleep disruption. Sleep disruption, in turn, may further impair EF in already vulnerable individuals, setting the stage for additional stress exposure, enhanced reactivity, and prolonged recovery. Thus, individuals with poor EF may be at risk for a trajectory of compounding and escalating stress regulation difficulty. Importantly, the presence of chronic illness and/or psychopathology can produce further decrements in EF via disease processes or medical treatments.

In conclusion, the endeavor of identifying individual differences in stress risk and resilience may be informed by considering EF. Focusing the research "lens" on EF will help us answer important questions about stress risk and resilience, including the further identification of mechanisms for stress-health associations.

NOTES

1. As already stated in Chapter 10, *stress* does not refer to an external context, but rather to internal psychological and physiological processes.

2. See Chapter 7 for more detailed discussion of emotion regulation strategies.
3. Spectral analysis is used to decompose heart rate variability at specific frequency components. The frequency component of RSA is the parasympathetically driven oscillations that corresponded to the high-frequency (HF) portion of the respiration cycle (0.15–0.40 Hz).
4. Also see Chapter 10.

CHAPTER 13

Future Directions for Clinical Neuropsychology of Emotion

As already outlined in the general introductory section (see "About This Book"), among the principal goals of this text was to demonstrate the clinical utility of assessing various domains of emotional processing as part of neuropsychological evaluations. The purpose of this chapter is to highlight some future directions that would further help incorporate the neuropsychology of emotion into mainstream neuropsychological research and practice. In particular, more work is needed in the following areas: (1) development of clinical measures for assessment of individual emotional domains; (2) use of assessment of emotional domains toward the improvement of the diagnostic sensitivity and specificity of extant methods; and (3) greater integration of neuropsychological research and practice with other allied disciplines toward continued prominence and prosperity of clinical neuropsychology. These are examined in turn below.

DEVELOPMENT OF CLINICAL TOOLS

Currently, there are very few clinical instruments for assessing the various domains of emotional processing. These are reviewed in the relevant chapters throughout the book. Whereas some emotional domains lend themselves to self-report assessments (e.g., feeling awareness, affective styles), others require performance-based assessments. It is this latter category that represents the greatest challenge for future development. Four areas of affective processing that are particularly relevant for a neuropsychological evaluation and that lend themselves to objective behavioral assessment are (1) emotion regulation, (2) affective communication, (3) sensitivity to rewards and punishments, and (4) the sensitivity of the trigger mechanism.

Emotion Regulation

Emotion regulation (ER) represents a domain of affective processing that seems particularly relevant for clinical neuropsychology. Evaluation of ER in current clinical assessments relies on qualitative behavioral observations, patient self-report, and reports from collateral sources. These qualitative observations and reports are typically given further weight if corroborated by objectively assessed deficits in EF and attentional control, consistent with the well-recognized relationship between EF and ER reviewed in Chapter 7. However, for many patients, difficulties in ER are not readily apparent, emerging only under certain conditions, such as during periods of stress, cognitive fatigue, or physical discomfort. These elusive "now you see it, now you don't" types of a problems represent the greatest challenge for clinicians, and parallel the equally challenging subtle weaknesses in EF that can also be situation-specific. It is of course well recognized that these types of subtle problems in both EF and ER are often obscured by the highly structured environment of a clinical evaluation.

The highly structured format employed in typical clinical settings is a vestige of the earliest impetus for psychological assessments, that is, cognitive evaluations of schoolchildren with academic problems. Briefly, cognitive and intellectual assessment originally emerged in France and in the United States in the early 20th century for the purpose of determining whether children who experienced academic difficulties were truly intellectually impaired, or whether other psychological or environmental issues masked these children's true potential. Put differently, the focus of assessment was on determining how a child could function under ideal circumstances. Unfortunately, this testing tradition does not lend itself to answering some of the questions that are of interest in neuropsychological evaluations, where clinicians are interested *not only* in how a patient functions under ideal circumstances, but also in how that patient negotiates complex real-life situations, interpersonally stressful events, or even just annoying daily hassles. In other words, clinicians are often charged with determining whether a patient's EF and ER resources are sufficient for handling the typical demands of daily life.

In order to address these types of referral questions, some aspects of neuropsychological evaluations must abandon the model of determining the patient's potential under ideal circumstances and instead aim to identify the opposite end of the spectrum. A model for this type of assessment exists in cardiology, where the functioning of the heart is assessed not only in a relaxed circumstance (i.e., resting heart rate and blood pressure), but also under stress (i.e., the treadmill stress test). The challenge for clinical neuropsychology is to elicit ecologically valid stress in a clinical setting without jeopardizing rapport, violating ethical standards, or compromising the validity of other cognitive performances. Creative solutions are needed that would allow us, as clinicians, to appropriately and safely remove both the cognitive and the emotional scaffolding that we normally provide to our patients. Removal of such structure would then allow us to *quantify* the functional *decrements* exhibited by patients under less than ideal circumstances, which would in turn improve the ecological validity of not only the assessment of ER, but also the assessment of EF.

Affective Communication

It is now well understood that a wide array of neuropsychiatric, neurodevelopmental, and neurodegenerative disorders are associated with deficits in affective communication that lead to interpersonal problems, decreased effectiveness at work, and reduced quality of life. Additionally, some circumscribed deficits in affective communication appear to be unique to certain populations (e.g., the dissociation of Huntington's and Alzheimer's dementias with respect to disgust recognition) (Hayes et al., 2007; Henry et al., 2008; also see Chapter 6), and as such may aid differential diagnosis. For these reasons, assessing affective communication routinely as part of neuropsychological evaluations should be of interest to the clinical neuropsychologist.

Fortunately, from among the various domains of emotional processing discussed in this book, affective communication is the most advanced when it comes to objective behavioral assessment. In fact, a number of excellent experimental batteries of emotional communication have been developed over the last several decades[1] that have contributed to the large body of knowledge that now exists in this area. Relatively recently, tests appropriate for clinical use have begun to emerge and are now commercially available.[2] The challenge for the future is for clinical neuropsychologists to begin to incorporate these tests routinely into their own assessment batteries, and for the field to move toward the expectation that assessment of emotional communication become a standard of practice.

Sensitivity to Rewards and Punishments

In the area of sensitivity to rewards and punishment, considerable strides have been made with the development of the Iowa Gambling Task

(IGT) (Bechara et al., 1997) as a measure of emotional decision making (described in more detail in Chapter 9). Now commercially available as a clinical instrument (Bechara, 2007), the IGT represents a true paradigm shift in neuropsychological evaluations in that it draws upon preconscious processes. Admittedly, the test has a number of limitations (reviewed in more detail in Chapter 9), and more work is needed. Thus, arguably, the principal contribution of the IGT is that it introduced a new paradigm in a fashion that is highly visible and therefore reaches many practicing neuropsychologists. Future research needs to focus on further refinement of the IGT (or similar measures) to make it maximally effective for clinical use, as well as on additional inquiries into how excessive sensitivity to rewards or diminished sensitivity to punishments affects cognitive performance and daily functioning.

Sensitivity of the Trigger Mechanism

Finally, despite the well-documented dissociation between memory for affective versus neutral stimuli and the relatively clear impact of amygdalar dysfunction on formation of emotional memories, mainstream clinical neuropsychology has thus far all but ignored this important phenomenon. This is all the more surprising given how elaborate and sophisticated memory assessment has become. Mainstream memory measures such as the Wechsler batteries or various verbal learning tests have become increasingly complex, offering a variety of composite scores and contrast scores that allow examination of clinically relevant memory profiles. Immediate versus delayed, visual versus auditory, and structured versus unstructured—these represent only a few examples of the types of comparisons that are made by practicing neuropsychologists on a daily basis. Taking this tradition a step further to include contrasts between memory for neutral versus memory for emotional stimuli seems like a fairly straightforward endeavor. Here, the challenge is not in designing a workable paradigm (as such a paradigm is self-evident), but rather in convincing test companies to include such tests as part of the next edition of their batteries. Additional research focusing on the diagnostic utility of contrasting memory for neutral and memory for emotional content would likely move this process further along.

IMPROVING DIAGNOSTIC SENSITIVITY AND SPECIFICITY

In clinical neuropsychology, the ability to link assessment results to neuropathology depends, to a great extent, on the ability to account for as much systematic variance that is *not* related to neuropathology as possible. Over the years, clinical neuropsychology has become quite sophisticated at doing just that. Systematic variance is now routinely removed by stratifying normative tables according to not only age, but also a number of other demographic characteristics that affect performance. Additionally, improved methods for estimating premorbid intelligence exist. Last but not least, neuropsychology now places considerable premium on assessment of effort and veracity of performance.

In addition to objective, formal ways of reducing noise in the test data, practicing neuropsychologists are keen on understanding a patient's psychological status, including the potentially deleterious effects of anxiety and depression, stressful life circumstance, and obsessive or oppositional personality characteristics. Unfortunately, the estimates of the relative contributions of these factors are typically based on subjective clinical judgments and simple "eyeballing" of test results. An additional limitation is the fact that psychiatric and personality factors are typically considered only if falling into the extremes of the trait continua. Yet, predictable relationships exist between cognition and various affective factors (whether pathological or within the range of normal individual differences), and these relationships could (and should) be formally quantified. Consider, for example, that certain types of criminal offenders exhibit lower verbal intelligence than their noncriminal counterparts despite comparable levels of education (Suchy, Whittaker, et al., 2009). Such systematic biases create a bit of a problem as far as applicability of existing demographically corrected norms, but could be addressed by subjecting normative data to regression formulas employing easily assessed characteristics, such as positive and negative affectivity, as assessed by the PANAS (Watson et al., 1988; also see Chapter 8); levels of neuroticism and openness to experience, as assessed by the NEO-PI (Costa & McCrae, 1992; also see Chapter 11); or levels of alexithymia, as assessed by the TAS-20 (Bagby, Parker, & Taylor, 1994; also see Chapter 5). Additionally, given that fluctuations in mood have been shown to affect test performance in experimental settings (Chapter 8), it may be worthwhile to determine whether such fluctuations could be corrected for by factoring in mood *states* (assessed via self-report) during clinical assessments.

In addition to integrating affective information into the normative tables or formulas, it may be particularly informative to determine the degree to which deficits in affective processing differentially impact affectively loaded stimuli in extant clinical instruments. This could be accomplished by determining the degree to which strengths and weaknesses in affective communication predict performance differences on affective versus neutral test items.

INTERDISCIPLINARY IMPLICATIONS

Just as the mid-20th century witnessed a proliferation of increasingly narrower subspecialties in many areas of science, recent years have been witnessing an increase in the numbers of cross-disciplines that span disparate fields. This interest in interdisciplinary research has many causes that are beyond the scope of this volume. One of the causes, however, is central to the topic of this book—the ever-growing interest in affective neuroscience. Social neuroscience, neuroecology, and neuroeconomics represent only a few from among the many possible examples of this growing incorporation of neuroscience, in general, and affective neuroscience, in particular, into a variety of disciplines.

Clinical neuropsychology has a rich tradition of interdisciplinary research and clinical practice that draws upon a number of allied disciplines. From its inception, clinical neuropsychology has seamlessly interfaced with neurology, psychiatry, and clinical psychology, and research findings from cognitive, behavioral, and affective neurosciences have influenced both theory and practice. Over the years, linkages with a wide array of additional medical subspecialties have also taken hold, including cardiology, nephrology, and oncology, to name a few. Given these traditions, clinical neuropsychology is well versed in the terminology, milieu, and culture, as well as up-and-coming clinical research questions across a variety disciplines. As such, clinical neuropsychology is well positioned to be at the forefront of increasingly interdisciplinary research and clinical practice.

Clinical neuropsychology now has the opportunity to expand its area of expertise beyond the understanding of how physical and mental illnesses lead to declines in cognition, to also include how cognitive weaknesses interact with personality and temperament, conferring a vulnerability to stress and the development of illness (see Chapters 11 and 12). In collaboration with health psychologists and personality theorists, clinical neuropsychology could position itself to be in the business of not only assessing the outcomes of an illness or an injury, but also evaluating risk factors for future physical, mental, or cognitive declines. This ability will likely become all the more important as medical reforms continue to shift the focus from treatment to prevention.

NOTES

1. Prominent examples include the New York Emotion Battery (NYEB; Borod, Welkowitz, & Obler, 1992) and the Florida Affect Battery (FAB; Bowers et al., 1999).

2. For example, The Awareness of Social Inference Test (TASIT; McDonald, Flanagan, & Rollins, 2002) and the Social Cognition Test (Pearson, 2009). Also see Chapter 6.

APPENDIX A

Affective Deficits, Symptoms, and Syndromes Associated with Select Clinical Populations

Disorder/ population	Symptoms/syndromes	Additional remarks	Chapter
Addiction disorders	• Alexithymia	• Especially among dual-diagnosis patients	5
	• AR deficits	• Similar to deficits seen in criminal offenders/ psychopaths	6
	• ER deficits		7
	• Incentive sensitivity deficits	• Relatively stronger responsiveness to rewards than punishments; deficient emotional decision making	9
ADHD	• Autonomic hypoactivation	• Likely secondary to right-hemisphere and ACC dysfunction	4
	• AR deficits	• Fear and disgust are most affected	6
	• Poor ER	• Sometimes considered more central than cognitive deficits	7
	• Incentive sensitivity deficits	• Greater sensitivity to rewards than punishments; this is also true of conduct disorder and externalizing tendencies	9
Agenesis of corpus callosum	• Alexithymia	• Alexithymia is typically accompanied by deficits in empathy	5
ALS	• PBA • Mild autonomic dysregulation	• PBA present only in the bulbar variant of ALS	4
	• AR deficits		6
AD	• Capgras syndrome • Human Klüver–Bucy syndrome	• Human Klüver–Bucy syndrome has only been associated with the amygdaloid variant of AD	3

Disorder/ population	Symptoms/syndromes	Additional remarks	Chapter
AD *(cont.)*	• PBA	• Rare	4
	• Facial AR deficits • Empathy deficits	• Recognition of facial disgust is usually spared	6
	• Poor ER	• Primarily physical and verbal aggression	7
	• Depression, negative affectivity	• Predicts future cognitive decline	8
	• Incentive sensitivity deficits, apathy, anhedonia	• Associated with dysfunction in the ACC and orbitofrontal cortex in this population • Anhedonia is fairly common; present in about one-third of AD cases	9
	• HPA axis hyperactivity		10
Anoxic injury	• PAID		4
	• PBA	• Rare	4
Autism	• Detection/recognition of social affective cues	• Although structural abnormalities in the amygdala have been found, amygdala-mediated abilities (e.g., fear conditioning and to *non*social affective cues) are spared	3
	• Facial AR deficits	• These are presumed to be driven by amygdalar dysfunction	6
CVA	• Capgras syndrome	• Usually right frontal–temporal lesions	3
	• AF, PBA • Fou rire prodromique syndrome • Foix–Chavany–Marie syndrome	• A variety of lesion locations have been associated with these syndromes	4
	• Alexithymia	• Usually right-hemisphere and frontal lesions	5
	• Affective communication deficits (receptive and expressive)	• Primarily right frontal and basal ganglia lesions for both receptive and expressive problems	6
	• Poor ER	• Poststroke depression is the most common example of poor affect regulation in this population, often following left frontal lesions	7
	• Apathy, abulia, akinetic mutism	• Typically lesions in the mesolimbic dopamine system, ACC, or ventral pallidum	8

Disorder/ population	Symptoms/syndromes	Additional remarks	Chapter
Dementia with Lewy bodies	• Capgras syndrome		3
	• PBA, AF		4
	• Anhedonia, apathy	• Anhedonia and apathy are extremely common in this population, with base rates ranging from 50 to 75%	9
Down syndrome	• Facial AR deficits		6
Fetal alcohol syndrome	• Facial AR deficits		6
FXTAS	• Abnormal detection and recognition of affective stimuli	• Broad range of deficits related to amygdalar dysfunction, including deficient recognition of facial affect, poor fear conditioning, poor memory for affective stimuli, etc.	3
Fragile X syndrome	• Avoidance of eye contact	• Enlarged amygdala and hippocampus; increased amygdalar and hippocampal activation in response to eye contact	3
Frontotemporal-lobar degeneration	• Human Klüver–Bucy syndrome	• Anterior temporal and ventral frontal atrophy	3
	• AR deficits • Impaired cognitive empathy	• Greater impairment in frontal, as compared to temporal, variant; temporal (semantic) variant is associated with greater deficits in both cognitive and emotional empathy	6
	• Poor ER	• Primarily disinhibition	7
	• Apathy	• Apathy in patients is particularly troublesome for caregivers	8
	• Incentive sensitivity deficits • Anhedonia	• Diminished sensitivity to rewards and punishments, presenting as disinhibition in this population	9
Huntington's dementia	• AR deficits	• Primarily disgust, due to basal ganglia involvement in this disorder	6
	• Apathy		8

Disorder/ population	Symptoms/syndromes	Additional remarks	Chapter
Major depression	• Alexithymia	• Alexithymia is typically accompanied by deficits in empathy	5
	• Facial AR deficits		6
	• ER deficits	• Poor reappraisal	7
	• Apathy, anhedonia		5, 8, 9
	• HPA axis dysregulation	• May represent the mechanism behind psedodementia	10
MS	• AF • PBA • Human Klüver–Bucy syndrome • Fou rire prodromique	• AF is related to greater reports of fatigue	4
	• Alexithymia	• Predicts depression and greater fatigue complaints	5
	• Poor regulation of affect	• May present as depression, which is sometimes associated with a greater lesion load in the left hemisphere	7
	• Depression/negative affectivity	• Predicts future cognitive declines; correlates with fatigue complaints	8
	• HPA axis hyperactivity	• Stress is a precursor of relapses, likely due to the changes in the immune receptor function secondary to chronic cortisol releases	10
MSA	• AF	• Greater AF symptoms predict shorted disease duration and greater risk of sudden death	4
PD	• AF	• Milder than in MSA; can be used to dissociate MSA and PD	4
	• Alexithymia	• Usually associated with depression in this population	5
	• Facial AR deficits		6
	• Apathy, anhedonia • Incentive sensitivity deficits	• Diminished responsiveness to rewards	9
Progessive supranuclear palsy	• PBA • Autonomic dysregulation		4
	• Apathy		8

Disorder/ population	Symptoms/syndromes	Additional remarks	Chapter
Psychopathy	• Reduced sensitivity to affective stimuli	• Reduced amygdalar volume; associated with impaired fear conditioning, startle response, AR, reduced memory for affective stimuli, etc.	3
	• Alexithymia	• Alexithymia is typically accompanied by deficits in empathy	5
	• AR deficits • Lexical affective deficits	• Mostly fear; tendency to mislabel other emotions as anger	6
	• Incentive sensitivity deficits • Impaired emotional decision making	• Relatively stronger responsiveness to rewards than punishments	9
PTSD	• Excessive responsiveness to threats	• Unmitigated by nonthreatening contexts, presumably due to hippocampal atrophy	3
	• Alexithymia	• Alexithymia is typically accompanied by deficits in empathy	5
	• HPA axis dysregulation	• HPA dysregulation results, among others, in an increased amygdalar volume	10
Schizophrenia	• Alexithymia	• Unrelated to severity of negative symptoms	5
	• AR deficits	• Normal recognition of genuine, but not posed, facial expressions among individuals with paranoid schizophrenia	6
	• Apathy, anhedonia		5, 8, 9
	• HPA axis hyperactivity	• Enlarged pituitary gland and higher levels of ACTH	10
Seizure disorder	• Mild decrease in processing of affective stimuli • Human Klüver–Bucy syndrome	• Prolonged febrile seizures lead to about 30% volume loss in the amygdala	3
	• Autonomic seizures and auras • Gelastic seizures		4
	• Poor ER	• Particularly in frontal seizures or frontal lobectomies	7

Disorder/ population	Symptoms/syndromes	Additional remarks	Chapter
TBI	• Human Klüver–Bucy syndrome	• Rare	3
	• PAID		4
	• PBA		
	• Alexithymia	• Unrelated to severity of injury or cognitive deficits	5
	• Facial AR deficits • Empathy deficits		6
	• Poor ER	• Primarily suppression of behavioral responses; secondary to ventral frontal lesions	7
	• Apathy • Decrease in positive affectivity		8
	• Incentive sensitivity deficits • Impaired emotional decision making	• Poor processing of rewards leads to an inability to benefit from reinforcement	9
	• PTHP • Alterations in cortisol levels	• Patients exhibit decreases in cortisol levels following a severe TBI, but increases following a mild TBI	10
Tumors	• Gelastic seizures • Appetite abnormalities • Endocrine abnormalities	• Hypothalamic tumors	4
	• AF	• Hypothalamus, brainstem	
	• Affective communication deficits	• Particularly frontal, right-hemisphere, and basal ganglia tumors	6
	• HPA axis hyperactivity	• ACTH released by many types of tumors (central and peripheral)	10
Turner syndrome	• Facial AR deficits	• Structural and functional amygdalar abnormalities	3
Urbach–Wiethe disease	• Abnormal responsiveness to affective stimuli	• Bilateral amygdalar calcification in second half of life in 50% of patients	3

Disorder/ population	Symptoms/syndromes	Additional remarks	Chapter
Vascular dementia	• Capgras syndrome		3
	• Anhedonia		5
	• Facial AR deficits		6
	• Poor ER	• Presents primarily as depression	7
	• HPA axis hyperactivity		10

Note. ACC, anterior cingulate cortex; AD, Alzheimer's disease; ADHD, attention-deficit/hyperactivity disorder; AF, autonomic failure; ALS, amyotrophic lateral sclerosis; AR, affect recognition; CVA, cerebral vascular accident; ER, emotion regulation; FXTAS, fragile X–associated tremor and ataxia syndrome; MS, multiple sclerosis; PAID, paroxysmal autonomic instability with dystonia; PBA, pseudobulbar affect; PD, Parkinson's disease; PTHP, posttraumatic hypopituitarism; PTSD, posttraumatic stress disorder; TBI, traumatic brain injury.

APPENDIX B

Disorders and Populations Associated with Select Affective Deficits, Symptoms, or Syndromes

Affective deficits, symptoms, or syndromes	Disorder/population	Chapter
Affective communication deficits (i.e., facial or prosodic affect recognition or expression) and deficits in processing of affective stimuli	• Addiction disorders • AD • ALS • Autism • ADHD • CVA • Down syndrome • Fetal alcohol syndrome • Fragile X syndrome • FXTAS • Frontotemporal-lobar degeneration • Huntington's disease • Major depression • Mild cognitive impairment • PD • Psychopathy • Schizophrenia • Seizure disorder • Substance abuse • Turner syndrome • TBI • Tumors • Urbach–Wiethe disease • Vascular dementia	3, 6
Alexithymia	• Addiction disorders • Agenesis of corpus callosum • CVA • Major depression • MS • PD • PTSD • Psychopathy • Schizophrenia • TBI	5

Affective deficits, symptoms, or syndromes	Disorder/population	Chapter
Anhedonia, apathy, abulia, akinetic mutism	• AD • Dementia with Lewy bodies • Frontotemporal-lobar degeneration • Major depression • PD • Progressive supranuclear palsy • Schizophrenia • TBI • Vascular dementia	5, 9
Autonomic failure or dysregulation	• ALS • ADHD • CVA • Dementia with Lewy bodies • MS • MSA • PD • Progressive supranuclear palsy • Tumors	4
Autonomic seizures and auras	• Seizure disorders	4
Capgras syndrome	• AD • CVA • Dementia with Lewy bodies • Vascular dementia	3
Empathy deficits	• AD • Frontotemporal-lobar degeneration • Psychopathy • Semantic dementia • TBI	6
Emotion regulation deficits	• Addiction disorders • AD • ADHD • CVA • Epilepsy • Frontotemporal-lobar degeneration • Major depression • MS • Seizure disorder • TBI • Vascular dementia	7
Emotional decision-making deficits	• Addiction disorders • Amygdalar dysfunction • Major depression • Psychopathy • TBI	9

Affective deficits, symptoms, or syndromes	Disorder/population	Chapter
Foix–Chavany–Marie syndrome	• CVA	4
Fou rire prodromique syndrome	• CVA • MS	4
Gelastic seizures	• Hypothalamic hamartoma • Seizure disorder • Tumors	4
HPA axis dysregulation	• AD • Major depression • MS • PTSD • Schizophrenia • TBI • Tumors • VD	10
Incentive sensitivity dysregulation/deficit	• Addiction disorders • AD • Anxiety disorders • ADHD • Frontotemporal-lobar degeneration • PD • PTSD • Psychopathy • TBI	9
Klüver–Bucy syndrome	• AD • Frontotemporal-lobar degeneration • MS • Seizure disorders • TBI	3
PAID	• Anoxic injury • TBI	4
PTHP	• TBI	
PBA	• ALS • AD • Anoxic injury • CVA • Dementia with Lewy bodies • MS • Progressive supranuclear palsy • TBI	4

Note. Abbreviations as in Appendix A.

APPENDIX C

Select Measures for Assessment of Affective Deficits, Symptoms, or Syndromes

Affective deficits, symptoms, or syndromes	Measure	References	Chapter
Pseudobulbar affect	Pathological Laughter and Crying Scale (PLACS)	Robinson, Parikh, Lipsey, & Starkstein (1993)	4
Autonomic/endocrine dysfunction	Composite Autonomic Symptom Scale (COMPASS)	Suarez, Opfer-Gehrking, Offord, Atkinson, O'Brien, & Low (1999)	4
Alexithymia	Toronto Alexithymia Scale (TAS-20)	Bagby, Parker, & Taylor (1994)	5
Affective communication	The Awareness of Social Inference Test (TASIT)	McDonald, Flanagan, & Rollins (2002)	6
	Social Cognition Test	Pearson (2009)	6
Emotion regulation styles	Emotion Regulation Questionnaire (ERQ)	Gross & John (2003)	7
Affective styles	Positive and Negative Affect Schedule (PANAS)	Watson, Clark, & Tellegen (1988)	8
Anhedonia	Snaith–Hamilton Pleasure Scale (SHAPS)	Snaith, Hamilton, Morley, & Humayan (1995)	9
	Chapman Physical Anhedonia Scale (CPAS)	Chapman, Chapman, & Raulin (1976)	
	Fawcett–Clark Pleasure Scale (FCPS)	Fawcett, Clark, Scheftner, & Gibbons (1983)	
Apathy	Apathy Evaluation Scale (AES)	Marin, Biedrzycki, & Firinciogullari (1991)	9

Affective deficits, symptoms, or syndromes	Measure	References	Chapter
Emotional decision making	Iowa Gambling Task (IGT)	Bechara (2007)	9
Sensitivity to rewards/ punishments	BIS/BAS scale	Carver & White (1994)	9

References

Abe, J. A. (2005). The predictive validity of the five-factor model of personality with preschool age children: A 9-year follow-up study. *Journal of Research in Personality, 39*(4), 423–442.

Abely, P. (1951). Hypothalamus et troubles psychiques. *Annales Médico-Psychologiques, 109*, 417–434.

Abler, B., Hofer, C., & Viviani, R. (2008). Habitual emotion regulation strategies and baseline brain perfusion. *NeuroReport, 19*(1), 21–24.

Abler, B., & Kessler, H. (2009). Emotion Regulation Questionnaire: Eine deutschsprachige Fassung des ERQ von Gross und John. *Diagnostica, 55*(3), 144–152.

Abrahamson, A. C., Baker, L. A., & Caspi, A. (2002). Rebellious teens?: Genetic and environmental influences on the social attitudes of adolescents. *Journal of Personality and Social Psychology, 83*(6), 1392–1408.

Achari, A. N., & Colover, J. (1976). Posterior fossa tumors with pathological laughter. *Journal of the American Medical Association, 235*, 1469–1471.

Addington, J., & Addington, D. (1998). Facial affect recognition and information processing in schizophrenia and bipolar disorder. *Schizophrenia Research, 32*(3), 171–181.

Adelmann, P. K., & Zajonc, R. B. (1989). Facial efference and the experience of emotion. *Annual Review of Psychology, 40*, 249–280.

Ader, R., Felten, D. L., & Cohen, N. (Eds.). (2001). *Psychoneuroimmunology* (3rd ed.). New York: Academic Press.

Adolphs, R. (2002). Neural systems for recognizing emotion. *Current Opinion in Neurobiology, 12*(2), 169–177.

Adolphs, R., Baron-Cohen, S., & Tranel, D. (2002). Impaired recognition of social emotions following amygdala damage. *Journal of Cognitive Neuroscience, 14*(8), 1264–1274.

Adolphs, R., Cahill, L., Schul, R., & Babinsky, R. (1997). Impaired declarative memory for emotional material following bilateral amygdala damage in humans. *Learning and Memory, 4*(3), 291–300.

Adolphs, R., Damasio, H., & Tranel, D. (2002). Neural systems for recognition of emotional prosody: A 3-D lesion study. *Emotion, 2*(1), 23–51.

Adolphs, R., Gosselin, F., Buchanan, T. W., Tranel, D., Schyns, P., & Damasio, A. R. (2005). A mechanism for impaired fear recognition after amygdala damage. *Nature, 433*(7021), 68–72.

Adolphs, R., Russell, J. A., & Tranel, D. (1999). A role for the human amygdala in recognizing emotional arousal from unpleasant stimuli. *Psychological Science, 10*(2), 167–171.

Adolphs, R., & Tranel, D. (2003). Amygdala damage impairs emotion recognition from scenes only when they contain facial expressions. *Neuropsychologia, 41*(10), 1281–1289.

Adolphs, R., & Tranel, D. (2004). Impaired judgments of sadness but not happiness following bilateral amygdala damage. *Journal of Cognitive Neuroscience, 16*(3), 453–462.

Adolphs, R., Tranel, D., Damasio, H., & Damasio, A. R. (1995). Fear and the human amygdala. *Journal of Neuroscience, 15*(9), 5879–5891.

Adolphs, R., Tranel, D., Hamann, S., Young, A. W., Calder, A. J., Phelps, E. A., et al. (1999). Recognition of facial emotion in nine individuals with bilateral amygdala damage. *Neuropsychologia, 37*(10), 1111–1117.

Aggleton, J. P. (Ed.). (2000). *The amygdala: A functional analysis*. Oxford, UK: Oxford University Press.

Ahadi, S. A., & Rothbart, M. K. (1994). Temperament, development and the Big Five. In C. F. Halverson, Jr., G. A. Kohnstamm, & R. P. Martin (Eds.), *The developing structure of temperament and personality from infancy to adulthood* (pp. 189–207). Hillsdale, NJ: Erlbaum.

Airaksinen, E., Larsson, M., Lundberg, I., & Forsell, Y. (2004). Cognitive functions in depressive disorders: Evidence from a population-based study. *Psychological Medicine, 34*(1), 83–91.

Aldao, A., Nolen-Hoeksema, S., & Schweizer, S. (2010). Emotion-regulation strategies across psychopathology: A meta-analytic review. *Clinical Psychology Review, 30*(2), 217–237.

Alexopoulos, G. S., Meyers, B. S., Young, R. C., Kalayam, B., Kakuma, T., Gabrielle, M., et al. (2000). Executive dysfunction and long-term outcomes of geriatric depression. *Archives of General Psychiatry, 57*(3), 285–290.

Allen, V. L., & Atkinson, M. L. (1981). Identification of spontaneous and deliberate behavior. *Journal of Nonverbal Behavior, 5*(4), 224–237.

Amat, J. A., Bansal, R., Whiteman, R., Haggerty, R., Royal, J., & Peterson, B. S. (2008). Correlates of intellectual ability with morphology of the hippocampus and amygdala in healthy adults. *Brain and Cognition, 66*(2), 105–114.

American Congress of Rehabilitation Medicine. (1995). Recommendations for use of uniform nomenclature pertinent to patients with severe alterations in consciousness. *Archives of Physical Medicine and Rehabilitation, 76*, 205–209.

American Psychiatric Association. (2000). *Diagnostic and statistical manual of mental disorders* (4th ed., text rev.). Washington, DC: Author.

Amodio, D. M., Master, S. L., Yee, C. M., & Taylor, S. E. (2008). Neurocognitive components of the behavioral inhibition and activation systems: Implications for theories of self-regulation. *Psychophysiology, 45*(1), 11–19.

Anderson, A. K., & Phelps, E. A. (2000). Expression without recognition: Contributions of the human amygdala to emotional communication. *Psychological Science, 11*(2), 106–111.

Anderson, A. K., & Phelps, E. A. (2001). Lesions of the human amygdala impair enhanced perception of emotionally salient events. *Nature, 411*, 305–309.

Anderson, A. K., & Phelps, E. A. (2002). Is the human amygdala critical for the subjective experience of emotion?: Evidence of intact dispositional affect in patients with amygdala lesions. *Journal of Cognitive Neuroscience, 14*(5), 709–720.

Andersson, E. H., Bjorklund, R., Emanuselson, I., & Stalhammar, D. (2003). Epidemiology of traumatic brain injury: A population based study in western Sweden. *Acta Neurologica Scandinavica, 107*(4), 256–259.

Andersson, S., & Bergedalen, A.-M. (2002). Cognitive correlates of apathy in traumatic brain injury. *Neuropsychiatry, Neuropsychology, and Behavioral Neurology, 15*(3), 184–191.

Andersson, S., & Finset, A. (1998). Heart rate and skin conductance reactivity to brief psychological stress in brain-injured patients. *Journal of Psychosomatic Research, 44*(6), 645–656.

Anglin, R. E., Rosebush, P. I., & Mazurek, M. F. (2006). The neuropsychiatric profile of Addison's disease: Revisiting a forgotten phenomenon. *Journal of Neuropsychiatry and Clinical Neurosciences, 18*(4), 450–459.

Anokhin, A. P., Heath, A. C., & Ralano, A. (2003). Genetic influences on frontal brain function: WCST performance in twins. *NeuroReport, 14*(15), 1975–1978.

Appleton, R., & Baldwin, T. (2006). Epidemiology: Incidence, causes, severity and outcome. In R. Appleton & T. Baldwin (Eds.), *Management of brain injured children* (2nd ed., pp. 1–19). New York: Oxford University Press.

Archer, N., Brown, R. G., Reeves, S., Nicholas, H., Boothby, H., & Lovestone, S. (2009). Midlife neuroticism and the age of onset of Alzheimer's disease. *Psychological Medicine: A Journal of Research in Psychiatry and the Allied Sciences, 39*(4), 665–673.

Archer, N., Brown, R. G., Reeves, S. J., Boothby, H., Nicholas, H., Foy, C., et al. (2007). Premorbid personality and behavioral and psychological symptoms in probable Alzheimer disease. *American Journal of Geriatric Psychiatry, 15*(3), 202–213.

Arendash, G. W., & Gorski, R. A. (2007). *Effects of discrete lesions of the sexually dimorphic nucleus of the preoptic area or other medial preoptic regions on the sexual behavior of male rats.* Cambridge, MA: MIT Press.

Arikha, N. (2007). *Passions and tempers: A history of the humours.* New York: HarperPerennial.

Arnett, P. A., Smith, S. S., & Newman, J. P. (1997). Approach and avoidance motivation in psychopathic criminal offenders during passive avoidance. *Journal of Personality and Social Psychology, 72*(6), 1413–1428.

Ashby, F. G., Isen, A. M., & Turken, A. U. (1999). A neuropsychological theory of positive affect and its influence on cognition. *Psychological Review, 106*(3), 529–550.

Ashby, F. G., Valentin, V. V., Turken, U., Moore, S. C., & Oaksford, M. (2002). The effects of positive affect and arousal and working memory and executive attention: Neurobiology and computational models. In S. Moore & M. Oaksford

(Eds.), *Emotional cognition: From brain to behaviour* (pp. 245–287). Amsterdam: Benjamins.

Aslaksen, P. M., Myrbakk, I. N., Hoifodt, R. S., & Flaten, M. A. (2007). The effect of experimenter gender on autonomic and subjective responses to pain stimuli. *Pain, 129*(3), 260–268.

Aszalos, Z., Barsi, P., Vitrai, J., & Nagy, Z. (2002). Lateralization as a factor in the prognosis of middle cerebral artery territorial infarct. *European Neurology, 48*(3), 141–145.

Atchley, R. A., Stringer, R., Mathias, E., Ilardi, S. S., & Minatrea, A. D. (2007). The right hemisphere's contribution to emotional word processing in currently depressed, remitted depressed, and never-depressed individuals. *Journal of Neurolinguistics, 20*(2), 145–160.

Baas, D., Aleman, A., & Kahn, R. S. (2004). Lateralization of amygdala activation: A systematic review of functional neuroimaging studies. *Brain Research Reviews, 45*(2), 96–103.

Bacalman, S., Farzin, F., Bourgeois, J. A., Cogswell, J., Goodlin-Jones, B. L., Gane, L. W., et al. (2006). Psychiatric phenotype of the fragile X–associated tremor/ataxia syndrome (FXTAS) in males: Newly described fronto-subcortical dementia. *Journal of Clinical Psychiatry, 67*(1), 87–94.

Bach, M., & Bach, D. (1996). Alexithymia in somatoform disorder and somatic disease: A comparative study. *Psychotherapy and Psychosomatics, 65*(3), 150–152.

Baeken, C., De Raedt, R., Ramsey, N., Van Schuerbeek, P., Hermes, D., Bossuyt, A., et al. (2009). Amygdala responses to positively and negatively valenced baby faces in healthy female volunteers: Influences of individual differences in harm avoidance. *Brain Research, 1296*, 94–103.

Baer, R. A., Smith, G. T., & Allen, K. B. (2004). Assessment of mindfulness by self-report: The Kentucky Inventory of Mindfulness Skills. *Assessment, 11*, 191–206.

Bagby, R. M., Parker, J. D. A., & Taylor, G. J. (1994). The twenty-item Toronto Alexithymia Scale: I. Item selection and cross-validation of the factor structure. *Journal of Psychosomatic Research, 38*(1), 23–32.

Bagby, R. M., Taylor, G. J., & Parker, J. D. A. (1994). The twenty-item Toronto Alexithymia Scale: II. Convergent, discriminant, and concurrent validity. *Journal of Psychosomatic Research, 38*(1), 33–40.

Baguley, I. J., Heriseanu, R. E., Felmingham, K. L., & Cameron, I. D. (2006). Dysautonomia and heart rate variability following severe traumatic brain injury. *Brain Injury, 20*(4), 437–444.

Baguley, I. J., Slewa-Younan, S., Heriseanu, R. E., Nott, M. T., Mudaliar, Y., & Nayyar, V. (2007). The incidence of dysautonomia and its relationship with autonomic arousal following traumatic brain injury. *Brain Injury, 21*(11), 1175–1181.

Bahroo, L. B., & Appleby, B. S. (2009). Behind the masked face: Depression and Parkinson's disease. *Minerva Psichiatrica, 50*(1), 45–53.

Baker, S. C., Frith, C. D., & Dolan, R. J. (1997). The interaction between mood and cognitive function studied with PET. *Psychological Medicine, 27*(3), 565–578.

Bala, P. (2009). *Medicine and medical policy in India: Social and historical perspectives*. Lanham, MD: Lexington Books.

Balfour, D. (2001). The role of mesolimbic dopamine in nicotine dependence. *Psycoloquy, 12*(1).

Ballmaier, M., Narr, K. L., Toga, A. W., Elderkin-Thompson, V., Thompson, P. M.,

Hamilton, L., et al. (2008). Hippocampal morphology and distinguishing late-onset from early-onset elderly depression. *American Journal of Psychiatry, 165*(2), 229–237.

Balzarotti, S., John, O. P., & Gross, J. J. (2010). An Italian adaptation of the Emotion Regulation Questionnaire. *European Journal of Psychological Assessment, 26*(1), 61–67.

Barahal, H. S. (1958). 1,000 prefrontal lobotomies: A five to ten year follow-up study. *Psychiatric Quarterly, 32*, 653–690.

Bard, P. (1928). A diencephalic mechanism for the expression of rage with special reference to the sympathetic nervous system. *American Journal of Physiology, 84*, 490–515.

Bard, P. (1929). Emotion: I. The neuro-humoral basis of emotional reactions. In C. Marchison (Ed.), *The foundations of experimental psychology* (pp. 449–487). Oxford, UK: Clark University Press.

Bard, P. (1934). On emotional expression after decortication with some remarks on certain theoretical views: Part II. *Psychological Review, 41*(5), 424–449.

Barisnikov, K., Hippolyte, L., & Van der Linden, M. (2008). Face processing and facial emotion recognition in adults with Down syndrome. *American Journal on Mental Retardation, 113*(4), 292–306.

Barrett, J., Pike, G. B., & Paus, T. A. (2004). The role of the anterior cingulate cortex in pitch variation during sad affect. *European Journal of Neuroscience, 19*(2), 458–464.

Barry, R. J., Clarke, A. R., McCarthy, R., Selikowitz, M., & Rushby, J. A. (2005). Arousal and activation in a continuous performance task: An exploration of state effects in normal children. *Journal of Psychophysiology, 19*(2), 91–99.

Bastien, C. H., St.-Jean, G., Morin, C. M., Turcotte, I., & Carrier, J. (2008). Chronic psychophysiological insomnia: Hyperarousal and/or inhibition deficits?: An ERPs investigation. *Sleep, 31*(6), 887–898.

Baum, S. R., & Pell, M. D. (1999). The neural bases of prosody: Insights from lesion studies and neuroimaging. *Aphasiology, 13*(8), 581–608.

Baxter, M. G., & Murray, E. A. (2002). The amygdala and reward. *Nature Review of Neuroscience, 3*, 563–573.

Bazett, H. C., & Penfield, W. G. (1922). A study of the Sherrington decerebrate animal in the chronic as well as the acute condition. *Brain: A Journal of Neurology, 45*, 185–265.

Beaucousin, V., Lacheret, A., Turbelin, M.-R., Morel, M., Mazoyer, B., & Tzourio-Mazoyer, N. (2007). fMRI study of emotional speech comprehension. *Cerebral Cortex, 17*(2), 339–352.

Becerra, R., Amos, A., & Jongenelis, S. (2002). Organic alexithymia: A study of acquired emotional blindness. *Brain Injury, 16*(7), 633–645.

Bechara, A. (2004). The role of emotion in decision-making: Evidence from neurological patients with orbitofrontal damage. *Brain and Cognition, 55*(1), 30–40.

Bechara, A. (2007). *Iowa Gambling Task professional manual.* Lutz, FL: Psychological Assessment Resources.

Bechara, A., & Damasio, A. R. (2005). The somatic marker hypothesis: A neural theory of economic decision. *Games and Economic Behavior, 52*(2), 336–372.

Bechara, A., Damasio, A. R., Damasio, H., & Anderson, S. W. (1994). Insensitivity to future consequences following damage to human prefrontal cortex. *Cognition, 50*(1), 7–15.

Bechara, A., Damasio, H., Tranel, D., & Damasio, A. R. (1997). Deciding advantageously before knowing the advantageous strategy. *Science, 275*, 1293–1294.

Bechara, A., Damasio, H., Tranel, D., & Damasio, A. R. (2005). The Iowa Gambling Task and the somatic marker hypothesis: Some questions and answers. *Trends in Cognitive Sciences, 9*(4), 159–162.

Bechara, A., Tranel, D., & Damasio, A. R. (2000). *Poor judgment in spite of high intellect: Neurological evidence for emotional intelligence.* San Francisco: Jossey-Bass.

Beck, I., Smits, D. J. M., Claes, L., Vandereycken, W., & Bijttebier, P. (2009). Psychometric evaluation of the Behavioral Inhibition/Behavioral Activation System Scales and the Sensitivity to Punishment and Sensitivity to Reward Questionnaire in a sample of eating disordered patients. *Personality and Individual Differences, 47*(5), 407–412.

Bediou, B., Krolak-Salmon, P., Saoud, M., Henaff, M.-A., Burt, M., Dalery, J., et al. (2005). Facial expression and sex recognition in schizophrenia and depression. *Canadian Journal of Psychiatry/La Revue Canadienne de Psychiatrie, 50*(9), 525–533.

Behan, L. A., Phillips, J., Thompson, C. J., & Agha, A. (2008). Neuroendocrine disorders after traumatic brain injury. *Journal of Neurology, Neurosurgery, and Psychiatry, 79*(7), 753–759.

Bell, M. A., & Fox, N. A. (2003). Cognition and affective style: Individual differences in brain electrical activity during spatial and verbal tasks. *Brain and Cognition, 53*(3), 441–451.

Benarroch, E. E., Schmeichel, A. M., Low, P. A., Boeve, B. F., Sandroni, P., & Parisi, J. E. (2005). Involvement of medullary regions controlling sympathetic output in Lewy body disease. *Brain: A Journal of Neurology, 128*(2), 338–344.

Bennett, C. M. (2009). *The integration of higher cognition and internal state across development.* Ann Arbor, MI: ProQuest Information & Learning.

Benuzzi, F., Meletti, S., Zamboni, G., Calandra-Buonaura, G., Serafini, M., Lui, F., et al. (2004). Impaired fear processing in right mesial temporal sclerosis: A fMRI study. *Brain Research Bulletin, 63*(4), 269–281.

Benvenga, S. (2003). Brain injury and hypopituitarism: The historical background. *Pituitary, 8*, 193–195.

Berg, D., Supprian, T., Thomas, J., Warmuth-Metz, M., Horowski, A., & Zeiler, B. (2000). Lesion pattern in patients with multiple sclerosis and depression. *Multiple Sclerosis, 6*, 156–162.

Berkovic, S. F., Arzimanoglou, A., Kuzniecky, R., Harvey, A. S., Palmini, A., & Andermann, F. (2003). Hypothalamic hamartoma and seizures: A treatable epileptic encephalopathy. *Epilepsia, 44*(7), 969–973.

Berlin, L., Bohlin, G., Nyberg, L., & Janols, L.-O. (2004). How well do measures of inhibition and other executive functions discriminate between children with ADHD and controls? *Child Neuropsychology, 10*(1), 1–13.

Bernier, R., Dawson, G., Panagiotides, H., & Webb, S. (2005). Individuals with autism spectrum disorder show normal responses to a fear potential startle paradigm. *Journal of Autism and Developmental Disorders, 35*(5), 575–583.

Berntson, G. G., Bechara, A., Damasio, H., Tranel, D., & Cacioppo, J. T. (2007). Amygdala contribution to selective dimensions of emotion. *Social Cognitive and Affective Neuroscience, 2*(2), 123–129.

Berridge, K. C. (1996). Food reward: Brain substrates of wanting and liking. *Neuroscience and Biobehavioral Reviews, 20*(1), 1–25.

Berridge, K. C., & Kringelbach, M. L. (2008). Affective neuroscience of pleasure: Reward in humans and animals. *Psychopharmacology, 199*(3), 457–480.

Berridge, K. C., & Robinson, T. E. (1998). What is the role of dopamine in reward: Hedonic impact, reward learning, or incentive salience? *Brain Research Reviews, 28*(3), 309–369.

Berrios, G. E. (1997). The origins of psychosurgery: Shaw, Burckhardt and Moniz. *History of Psychiatry, 8*(29, Pt. 1), 61–81.

Berthoz, S., Blair, R. J. R., Le Clec'h, G., & Martinot, J.-L. (2002). Emotions: From neuropsychology to functional imaging. *International Journal of Psychology, 37*(4), 193–203.

Besel, L. D. S. (2007). *Empathy: The role of facial expression recognition.* Ann Arbor, MI: ProQuest Information & Learning.

Beyerstein, B. L. (1999). Whence cometh the myth that we only use 10% of the brain? In S. Della Sala (Ed.), *Mind myths: Exploring popular assumptions about the mind and brain* (pp. 3–24). Chichester, UK: Wiley.

Bhatt, S., Bhatt, R., Zalcman, S. S., & Siegel, A. (2008). Role of IL1 beta and 5-HT2 receptors in midbrain periaqueductal gray (PAG) in potentiating defensive rage behavior in cat. *Brain, Behavior, and Immunity, 22*(2), 224–233.

Bhogal, S. K., Teasell, R., Foley, N., & Speechley, M. (2005). Heterocyclics and selective serotonin reuptake inhibitors in the treatment and prevention of poststroke depression. *Journal of the American Geriatrics Society, 53*(6), 1051–1057.

Biederman, J., Faraone, S. V., Spencer, T., Wilens, T., Norman, D., Lapey, K. A., et al. (1993). Patterns of psychiatric comorbidity, cognition, and psychosocial functioning in adults with attention deficit hyperactivity disorder. *American Journal of Psychiatry, 150*(12), 1792–1798.

Bigelow, H. J. (1850). Dr. Harlow's case of recovery from the passage of an iron bar through the head. *American Journal of the Medical Science, 20*, 13–22.

Biggio, G., Dazzi, L., Serra, M., & Smith, S. S. (2004). Allopregnanolone modulates the action of ethanol and stress on the activity of mesocortical dopaminergic neurons and HPA axis. In S. S. Smith (Ed.), *Neurosteroid effects in the central nervous system: The role of the* $GABA_A$ receptor (pp. 247–264). Boca Raton, FL: CRC Press.

Bigler, E. D. (2004). Neuropsychological results and neuropathological findings at autopsy in a case of mild traumatic brain injury. *Journal of the International Neuropsychological Society, 10*(5), 794–806.

Birbaumer, N., Veit, R., Lotze, M., Erb, M., Hermann, C., Grodd, W., et al. (2005). Deficient fear conditioning in psychopathy: A functional magnetic resonance imaging study. *Archives of General Psychiatry, 62*(7), 799–805.

Bishop, S. J., Cohen, J. D., Fossella, J., Casey, B. J., & Farah, M. J. (2006). COMT genotype influences prefrontal response to emotional distraction. *Cognitive, Affective and Behavioral Neuroscience, 6*(1), 62–70.

Bjornebekk, G. (2009). Psychometric properties of the scores on the behavioral inhibition and activation scales in a sample of Norwegian children. *Educational and Psychological Measurement, 69*(4), 636–654.

Blackman, J. A., Patrick, P. D., Buck, M. L., & Rust, R. S. (2004). Paroxysmal autonomic instability with dystonia after brain injury. *Archives of Neurology, 61*, 321–328.

Blair, C. (2003). Behavioral inhibition and behavioral activation in young children: Relations with self-regulation and adaptation to preschool in children attending Head Start. *Developmental Psychobiology, 42*(3), 301–311.

Blair, C., Peters, R., & Granger, D. (2004). Physiological and neuropsychological correlates of approach/withdrawal tendencies in preschool: Further examination of the behavioral inhibition system/behavioral activation system scales for young children. *Developmental Psychobiology, 45*(3), 113–124.

Blair, E. A., & Erlanger, J. (1936). Temporal summation in peripheral nerve fibers. *American Journal of Physiology, 117*, 355–365.

Blair, K. S., Morton, J., Leonard, A., & Blair, R. J. R. (2006). Impaired decision-making on the basis of both reward and punishment information in individuals with psychopathy. *Personality and Individual Differences, 41*(1), 155–165.

Blair, R. J. R. (2001). Neurocognitive models of aggression, the antisocial personality disorders, and psychopathy. *Journal of Neurology, Neurosurgery, and Psychiatry, 71*(6), 727–731.

Blair, R. J. R., & Cipolotti, L. (2000). Impaired social response reversal. A case of "acquired sociopathy." *Brain: A Journal of Neurology, 123*(6), 1122–1141.

Blair, R. J. R., Mitchell, D. G. V., Leonard, A., Budhani, S., Peschardt, K. S., & Newman, C. (2004). Passive avoidance learning in individuals with psychopathy: Modulation by reward but not by punishment. *Personality and Individual Differences, 37*(6), 1179–1192.

Blanchard, D. C., & Blanchard, R. J. (1972). Innate and conditional reactions to threat in rats with amygdaloid lesions. *Journal of Comparative and Physiological Psychology, 81*(2), 281–290.

Blanchard, R. J., & Blanchard, D. C. (1994). Opponent environmental targets and sensorimotor systems in aggression and defence. In J. C. Cooper & C. A. Hedrie (Eds.), *Ethology and psychopharmacology* (pp. 133–157). Chichester, UK: Wiley.

Blasi, G., Mattay, V. S., Bertolino, A., Elvevag, B., Callicott, J. H., Das, S., et al. (2005). Effect of catechol-O-methyltransferase val158met genotype on attentional control. *Journal of Neuroscience, 25*, 5038–5045.

Blass, D. M., & Rabins, P. V. (2009). Depression in frontotemporal dementia. *Psychosomatics, 50*(3), 239–247.

Blonder, L. X., Burns, A. F., Bowers, D., Moore, R. W., & Heilman, K. M. (1993). Right hemisphere facial expressivity during natural conversation. *Brain and Cognition, 21*(1), 44–56.

Blonder, L. X., Heilman, K. M., Ketterson, T., Rosenbek, J., Raymer, A., Crosson, B., et al. (2005). Affective facial and lexical expression in aprosodic versus aphasic stroke patients. *Journal of the International Neuropsychological Society, 11*(6), 677–685.

Blood, A. J., Zatorre, R. J., Bermudez, P., & Evans, A. C. (1999). Emotional responses to pleasant and unpleasant music correlate with activity in paralimbic brain regions. *Nature Neuroscience, 2*(4), 382–387.

Blume, A. W., & Marlatt, G. A. (2009). The role of executive cognitive functions in changing substance use: What we know and what we need to know. *Annals of Behavioral Medicine, 37*, 117–125.

Boakes, J., Chapman, E., Houghton, S., & West, J. (2008). Facial affect interpretation in boys with attention deficit/hyperactivity disorder. *Child Neuropsychology, 14*(1), 82–96.

Boccardi, E., Della Sala, S., Motto, C., & Spinnler, H. (2002). Utilisation behaviour consequent to bilateral SMA softening. *Cortex, 38*(3), 289–308.

Bodini, B., Mandarelli, G., Tomassini, V., Tarsitani, L., Pestalozza, I., Gasperini, C., et al. (2008). Alexithymia in multiple sclerosis: Relationship with fatigue and depression. *Acta Neurologica Scandinavica, 118*(1), 18–23.

Boelte, S., & Poustka, F. (2003). The recognition of facial affect in autistic and schizophrenic subjects and their first-degree relatives. *Psychological Medicine, 33*(5), 907–915.

Boiten, F. (1996). Autonomic response patterns during voluntary facial action. *Psychophysiology, 33*(2), 123–131.

Bol, Y., Duits, A. A., Vertommen-Mertens, C. E., Hupperts, R. M., Romberg-Camps, M. J., Verhey, F. R., et al. (2010). The contribution of disease severity, depression, and negative affectivity to fatigue in multiple sclerosis: A comparison with ulcerative colitis. *Journal of Psychosomatic Research, 69*, 43–44.

Bonatti, E., Zamarian, L., Wagner, M., Benke, T., Hollosi, P., Strubreither, W., et al. (2008). Making decisions and advising decisions in traumatic brain injury. *Cognitive and Behavioral Neurology, 21*(3), 164–175.

Bornke, C., Postert, T., Przuntek, H., & Buttner, T. (1998). Acute mania due to a right hemisphere infarction. *European Journal of Neurology, 5*(4), 407–409.

Borod, J. C., Bloom, R. L., Brickman, A. M., Nakhutina, L., & Curko, E. A. (2002). Emotional processing deficits in individuals with unilateral brain damage. *Applied Neuropsychology, 9*(1), 23–36.

Borod, J. C., Bloom, R. L., Haywood, C. S., Beeman, M., & Chiarello, C. (1998). Verbal aspects of emotional communication. In M. Beeman & C. Chiarello (Eds.), *Right hemisphere language comprehension: Perspectives from cognitive neuroscience* (pp. 285–307). Mahwah, NJ: Erlbaum.

Borod, J. C., Cicero, B. A., Obler, L. K., Welkowitz, J., Erhan, H. M., Santschi, C., et al. (1998). Right hemisphere emotional perception: Evidence across multiple channels. *Neuropsychology, 12*(3), 446–458.

Borod, J. C., Koff, E., Yecker, S., Santschi, C., & Schmidt, J. M. (1998). Facial asymmetry during emotional expression: Gender, valence, and measurement technique. *Neuropsychologia, 36*(11), 1209–1215.

Borod, J. C., Pick, L. H., Hall, S., Sliwinski, M., Madigan, N., Obler, L. K., et al. (2000). Relationships among facial, prosodic, and lexical channels of emotional perceptual processing. *Cognition and Emotion, 14*(2), 193–211.

Borod, J. C., Tabert, M. H., Santschi, C., & Strauss, E. H. (2000). Neuropsychological assessment of emotional processing in brain-damaged patients. In J. C. Borod (Ed.), *The neuropsychology of emotion* (pp. 80–105). New York: Oxford University Press.

Borod, J. C., Welkowitz, J., & Obler, L. K. (1992). *The New York Emotion Battery.* New York: Mount Sinai Medical Center.

Borroni, B., Turla, M., Bertasi, V., Agosti, C., Gilberti, N., & Padovani, A. (2008). Cognitive and behavioral assessment in the early stages of neurodegenerative extrapyramidal syndromes. *Archives of Gerontology and Geriatrics, 47*(1), 53–61.

Botvinick, M. M., Braver, T. S., Barch, D. M., Carter, C. S., & Cohen, J. D. (2001). Conflict monitoring and cognitive control. *Psychological Review, 108*(3), 624–652.

Boucher, J., Lewis, V., & Collis, G. M. (2000). Voice processing abilities in children with autism, children with specific language impairments, and young typically developing children. *Journal of Child Psychology and Psychiatry, 41*(7), 847–857.

Bourdeau, I., Bard, C., Forget, H., Boulanger, Y., Cohen, H., & Locroix, A. (2005). Cognitive function and cerebral assessment in patients who have Cushing's syndrome. *Endocrinology and Metabolism Clinics of North America, 34*, 357–369.

Bowers, D., Bauer, R. M., Coslett, H. B., & Heilman, K. M. (1985). Processing of faces by patients with unilateral hemisphere lesions: I. Dissociation between judgments of facial affect and facial identity. *Brain and Cognition, 4*(3), 258–272.

Bowers, D., Bauer, R. M., & Heilman, K. M. (1993). The nonverbal affect lexicon: Theoretical perspectives from neuropsychological studies of affect perception. *Neuropsychology, 7*(4), 433–444.

Bowers, D., Blonder, L. X., & Heilman, K. M. (1999). *Florida Affect Battery*. Gainesville: Center for Neuropsychological Studies, Cognitive Neuroscience Laboratory, University of Florida.

Bowers, D., Coslett, H. B., Bauer, R. M., & Speedie, L. J. (1987). Comprehension of emotional prosody following unilateral hemispheric lesions: Processing defect versus distraction defect. *Neuropsychologia, 25*(2), 317–328.

Bowers, D., Miller, K., Bosch, W., Gokcay, D., Pedraza, O., Springer, U., et al. (2006). Faces of emotion in Parkinson's disease: Micro-expressivity and bradykinesia during voluntary facial expressions. *Journal of the International Neuropsychological Society, 12*(6), 765–773.

Bozikas, V. P., Kosmidis, M. H., Anezoulaki, D., Giannakou, M., Andreou, C., & Karavatos, A. (2006). Impaired perception of affective prosody in schizophrenia. *Journal of Neuropsychiatry and Clinical Neuroscience, 18*(1), 81–85.

Bozikas, V. P., Kosmidis, M. H., Anezoulaki, D., Giannakou, M., & Karavatos, A. (2004). Relationship of affect recognition with psychopathology and cognitive performance in schizophrenia. *Journal of the International Neuropsychological Society, 10*(4), 549–558.

Bozikas, V. P., Tonia, T., Fokas, K., Karavatos, A., & Kosmidis, M. H. (2006). Impaired emotion processing in remitted patients with bipolar disorder. *Journal of Affective Disorders, 91*(1), 53–56.

Bradvik, B., Dravins, C., Holtas, S., & Rosen, I. (1991). Disturbances of speech prosody following right hemisphere infarcts. *Acta Neurologica Scandinavica, 84*(2), 114–126.

Brand, M., Franke-Sievert, C., Jacoby, G. E., Markowitsch, H. J., & Tuschen-Caffier, B. (2007). Neuropsychological correlates of decision making in patients with bulimia nervosa. *Neuropsychology, 21*, 742–750.

Brand, M., Grabenhorst, F., Starcke, K., Vandekerckhove, M. M. P., & Markowitsch, H. J. (2007). Role of the amygdala in decisions under ambiguity and decisions under risk: Evidence from patients with Urbach–Wiethe disease. *Neuropsychologia, 45*(6), 1305–1317.

Braun, C. M. J. (2007). Evolution of hemispheric specialisation of antagonistic systems of management of the body's energy resources. *Laterality, 12*(5), 397–427.

Breen, N., Caine, D., & Coltheart, M. (2000). Models of face recognition and delusional misidentification: A critical review. *Cognitive Neuropsychology, 17*(1), 55–71.

Breitenstein, C., Daum, I., & Ackermann, H. (1998). Emotional processing following cortical and subcortical brain damage: Contribution of the fronto-striatal circuitry. *Behavioural Neurology, 11*(1), 29–42.

Bremner, J. D., Randall, P., Vermetten, E., & Staib, L. (1997). Magnetic resonance imaging-based measurement of hippocampal volume in posttraumatic stress disorder related to childhood physical and sexual abuse: A preliminary report. *Biological Psychiatry, 41*(1), 23–32.

Bremner, J. D., Vermetten, E., Afzal, N., & Vythilingam, M. (2004). Deficits in verbal declarative memory function in women with childhood sexual abuse-related posttraumatic stress disorder. *Journal of Nervous and Mental Disease, 192*(10), 643–649.

Bremner, J. D., Vythilingam, M., Vermetten, E., Charney, D. S., & Vaccarino, V. (2004). Deficits in hippocampal and anterior cingulate functioning during verbal declarative memory encoding in midlife major depression. *American Journal of Psychiatry, 161*(4), 637–645.

Bremner, J. D., Vythilingam, M., Vermetten, E., Khan, S., Afzal, N., Elzinga, B., et al. (2003). Cortisol response to a cognitive stress challenge in posttraumatic stress disorder (PTSD) related to childhood abuse. *Psychoneuroendocrinology, 28*(6), 733–750.

Bremner, J. D., Vythilingam, M., Vermetten, E., McGlashan, T., Khan, S., Soufer, R., et al. (2003). MRI and PET study of deficits in hippocampal structure and function in women with childhood sexual abuse and posttraumatic stress disorder. *American Journal of Psychiatry, 160*(5), 924–932.

Brooks, B. R., Thisted, R. A., Appel, S. H., Bradley, W. G., Olney, R. K., Berg, J. E., et al. (2004). Treatment of pseudobulbar affect in ALS with dextromethorphan/quinidine: A randomized trial. *Neurology, 63*(8), 1364–1370.

Brosschot, J. F., Gerin, W., & Thayer, J. F. (2006). The perseverative cognition hypothesis: A review of worry, prolonged stress-related physiological activation, and health. *Journal of Psychosomatic Research, 60*, 113–124.

Brotman, M. A., Guyer, A. E., Lawson, E. S., Horsey, S. E., Rich, B. A., Dickstein, D. P., et al. (2008). Facial emotion labeling deficits in children and adolescents at risk for bipolar disorder. *American Journal of Psychiatry, 165*(3), 385–389.

Brown, J. S. (1961). *The motivation of behavior.* New York: McGraw-Hill.

Brown, W. A., Kesler, S. R., Eliez, S., Warsofsky, I. S., Haberecht, M., Patwardhan, A., et al. (2002). Brain development in Turner syndrome: A magnetic resonance imaging study. *Psychiatry Research: Neuroimaging, 116*(3), 187–196.

Buchanan, D. C., Waterhouse, G. J., & West, S. C. (1980). A proposed neurophysiological basis of alexithymia. *Psychotherapy and Psychosomatics, 34*(4), 248–255.

Buchanan, T. W., Denburg, N. L., Tranel, D., & Adolphs, R. (2001). Verbal and nonverbal emotional memory following unilateral amygdala damage. *Learning and Memory, 8*(6), 326–335.

Buchanan, T. W., Lutz, K., Mirzazade, S., Specht, K., Shah, N. J., Zilles, K., et al. (2000). Recognition of emotional prosody and verbal components of spoken language: An fMRI study. *Cognitive Brain Research, 9*(3), 227–238.

Buckholtz, J. W., & Meyer-Lindenberg, A. (2008). MAOA and the neurogenetic architecture of human aggression. *Trends in Neurosciences, 31*(3), 120–129.

Buelow, M. T., & Suhr, J. A. (2009). Construct validity of the Iowa Gambling Task. *Neuropsychology Review, 19*(1), 102–114.

Burgdorf, J., & Panksepp, J. (2006). The neurobiology of positive emotions. *Neuroscience and Biobehavioral Reviews, 30*(2), 173–187.

Burns, J., Jr., & Hauser, W. A. (2003). The epidemiology of traumatic brain injury: A review. *Epilepsia, 44*, 2–10.

Burton, C. L., Strauss, E., Hultsch, D. F., & Hunter, M. A. (2006). Cognitive functioning and everyday problem solving in older adults. *Clinical Neuropsychologist, 20*(3), 432–452.

Busch, C. R., & Alpern, H. P. (1998). Depression after mild traumatic brain injury: A review of current research. *Neuropsychology Review, 8*(2), 95–108.

Bushnik, T., Englander, J., & Katznelson, L. (2007). Fatigue after TBI: Association with neuroendocrine abnormalities. *Brain Injury, 21*(6), 559–566.

Caci, H., Deschaux, O., & Bayle, F. J. (2007). Psychometric properties of the French versions of the BIS/BAS scales and the SPSRQ. *Personality and Individual Differences, 42*(6), 987–998.

Cacioppo, J. T., & Berntson, G. G. (2007). The brain, homeostasis, and health: Balancing demands of the internal and external milieu. In H. S. Friedman & R. Cohen Silver (Eds.), *Foundations of health psychology* (pp. 73–91). New York: Oxford University Press.

Cadesky, E. B., Mota, V. L., & Schachar, R. J. (2000). Beyond words: How do problem children with ADHD and/or conduct problems process nonverbal information about affect? *Journal of the American Academy of Child and Adolescent Psychiatry, 39*(9), 1160–1167.

Cahill, L. (1996). Amygdala activity at encoding correlated with long-term, free recall of emotional information. *Proceedings of National Society of Sciences, 93*, 8016–8021.

Cahill, L. T., Kaminer, R. K., & Johnson, P. G. (1999). Developmental, cognitive, and behavioral sequelae of child abuse. *Child and Adolescent Psychiatric Clinics of North America, 8*(4), 827–843.

Cahn-Weiner, D. A., Farias, S. T., Julian, L., Harvey, D. J., Kramer, J. H., Reed, B. R., et al. (2007). Cognitive and neuroimaging predictors of instrumental activities of daily living. *Journal of the International Neuropsychological Society, 13*(5), 747–757.

Calder, A. J., Keane, J., Manly, T., Sprengelmeyer, R., Scott, S., Nimmo-Smith, I., et al. (2003). Facial expression recognition across the adult life span. *Neuropsychologia, 41*(2), 195–202.

Cameron, O. G., & Minoshima, S. (2002). Regional brain activation due to pharmacologically induced adrenergic interoceptive stimulation in humans. *Psychosomatic Medicine, 64*(6), 851–861.

Campbell, S., Marriott, M., Nahmias, C., & MacQueen, G. M. (2004). Lower hippocampal volume in patients suffering from depression: A meta-analysis. *American Journal of Psychiatry, 161*(4), 598–607.

Campbell-Sills, L., Liverant, G. I., & Brown, T. A. (2004). Psychometric evaluation of the behavioral inhibition/behavioral activation scales in a large sample of outpatients with anxiety and mood disorders. *Psychological Assessment, 16*(3), 244–254.

Cancelliere, A. E., & Kertesz, A. (1990). Lesion localization in acquired deficits of emotional expression and comprehension. *Brain and Cognition, 13*(2), 133–147.

Canli, T., Omura, K., Haas, B. W., Fallgatter, A., Constable, R. T., & Lesch, K. P. (2005). Beyond affect: A role for genetic variation of the serotonin transporter in neural activation during a cognitive attention task. *Proceedings of the National Academy of Sciences of the United States of America, 102*(34), 12224–12229.

Cannon, W. B. (1915). *Bodily changes in pain, hunger, fear and rage: An account of recent researches into the function of emotional excitement.* New York: Appleton.

Cannon, W. B. (1927). The James–Lange theory of emotions: A critical examination and an alternative theory. *American Journal of Psychology, 39*, 106–124.
Cannon, W. B. (1929). *Bodily changes in pain, hunger, fear and rage.* Oxford, UK: Appleton.
Cannon, W. B. (1931). Again the James–Lange and the thalamic theories of emotion. *Psychological Review, 38*(4), 281–295.
Cannon, W. B., & Britton, S. W. (1925). Studies on the conditions of activity in endocrine glands. *American Journal of Physiology, 72*, 283–294.
Cappella, J. N. (1993). The facial feedback hypothesis in human interaction: Review and speculation. *Journal of Language and Social Psychology, 12*(1), 13–29.
Carlson, S. M., & Wang, T. S. (2007). Inhibitory control and emotion regulation in preschool children. *Cognitive Development, 22*(4), 489–510.
Carr, L., Iacoboni, M., Dubeau, M. C., Mazziotta, J. C., & Lenzi, G. L. (2003). Neural mechanisms of empathy in humans: A relay from neural systems for imitations to limbic areas. *Proceedings of the National Academy of Sciences, 100*, 5497–5502.
Carr, M. B., & Lutjemeier, J. A. (2005). The relation of facial affect recognition and empathy to delinquency in youth offenders. *Adolescence, 40*, 601–619.
Carran, M. A., Kohler, C. G., O'Connor, M. J., Bilker, W. B., & Sperling, M. R. (2003). Mania following temporal lobectomy. *Neurology, 61*(6), 770–774.
Carrington, S. J., & Bailey, A. J. (2009). Are there theory of mind regions in the brain?: A review of the neuroimaging literature. *Human Brain Mapping, 30*(8), 2313–2335.
Carter, E. J., & Pelphrey, K. A. (2008). Friend or foe?: Brain systems involved in the perception of dynamic signals of menacing and friendly social approaches. *Social Neuroscience, 3*(2), 151–163.
Carver, C. S., & White, T. L. (1994). Behavioral inhibition, behavioral activation, and affective responses to impending reward and punishment: The BIS/BAS Scales. *Journal of Personality and Social Psychology, 67*(2), 319–333.
Casey, B. J., Castellanos, F. X., Giedd, J. N., & Marsh, W. L. (1997). Implication of right frontostriatal circuitry in response inhibition and attention-deficit/hyperactivity disorder. *Journal of the American Academy of Child and Adolescent Psychiatry, 36*(3), 374–383.
Caspi, A., McClay, J., Moffitt, T., Mill, J., Martin, J., Craig, I. W., et al. (2002). Role of genotype in the cycle of violence in maltreated children. *Science, 297*, 851–854.
Castaneda, A. E., Tuulio-Henriksson, A., Marttunen, M., Suvisaari, J., & Loennqvist, J. (2008). A review of cognitive impairments in depressive and anxiety disorders with a focus on young adults. *Journal of Affective Disorders, 106*(1–2), 1–27.
Cataldo, M. G., Nobile, M., Lorusso, M. L., Battaglia, M., & Molteni, M. (2005). Impulsivity in depressed children and adolescents: A comparison between behavioral and neuropsychological data. *Psychiatry Research, 136*(2–3), 123–133.
Cavigelli, S. A., Stine, M. M., Kovacsics, C., Diep, M. N., Barrett, C. E., & Jefferson, A. (2007). Behavioral inhibition and glucocorticoid dynamics in a rodent model. *Physiology and Behavior, 92*(5), 897–905.
Celik, Y., Erdogan, E., Tuglu, C., & Utku, U. (2004). Post-stroke mania in late life due to right temporoparietal infarction. *Psychiatry and Clinical Neurosciences, 58*(4), 446–447.
Cendes, F., Andermann, F., Dubeau, F., Gloor, P., Evans, A., Jones-Gotman, M., et al. (1993). Early childhood prolonged febrile convulsions, atrophy and sclerosis of

mesial structrues, and temporal lobe epilepsy: An MRI volumentric study. *Neurology, 43*, 1083–1087.

Cendes, F., Andermann, F., Gloor, P., Evans, A., Jones-Gotman, M., Watson, C., et al. (1993). MRI volumentric measurement of amygdala and hippocampus in temporal lobe epilepsy. *Neurology, 43*, 719–725.

Cerrato, P., Imperiale, D., Bergui, M., Giraudo, M., Baima, C., Grasso, M., et al. (2003). Emotional facial paresis in a patient with a lateral medullary infarction. *Neurology, 60*, 723–724.

Chahraoui, K., Pinoit, J. M., Viegas, N., Adnet, J., Bonin, B., & Moreau, T. (2008). Alexithymie et liens avec la dépression et l'anxiété dans la sclérose en plaques. *Revue Neurologique, 164*(3), 242–245.

Chamorro-Premuzic, T., & Furnham, A. (2008). Personality, intelligence, and approaches to learning as predictors of academic performance. *Personality and Individual Differences, 44*(7), 1596–1603.

Chan, J., Parmenter, T., & Stancliffe, R. (2009). The impact of traumatic brain injury on the mental health outcomes of individuals and their family carers. *Australian e-Journal for the Advancement of Mental Health, 8*(2), 1–10.

Chapman, L. J., Chapman, J. P., & Raulin, M. L. (1976). Scales for physical and social anhedonia. *Journal of Abnormal Psychology, 85*(4), 374–382.

Chatfield, P. O., & Lyman, C. P. (1950). Circulatory changes during process of arousal in the hibernating hamster. *American Journal of Physiology, 163*, 566–574.

Cheung, A. M., Mitsis, E. M., & Halperin, J. M. (2004). The relationship of behavioral inhibition to executive functions in young adults. *Journal of Clinical and Experimental Neuropsychology, 26*(3), 393–404.

Chinet, L., Bolognini, M., Plancherel, B., Stephan, P., & Halfon, O. (1998). Is alexithymia a typical characteristic of addictive behaviours in adolescents and young adults? *Swiss Journal of Psychology/Schweizerische Zeitschrift fuer Psychologie/Revue Suisse de Psychologie, 57*(3), 145–152.

Chopra, M. P., Sullivan, J. R., Feldman, Z., Landes, R. D., & Beck, C. (2008). Self-, collateral- and clinician assessment of depression in persons with cognitive impairment. *Aging and Mental Health, 12*(6), 675–683.

Chow, K. L. (1952). Further studies on selective ablation of associative cortex in relation to visually mediated behavior. *Journal of Comparative Physiological Psychology, 45*, 109–118.

Christianson, B. A. (1992). Emotional stress and eyewitness memroy: A critical review. *Psychological Bulletin, 112*, 284–309.

Christodoulou, C., Melville, P., Scherl, W. F., MacAllister, W. S., Abensur, R. L., Troxell, R. M., et al. (2009). Negative affect predicts subsequent cognitive change in multiple sclerosis. *Journal of the International Neuropsychological Society, 15*(1), 53–61.

Christophe, V., Antoine, P., Leroy, T., & Delelis, G. (2009). Evaluation de deux strategies de regulation emotionnelle: La suppression expressive et la reevaluation cognitive. *European Review of Applied Psychology/Revue Européenne de Psychologie Appliquée, 59*(1), 59–67.

Chrousos, G. P., Kino, T., Judd, L. L., & Sternberg, E. M. (2009). Glucocorticoid signaling in the cell: Expanding clinical implications to complex human behavioral and somatic disorders. In L. L. Judd & E. M. Stenberg (Eds.), *Glucocorticoids and mood: Clinical manifestations, risk factors and molecular mechanisms* (pp. 153–166). Chichester, UK: Wiley-Blackwell.

Cicero, B. A., Borod, J. C., Santschi, C., Erhan, H. M., Obler, L. K., Agosti, R. M., et al. (1999). Emotional versus nonemotional lexical perception in patients with right and left brain damage. *Neuropsychiatry, Neuropsychology, and Behavioral Neurology, 12*(4), 255–264.

Claes, S. J., Nemeroff, C. B., Corveleyn, J., Luyten, P., & Blatt, S. J. (2005). Corticotropin releasing factor (CRF) and major depression: Towards an integration of psychology and neurobiology in depression research. In J. Corveleyn, P. Luyten, & S. J. Blatt (Eds.), *The theory and treatment of depression: Towards a dynamic interactionism model* (pp. 227–252). Mahwah, NJ: Erlbaum.

Clark, D. A., Steer, R. A., & Beck, A. T. (1994). Common and specific dimensions of self-reported anxiety and depression: Implications for the cognitive and tripartite models. *Journal of Abnormal Psychology, 103*(4), 645–654.

Clark, D. C., Fawcett, J., Salazar-Grueso, E., & Fawcett, E. (1984). Seven-month clinical outcome of anhedonic and normally hedonic depressed inpatients. *American Journal of Psychiatry, 141*(10), 1216–1220.

Clark, L., Cools, R., & Robbins, T. W. (2004). The neuropsychology of ventral prefrontal cortex: Decision-making and reversal learning. *Brain and Cognition, 55*(1), 41–53.

Clark, L., Manes, F., Antoun, N., Sahakian, B. J., & Robbins, T. W. (2003). The contributions of lesion laterality and lesion volume to decision-making impairment following frontal lobe damage. *Neuropsychologia, 41*(11), 1474–1483.

Clark, L. A., & Watson, D. (1991). Tripartite model of anxiety and depression: Psychometric evidence and taxonomic implications. *Journal of Abnormal Psychology, 100*(3), 316–336.

Clarke, D. E., van Reekum, R., Patel, J., Simard, M., Gomez, E., & Streiner, D. L. (2007). An appraisal of the psychometric properties of clinician version of the Apathy Evaluation Scale (AES-C). *International Journal of Methods in Psychiatric Research, 16*(2), 97–110.

Clarke, D. E., van Reekum, R., Simard, M., Streiner, D. L., Freedman, M., & Conn, D. (2007). Apathy in dementia: An examination of the psychometric properties of the Apathy Evaluation Scale. *Journal of Neuropsychiatry and Clinical Neurosciences, 19*(1), 57–64.

Cleckley, H. (1976). *The mask of sanity* (5th ed.). St. Louis, MO: Mosby.

Clifford, J. S., Boufal, M. M., & Kurtz, J. E. (2004). Personality traits and critical thinking skills in college students: Empirical tests of a two-factor theory. *Assessment, 11*, 169–176.

Cohen, L. H., Novick, R. G., & Ettleson, A. (1942). Frontal lobotomy in the treatment of chronic psychotic overactivity. *Psychosomatic Medicine, 4*, 96–103.

Cohen, S., Doyle, W. J., Alper, C. M., Janicki-Deverts, D., & Turner, M. D. (2009). Sleep habits and susceptibility to the common cold. *Archives of Internal Medicine, 169*(1), 62–67.

Colivicchi, F., Bassi, A., Santini, M., & Caltagirone, C. (2004). Prognostic implications of right-sided stroke with insular involvements. *Stroke, 35*, 2094–2098.

Colla, M., Ende, G., Alm, B., Deuschle, M., Heuser, I., & Kronenberg, G. (2008). Cognitive MR spectroscopy of anterior cingulate cortex in ADHD: Elevated choline signal correlates with slowed hit reaction times. *Journal of Psychiatric Research, 42*(7), 587–595.

Compton, R. J., Wirtz, D., Pajoumand, G., Claus, E., & Heller, W. (2004). Association between positive affect and attentional shifting. *Cognitive Therapy and Research, 28*(6), 733–744.

Connelly, M., & Denney, D. R. (2007). Regulation of emotions during experimental stress in alexithymia. *Journal of Psychosomatic Research, 62*(6), 649–656.

Cooke, D. J., Michie, C., Hart, S. D., & Hare, R. D. (1999). Evaluating the Screening Version of the Hare Psychopathy Checklist—Revised (PCL:SV): An item response theory analysis. *Psychological Assessment, 11*(1), 3–13.

Coolen, L. M., Allard, J., Truitt, W. A., & McKenna, K. E. (2004). Central regulation of ejaculation. *Physiology and Behavior, 83*(2), 203–215.

Coolidge, F. L., Segal, D. L., Stewart, S. E., & Ellett, J. A. C. (2000). Neuropsychological dysfunction in children with borderline personality disorder features: A preliminary investigation. *Journal of Research in Personality, 34*(4), 554–561.

Cooper, A., Gomez, R., & Aucote, H. (2007). The Behavioral Inhibition System and Behavioral Approach System (BIS/BAS) Scales: Measurement and structural invariance across adults and adolescents. *Personality and Individual Differences, 43*(2), 295–305.

Corbett, B., & Glidden, H. (2000). Processing affective stimuli in children with attention-deficit hyperactivity disorder. *Child Neuropsychology, 6*(2), 144–155.

Corcoran, C., Walker, E., Huot, R., Mittal, V., Tessner, K., Kestler, L., et al. (2003). The stress cascade and schizophrenia: Etiology and onset. *Schizophrenia Bulletin, 29*(4), 671–692.

Corden, B., Critchley, H. D., Skuse, D., & Dolan, R. J. (2006). Fear recognition ability predicts differences in social cognitive and neural functioning in men. *Journal of Cognitive Neuroscience, 18*(6), 889–897.

Cornblatt, B. A., Risch, N. J., Faris, G., Friedman, D., & Erlenmeyer-Kimling, L. (1988). The Continuous Performance Test, Identical Pairs version (CPT-IP): I. New findings about sustained attention in normal families. *Psychiatry Research, 26*(2), 223–228.

Costa, A., Peppe, A., Carlesimo, G. A., Pasqualetti, P., & Caltagirone, C. (2006). Alexithymia in Parkinson's disease is related to severity of depressive symptoms. *European Journal of Neurology, 13*(8), 836–841.

Costa, A., Peppe, A., Carlesimo, G. A., Salamone, G., & Caltagirone, C. (2007). Neuropsychological correlates of alexithymia in Parkinson's disease. *Journal of the International Neuropsychological Society, 13*(6), 980–992.

Costa, P. T., & McCrae, R. R. (1992). *Revised NEO Personality Inventory (NEO-PI-R) and NEO Five-Factor Inventory (NEO-FFI)*. Odessa, FL: Psychological Assessment Resources.

Cox, S. M. L., Andrade, A., & Johnsrude, I. S. (2005). Learning to like: A role for human orbitofrontal cortex in conditioned reward. *Journal of Neuroscience, 25*(10), 2733–2740.

Craig, J. B. (2008). *The relationship between the emotional intelligence of the principal and teacher job satisfaction*. Ann Arbor, MI: ProQuest Information & Learning.

Crawford, J. R., Garthwaite, P. H., Lawrie, C. J., Henry, J. D., MacDonald, M. A., Sutherland, J., et al. (2009). A convenient method of obtaining percentile norms and accompanying interval estimates for self-report mood scales (DASS, DASS-21, HADS, PANAS, and sAD). *British Journal of Clinical Psychology, 48*(2), 163–180.

Crawford, J. R., & Henry, J. D. (2004). The Positive and Negative Affect Schedule (PANAS): Construct validity, measurement properties and normative data in a large non-clinical sample. *British Journal of Clinical Psychology, 43*(3), 245–265.

Critchley, H. D. (2005). Neural mechanisms of autonomic, affective, and cognitive integration. *Journal of Comparative Neurology, 493*(1), 154–166.

Critchley, H. D., Elliott, R., Mathias, C. J., & Dolan, R. J. (2000). Neural activity relating to generation and representation of galvanic skin conductance responses: A functional magnetic resonance imaging study. *Journal of Neuroscience, 20*(8), 3033–3040.

Critchley, H. D., Mathias, C. J., Josephs, O., O'Doherty, J., Zanini, S., Dewar, B.-K., et al. (2003). Human cingulate cortex and autonomic control: Converging neuroimaging and clinical evidence. *Brain: A Journal of Neurology, 126*(10), 2139–2152.

Critchley, H. D., Wiens, S., Rotshtein, P., Ohman, A., & Dolan, R. J. (2004). Neural systems supporting interoceptive awareness. *Nature Neuroscience, 7*(2), 189–195.

Crouse, E. M. (2005). *Anna Thompson's starving children: Emotion regulation and verbal memory in borderline personality disorder.* Ann Arbor, MI: ProQuest Information & Learning.

Crowell, S. E., Beauchaine, T. P., Gatzke-Kopp, L., Sylvers, P., Mead, H., & Chipman-Chacon, J. (2006). Autonomic correlates of attention-deficit/hyperactivity disorder and oppositional defiant disorder in preschool children. *Journal of Abnormal Psychology, 115*(1), 174–178.

Csernansky, J. G., Dong, H., Fagan, A. M., Xiong, C., Morris, J. C., Holtzman, D. M., et al. (2006). Plasma cortisol and progression of dementia in subjects with Alzheimer-type dementia. *American Journal of Psychiatry, 163*(12), 2164–2169.

Cui, X., Lyness, J. M., Tu, X., King, D. A., & Caine, E. D. (2007). Does depression precede or follow executive dysfunction?: Outcomes in older primary care patients. *American Journal of Psychiatry, 164*(8), 1221–1228.

Cumberland-Li, A., Eisenberg, N., & Reiser, M. (2004). Relations of young children's agreeableness and resiliency to effortful control and impulsivity. *Social Development, 13*(2), 193–212.

Cunningham, W. A., Raye, C. L., & Johnson, M. K. (2004). Implicit and explicit evaluation: fMRI correlates of valence, emotional intensity, and control in the processing of attitudes. *Journal of Cognitive Neuroscience, 16*(10), 1717–1729.

Dadds, M. R., El Masry, Y., Wimalaweera, S., & Guastella, A. J. (2008). Reduced eye gaze explains "fear blindness" in childhood psychopathic traits. *Journal of the American Academy of Child and Adolescent Psychiatry, 47*(4), 455–463.

Dadds, M. R., Hawes, D. J., Frost, A. D. J., Vassallo, S., Bunn, P., Hunter, K., et al. (2009). Learning to "talk the talk": The relationship of psychopathic traits to deficits in empathy across childhood. *Journal of Child Psychology and Psychiatry, 50*(5), 599–606.

Dadds, M. R., & Salmon, K. (2003). Punishment insensitivity and parenting: Temperament and learning as interacting risks for antisocial behavior. *Clinical Child and Family Psychology Review, 6*(2), 69–86.

Da Fonseca, D., Seguier, V., Santos, A., Poinso, F. O., & Deruelle, C. (2009). Emotion understanding in children with ADHD. *Child Psychiatry and Human Development, 40*(1), 111–121.

Dalgleish, T., Yiend, J., Schweizer, S., & Dunn, B. D. (2009). Ironic effects of emotion suppression when recounting distressing memories. *Emotion, 9*(5), 744–749.

Dalton, E. J., & Heinrichs, R. W. (2005). Depression in multiple sclerosis: A quantitative review of the evidence. *Neuropsychology, 19*(2), 152–158.

Dalton, K. M., Holsen, L., Abbeduto, L., & Davidson, R. J. (2008). Brain function and gaze fixation during facial-emotion processing in fragile X and autism. *Autism Research, 1*(4), 231–239.

Daly, D. D., & Mulder, D. W. (1957). Gelastic seizures. *Neurology, 7*, 189–192.

Damsa, C., Maris, S., & Pull, C. B. (2005). New fields of research in posttraumatic stress disorder: Brain imaging. *Current Opinion in Psychiatry, 18*(1), 55–64.

da Rocha, F. F., Correa, H., & Teixeira, A. L. (2008). A successful outcome with valproic acid in a case of mania secondary to stroke of the right frontal lobe. *Progress in Neuro-Psychopharmacology and Biological Psychiatry, 32*(2), 587–588.

Darwin, C. (2009). *The expression of the emotions in man and animals* (3rd ed.). New York: Oxford University Press. (Original work published 1872)

Davidson, R. J. (1992a). Anterior cerebral asymmetry and the nature of emotion. *Brain and Cognition, 20*(1), 125–151.

Davidson, R. J. (1992b). Emotion and affective style: Hemispheric substrates. *Psychological Science, 3*(1), 39–43.

Davidson, R. J. (1993). Parsing affective space: Perspectives from neuropsychology and psychophysiology. *Neuropsychology, 7*(4), 464–475.

Davidson, R. J. (1998a). Affective style and affective disorders: Perspectives from affective neuroscience. *Cognition and Emotion, 12*(3), 307–330.

Davidson, R. J. (1998b). Anterior electrophysiological asymmetries, emotion, and depression: Conceptual and methodological conundrums. *Psychophysiology, 35*(5), 607–614.

Davidson, R. J. (2003). Affective neuroscience and psychophysiology: Toward a synthesis. *Psychophysiology, 40*(5), 655–665.

Davidson, R. J., Ekman, P., Saron, C. D., Senulis, J. A., & Friesen, W. V. (1990). Approach–withdrawal and cerebral asymmetry: Emotional expression and brain physiology: I. *Journal of Personality and Social Psychology, 58*(2), 330–341.

Davidson, R. J., & Fox, N. A. (1989). Frontal brain asymmetry predicts infants' response to maternal separation. *Journal of Abnormal Psychology, 98*(2), 127–131.

Davidson, R. J., & Irwin, W. (1999). The functional neuroanatomy of emotion and affective style. *Trends in Cognitive Sciences, 3*(1), 11–21.

Davidson, R. J., Jackson, D. C., & Kalin, N. H. (2000). Emotion, plasticity, context, and regulation: Perspectives from affective neuroscience. *Psychological Bulletin, 126*(6), 890–909.

Davidson, R. J., Lane, R. D., & Nadel, L. (2000). The functional neuroanatomy of affective style. In R. D. Lane & L. Nadel (Eds.), *Cognitive neuroscience of emotion* (pp. 371–388). New York: Oxford University Press.

Davidson, R. J., Rickman, M., Schmidt, L. A., & Schulkin, J. (1999). Behavioral inhibition and the emotional circuitry of the brain: Stability and plasticity during the early childhood years. In L. A. Schmidt & J. Schulkin (Eds.), *Extreme fear, shyness, and social phobia: Origins, biological mechanisms, and clinical outcomes* (pp. 67–87). New York: Oxford University Press.

Davis, J. I., Senghas, A., & Ochsner, K. N. (2009). How does facial feedback modulate emotional experience? *Journal of Research in Personality, 43*(5), 822–829.

Davis, K. D., Pope, G. E., Crawley, A. P., & Mikulis, D. J. (2004). Perceptual illusion of "paradoxical heat" engages the insular cortex. *Journal of Neurophysiology, 92*(2), 1248–1251.

Davis, M. (1997). Neurobiology of fear responses: The role of the amygdala. *Journal of Neuropsychiatry and Clinical Neurosciences, 9*, 382–402.

Davis, M., & Whalen, P. J. (2001). The amygdala: Vigilance and emotion. *Molecular Psychiatry, 6*(1), 13–34.

Davis, M. H., Hull, J. G., Young, R. D., & Warren, G. G. (1987). Emotional reactions to dramatic film stimuli: The influence of cognitive and emotional empathy. *Journal of Personality and Social Psychology, 52*(1), 126–133.

Davis, P. J., & Gibson, M. G. (2000). Recognition of posed and genuine facial expressions of emotion in paranoid and nonparanoid schizophrenia. *Journal of Abnormal Psychology, 109*(3), 445–450.

Davis, R. N., & Nolen-Hoeksema, S. (2000). Cognitive inflexibility among ruminators and nonruminators. *Psychological Medicine, 24*, 699–711.

Dawson, G., Frey, K., Self, J., Panagiotides, H., Hessl, D., Yamada, E., et al. (1999). Frontal brain electrical activity in infants of depressed and nondepressed mothers: Relation to variations in infant behavior. *Development and Psychopathology, 11*(3), 589–605.

Dawson, G., Webb, S. J., & McPartland, J. (2005). Understanding the nature of face processing impairment in autism: Insights from behavioral and electrophysiological studies. *Developmental Neuropsychology, 27*(3), 403–424.

De Bellis, M. D., Hooper, S. R., & Sapia (2005). Early trauma exposure and the brain. In J. J. Vasterling & R. Brewin (Eds.), *Neuropsychology of PTSD: Biological, cognitive, and clinical perspectives* (pp. 153–177). New York: Guilford Press.

Debener, S., Beauducel, A., Nessler, D., Brocke, B., Heilemann, H., & Kayser, J. (2000). Is resting anterior EEG alpha asymmetry a trait marker for depression?: Findings for healthy adults and clinically depressed patients. *Neuropsychobiology, 41*(1), 31–37.

De Berardis, D., Campanella, D., Gambi, F., La Rovere, R., Sepede, G., Core, L., et al. (2007). Alexithymia, fear of bodily sensations, and somatosensory amplification in young outpatients with panic disorder. *Psychosomatics: Journal of Consultation Liaison Psychiatry, 48*(3), 239–246.

de Frias, C. M., Annerbrink, K., Westberg, L., Eriksson, E., Adolfsson, R., & Nilsson, L. G. (2005). Catechol O-methyltransferase Val158Met polymorphism is associated with cognitive performance in nondemented adults. *Journal of Cognitive Neuroscience, 17*(7), 1018–1025.

de Gelder, B., Vroomen, J., Pourtois, G., & Weiskrantz, L. (1999). Non-conscious recognition of affect in the absence of striate cortex. *NeuroReport, 10*(18), 3759–3763.

de Gelder, B., Vroomen, J., Pourtois, G., & Weiskrantz, L. (2000). Affective blindsight: Are we blindly led by emotions?: Response to Heywood and Kentridge (2000). *Trends in Cognitive Sciences, 4*(4), 126–127.

de Kloet, E. R., & Oitzl, M. S. (2006). Cortisol and PTSD: Animal experiments and clinical perspectives. In N. Kato, M. Kawate, & R.K. Pitman (Eds.), *PTSD: Brain mechanisms and clinical implications* (pp. 13–28). Tokyo: Springer.

de Lacoste-Utamsing, C., & Holloway, R. L. (1982). Sexual dimorphism in the human corpus callosum. *Science, 216*, 1431–1432.

Delahunty, K. M., McKay, D. W., Noseworthy, D. E., & Storey, A. E. (2007). Prolactin responses to infant cues in men and women: Effects of parental experience and recent infant contact. *Hormones and Behavior, 51*(2), 213–220.

De La O, V. H. (2005, Spring). The Koko connections. *Santa Clara Magazine*. Retrieved from *www.scu.edu/scm/spring2005/koko.cfm*.

Delgado, J. M. R. (1955). Study of some cerebral structures related to transimission and elaboration of noxious stimulation. *Journal of Neurophysiology, 18*, 261–275.

Delgado, J. M. R., Rosvold, H. E., & Looney, E. (1956). Evoking conditioned fear by electrical stimulation of subcortical structures in the monkey brain. *Journal of Comparative and Physiological Psychology, 49*(4), 373–380.

Dellu, F., Mayo, W., Vallee, M., Maccari, S., & Piazza, P. V. (1996). Behavioral reactivity to novelty during youth as a predictive factor of stress-induced corticosterone secretion in the elderly: A life-span study in rats. *Psychoneuroendocrinology, 21*(5), 441–453.

Demakis, G. J. (2003). A meta-analytic review of the sensitivity of the Wisconsin Card Sorting Test to frontal and lateralized frontal brain damage. *Neuropsychology, 17*, 255–264.

Dembiec, J., LeDoux, J., Shiromani, P. J., Keane, T. M., & LeDoux, J. E. (2009). The amygdala and the neural pathways of fear. In P. J. Shiromani, T. M. Keane, & J. E. LeDoux (Eds.), *Post-traumatic stress disorder: Basic science and clinical practice* (pp. 23–38). Totowa, NJ: Humana Press.

Denburg, N. L., Buchanan, T. W., Tranel, D., & Adolphs, R. (2003). Evidence for preserved emotional memory in normal older persons. *Emotion, 3*(3), 239–253.

Denburg, N. L., Weller, J. A., Yamada, T. H., Shivapour, D. M., Kaup, A. R., LaLoggia, A., et al. (2009). Poor decision-making among older adults is related to elevated levels of neuroticism. *Annals of Behavioral Medicine, 37*, 164–172.

Dennis, T. A. (2007). Interactions between emotion regulation strategies and affective style: Implications for trait anxiety versus depressed mood. *Motivation and Emotion, 31*(3), 200–207.

Denollet, J., Nyklicek, I., Vingerhoets, A. J., & Vingerhoets, A. (2008). Introduction: Emotions, emotion regulation, and health. In A. J. Vingerhoets, I. Nyklicek, & J. Denollet (Eds.), *Emotion regulation: Conceptual and clinical issues* (pp. 3–11). New York: Springer Science+Business Media.

de Oca, B. M., & Fanselow, M. S. (2004). Amygdala and periaqueductal gray lesions only partially attenuate unconditional defensive reponses in rats exposed to a cat. *Integrative Physiological and Behavioral Science, 39*, 318–333.

Depue, R. A., & Collins, P. F. (1999). Neurobiology of the structure of personality: Dopamine, facilitation of incentive motivation, and extraversion. *Behavioral Brain Science, 22*(3), 491–517.

Derntl, B., Habel, U., Windischberger, C., Robinson, S., Kryspin-Exner, I., Gur, R. C., et al. (2009). General and specific responsiveness of the amygdala during explicit emotion recognition in females and males. *BMC Neuroscience, 10*, 91.

De Tanti, A., Gasperini, G., & Rossini, M. (2005). Paroxysmal episodic hypothalamic instability with hypothermia after traumatic brain injury. *Brain Injury, 19*(14), 1277–1283.

Dettmers, C., Fatepour, D., Faust, H., & Jerusalem, F. (1993). Sympathetic skin response abnormalities in amyotrophic lateral sclerosis. *Muscle and Nerve, 16*, 930–934.

Devinsky, O. (2004). Effects of seizures on autonomic and cardiovascular function. *Epilepsy Currents, 4*, 43–46.

Dew, M. A., Hoch, C. C., Buysse, D. J., Monk, T. H., Begley, A. E., Houck, P. R., et al. (2003). Healthy older adults' sleep predicts all-cause mortality at 4 to 19 years of follow-up. *Psychosomatic Medicine, 65*(1), 63–73.

DeYoung, C. G., Peterson, J. B., & Higgins, D. M. (2005). Sources of openness/intellect: Cognitive and neuropsychological correlates of the fifth factor of personality. *Journal of Personality, 73*(4), 825–858.

Diamond, A., Briand, L., Fossella, J., & Gehlbach, L. (2004). Genetic and neurochemical modulation of prefrontal cognitive functions in children. *American Journal of Psychiatry, 161(1), 125–132.*

Diamond, B. J., Johnson, S. K., Kaufman, M., & Graves, L. (2008). Relationships between information processing, depression, fatigue and cognition in multiple sclerosis. *Archives of Clinical Neuropsychology, 23*(2), 189–199.

Diaz, M. T., & McCarthy, G. (2007). Unconscious word processing engages a distributed network of brain regions. *Journal of Cognitive Neuroscience, 19*(11), 1768–1775.

Di Chiara, G., & Tanda, G. (1997). Blunting of reactivity of dopamine transmission to palatable food: A biochemical marker of anhedonia in the CMS model? *Psychopharmacology, 134*(4), 351–353.

Diehl-Schmid, J., Pohl, C., Ruprecht, C., Wagenpfeil, S., Foerstl, H., & Kurz, A. (2007). The Ekman 60 Faces Test as a diagnostic instrument in frontotemporal dementia. *Archives of Clinical Neuropsychology, 22*(4), 459–464.

Dietl, T., Herr, A., Brunner, H., & Friess, E. (2003). Capgras syndrome: Out of sight, out of mind? *Acta Psychiatrica Scandinavica, 108*(6), 460–463.

Dietrich, S., Hertrich, I., Alter, K., lschebeck, A., & Ackermann, H. (2008). Understanding the emotional expression of verbal interjections: A functional MRI study. *NeuroReport, 19*(18), 1751–1755.

DiGirolamo, G. J., Kramer, A. F., Barad, V., Cepeda, N. J., Weissman, D. H., Milham, M. P., et al. (2001). General and task-specific frontal lobe recruitment in older adults during executive processes: A fMRI investigation of task-switching. *NeuroReport, 12*, 2065–2071.

Digman, J. M. (1990). Personality structure: Emergence of the five-factor model. *Annual Review of Psychology, 41*, 417–440.

Dillon, D. G., Holmes, A. J., Jahn, A. L., Bogdan, R., Wald, L. L., & Pizzagalli, D. A. (2008). Dissociation of neural regions associated with anticipatory versus consummatory phases of incentive processing. *Psychophysiology, 45*(1), 36–49.

Dimitrovsky, L., Spector, H., & Levy-Shiff, R. (2000). Stimulus gender and emotional difficulty level: Their effect on recognition of facial expressions of affect in children with and without LD. *Journal of Learning Disabilities, 33*(5), 410–416.

Dimitrovsky, L., Spector, H., Levy-Shiff, R., & Vakil, E. (1998). Interpretation of facial expressions of affect in children with learning disabilities with verbal or nonverbal deficits. *Journal of Learning Disabilities, 31*(3), 286–292.

Doby, T. (1992). Cerebral angiography and Egas Moniz. *Americal Journal of Radiology, 159*, 364.

Docherty, A. R., & Sponheim, S. R. (2008). Anhedonia as a phenotype for the Val-158Met COMT polymorphism in relatives of patients with schizophrenia. *Journal of Abnormal Psychology, 117*(4), 788–798.

Doherty, R. W. (1997). The Emotional Contagion Scale: A measure of individual differences. *Journal of Nonverbal Behavior, 21*(2), 131–154.

Dolan, M. C., & Fullam, R. (2006). Face affect recognition deficits in personality-disordered offenders: Association with psychopathy. *Psychological Medicine, 36*(11), 1563–1569.

Dolan, M.C., & Fullam, R. (2010). Emotional memory and psychopathic traits in conduct disordered adolescents. *Personality and Individual Differences, 48*(3), 327–331.

Dorion, A. A., Capron, C., & Duyme, M. (2001). Measurement of the corpus callosum using magnetic resonance imaging: Analysis of methods and techniques. *Perceptual and Motor Skills, 92*(32), 1075–1094.

Dove, A., Pollmann, S., Schubert, T., Wiggins, C. J., & von Cramon, D. Y. (2000). Prefrontal cortex activation in task switching: An event-related fMRI study., *Cognitive Brain Research, 9*, 103–109.

Dreher, J.-C., & Grafman, J. (2003). Dissociating the roles of the rostral anterior cingulate and the lateral prefrontal cortices in performing two tasks simultaneously or successively. *Cerebral Cortex, 13*, 329–339.

Dreisbach, G., & Goschke, T. (2004). How positive affect modulates cognitive control: Reduced perseveration at the cost of increased distractibility. *Journal of Experimental Psychology: Learning, Memory, and Cognition, 30*(2), 343–353.

Drevets, W. C., Price, J. L., & Furey, M. L. (2008). Brain structural and functional abnormalities in mood disorders: Implications for neurocircuitry models of depression. *Brain Structure and Function, 213*(1), 93–118.

Dror, O. E. (2001). Techniques of the brain and the paradox of emotions, 1880–1930. *Science in Context, 14*(4), 643–660.

Duchek, J. M., Balota, D. A., Storandt, M., & Larsen, R. (2007). The power of personality in discriminating between healthy aging and early-stage Alzheimer's disease. *Journals of Gerontology: Series B: Psychological Sciences and Social Sciences, 62B*(6), P353–P361.

Duchenne, G. (1990). *The mechanism of human facial expression*. New York: Cambridge University Press. (Original work published 1862)

Duffy, J. D., Campbell, J. J., III, Salloway, S. P., & Malloy, P. F. (2001). Regional prefrontal syndromes: A theoretical and clinical overview. In S. P. Salloway, P. F. Malloy, & J. D. Duffy (Eds.), *The frontal lobes and neuropsychiatric illness* (pp. 113–123). Arlington, VA: American Psychiatric Publishing.

Dujardin, K., Blairy, S., Defebvre, L., Duhem, S. P., Noel, Y., Hess, U., et al. (2004). Deficits in decoding emotional facial expressions in Parkinson's disease. *Neuropsychologia, 42*(2), 239–250.

Dukewich, T. L., Borkowski, J. G., & Whitman, T. L. (1999). A longitudinal analysis of maternal abuse potential and developmental delays in children of adolescent mothers. *Child Abuse and Neglect, 23*(5), 405–420.

Dunn, B. D., Dalgleish, T., & Lawrence, A. D. (2006). The somatic marker hypothesis: A critical evaluation. *Neuroscience and Biobehavioral Reviews, 30*(2), 239–271.

Dusser de Barenne, J. G. (1915). Experimental researchers on sensory localization in the cerebral cortex. *Quarterly Journal of Experimental Physiology, 9*, 355–390.

Dutton, D. G., & Aron, A. P. (1974). Some evidence for heightened sexual attraction under conditions of high anxiety. *Journal of Personality and Social Psychology, 30*(4), 510–517.

Dux, M. C., Woodard, J. L., Calamari, J. E., Messina, M., Arora, S., Chik, H., et al. (2008). The moderating role of negative affect on objective verbal memory performance and subjective memory complaints in healthy older adults. *Journal of the International Neuropsychological Society, 14*(2), 327–336.

Dvir, Y., & Smallwood, P. (2008). Serotonin syndrome: A complex but easily avoidable condition. *General Hospital Psychiatry, 30*(3), 284–287.

Dziobek, I., Rogers, K., Fleck, S., Bahnemann, M., Heekeren, H. R., Wolf, O. T., et al. (2008). Dissociation of cognitive and emotional empathy in adults with Asperger syndrome using the Multifaceted Empathy Test (MET). *Journal of Autism and Developmental Disorders, 38*(3), 464–473.

Edelstyn, N. M. J., & Oyebode, F. (1999). A review of the phenomenology and cognitive neuropsychological origins of the Capgras syndrome. *International Journal of Geriatric Psychiatry, 14*(1), 48–59.

Edelstyn, N. M. J., Oyebode, F., & Barrett, K. (2001). The delusions of Capgras and intermetamorphosis in a patient with right-hemisphere white-matter pathology. *Psychopathology, 34*(6), 299–304.

Edmonds, B. K., & Edwards, G. L. (1998). Dorsomedial hindbrain participation in glucoprivic feeding response to 2DG but not 2DG-induced hyperglycemia or activation of the HPA axis. *Brain Research, 801*(1), 21–28.

Egeland, J., Lund, A., Landro, N. I., Rund, B. R., Sundet, K., Asbjornsen, A., et al. (2005). Cortisol level predicts executive and memory function in depression, symptom level predicts psychomotor speed. *Acta Psychiatrica Scandinavica, 112*(6), 434–441.

Egloff, B., Schmukle, S. C., Burns, L. R., & Schwerdtfeger, A. (2006). Spontaneous emotion regulation during evaluated speaking tasks: Associations with negative affect, anxiety expression, memory, and physiological responding. *Emotion, 6*(3), 356–366.

Ekman, P. (2009). *Telling lies: Clues to deceit in the marketplace, politics, and marriage.* New York: Norton.

Ekman, P., Hager, J. C., & Friesen, W. V. (1981). The symmetry of emotional and deliberate facial actions. *Psychophysiology, 18*(2), 101–106.

Ellen, S. R., Judd, F. K., Mijch, A. M., & Cockram, A. (1999). Secondary mania in patients with HIV infection. *Australian and New Zealand Journal of Psychiatry, 33*(3), 353–360.

Elliott, R., Dolan, R. J., & Frith, C. D. (2000). Dissociable functions in the medial and lateral orbitofrontal cortex: Evidence from human neuroimaging studies. *Cerebral Cortex, 10*(3), 308–317.

Ellis, A. (1985). Cognition and affect in emotional disturbance. *American Psychologist, 40*(4), 471–472.

Ellis, H. D., Lewis, M. B., Moselhy, H. F., & Young, A. W. (2000). Automatic without autonomic responses to familiar faces: Differential components of covert face recognition in a case of Capgras delusion. *Cognitive Neuropsychiatry, 5*(4), 255–269.

Ellis, H. D., & Young, A. W. (1990). Accounting for delusional misidentifications. *British Journal of Psychiatry, 157*, 239–248.

Ellsworth, P. C. (1994). William James and emotion: Is a century of fame worth a century of misunderstanding? *Psychological Review, 101*(2), 222–229.

El-Mallakh, R. S., Shrader, S. A., & Widger, E. (1987). Mania as a manifestation of end-stage renal disease. *Journal of Nervous and Mental Disease, 175*(4), 243–245.

Elmquist, J., Zigman, J., Lutter, M., & Tamminga, C. A. (2006). Molecular determinants of energy homeostasis. *American Journal of Psychiatry, 163*(7), 1137–1137.

Engelborghs, S., Maertens, K., Nagels, G., Vloeberghs, E., Marien, P., Symons, A., et al. (2005). Neuropsychiatric symptoms of dementia: Cross-sectional analysis from a prospective, longitudinal Belgian study. *International Journal of Geriatric Psychiatry, 20*(11), 1028–1037.

Engelen, U., De Peuter, S., Victoir, A., Van Diest, I., & Van Den Bergh, O. (2006). Verdere validering van de Positive and Negative Affect Schedule (PANAS) en vergelijking van twee Nederlandstalige versies [Further validation of the Positive and Negative Affect Schedule (PANAS) and comparison of two Dutch versions]. *Gedrag & Gezondheid: Tijdschrift voor Psychologie en Gezondheid, 34*(2), 89–102.

Ennis, R. H. (1987). A taxonomy of critical thinking dispositions and abilities. In J. B. Baron & R. J. Sternberg (Eds.), *Teaching thinking skills: Theory and practice* (pp. 9–26). New York: Freeman.

Erciyas, A. H., Topalkara, K., Topaktas, S., Akyuz, A., & Dener, S. (1999). Suppression of cardiac parasympathetic functions in patients with right hemisphere stroke. *European Journal of Neurology, 6*(6), 685–690.

Eren, I., Civi, I., & Yildiz, M. (2005). Capgras sendromunda frontopariyetal hipoperfuezyon: Olgu sunumu ve goezden gecirme [Frontoparietal hypoperfusion in Capgras syndrome: A case report and review]. *Tuerk Psikiyatri Dergisi, 16*(4), 284–290.

Ernst, H., Key, J. D., & Koval, M. S. (1999). Alexithymia in an adolescent with agenesis of the corpus callosum and chronic pain. *Journal of the American Academy of Child and Adolescent Psychiatry, 38*(10), 1212–1213.

Eslinger, P. J., Grattan, L. M., & Geder, L. (1996). Neurologic and neuropsychiatric aspects of frontal lobe impairments in postconcussive syndrome. In M. Rizzo & D. Tranel (Eds.), *Head injury and postconcussive syndrome* (pp. 415–440). New York: Churchill Livingstone.

Etkin, A., & Wager, T. D. (2007). Functional neuroimaging of anxiety: A meta-analysis of emotional processing in PTSD, social anxiety disorder, and specific phobia. *American Journal of Psychiatry, 164*(10), 1476–1488.

Evans, D. E., & Rothbart, M. K. (2007). Development of a model for adult temperament. *Journal of Research in Personality, 41*(4), 868–888.

Everitt, B. J., Cardinal, R. N., Parkinsons, J. A., & Robbins, T. W. (2003). Appetitive behavior: Impact of amydgala-dependent mechanisms of emotional learning. *Annals of the New York Academy of Sciences, 985*, 233–250.

Evren, C., Evren, B., & Dalbudak, E. (2009). Alexithymia and personality dimensions in relation to depression and anxiety in male alcohol-dependent inpatients. *International Journal of Psychiatry in Clinical Practice, 13*(1), 3–10.

Extremera, N., & Fernandez-Berrocal, P. (2002). Relation of perceived emotional intelligence and health-related quality of life of middle-aged women. *Psychological Reports, 91*(1), 47–59.

Eysenck, H. J., & Eysenck, M. W. (1958). *Personality and individual differences*. New York: Plenum Press.

Ezzat, S., Asa, S. L., Couldwell, W. T., Barr, C. E., Dodge, W. E., Vance, M. L., et al. (2004). The prevalence of pituitary adenomas: A systematic review. *Cancer, 101*(3), 613–619.

Faerden, A., Nesvag, R., Barrett, E. A., Agartz, I., Finset, A., Friis, S., et al. (2008). Assessing apathy: The use of the Apathy Evaluation Scale in first episode psychosis. *European Psychiatry, 23*(1), 33–39.

Fairchild, G., van Goozen, S. H. M., Stollery, S. J., Aitken, M. R. F., Savage, J., Moore, S. C., et al. (2009). Decision making and executive function in male adolescents with early-onset or adolescence-onset conduct disorder and control subjects. *Biological Psychiatry, 66*(2), 162–168.

Falkenbach, D., Poythress, N., & Creevy, C. (2008). The exploration of subclinical psychopathic subtypes and the relationship with types of aggression. *Personality and Individual Differences, 44*(4), 821–832.

Fan, J., Fossella, J., Sommer, T., Wu, Y., & Posner, M. I. (2003). Mapping genetic variation of executive attention onto brain activity. *Proceedings of the National Academy of Sciences of the United States of America, 100*(12), 7406–7411.

Fan, J., Wu, Y., Fossella, J. A., & Posner, M. I. (2001). Assessing the heritability of attentional networks. *BMC Neuroscience, 2*, 14–20.

Fann, J. R., Burington, B., Leonetti, A., Jaffe, K., Katon, W. J., & Thompson, R. S. (2004). Psychiatric illness following traumatic brain injury in an adult health maintenance organization population. *Archives of General Psychiatry, 61*(1), 53–63.

Farsides, T., & Woodfield, R. (2003). Individual differences and undergraduate academic success: The roles of personality, intelligence, and application. *Personality and Individual Differences, 34*(7), 1225–1243.

Fassbender, K., Schmidt, R., Moesssner, R., Kischka, U., Kuehnen, J., Schwartz, A., et al. (1998). Mood disorders and dysfunction of the hypothalamic–pituitary–adrenal axis in multiple sclerosis: Association with cerebral inflammation. *Archives of Neurology, 55*(1), 66–72.

Faure, A., Reynolds, S. M., Richard, J. M., & Berridge, K. C. (2008). Mesolimbic dopamine in desire and dread: Enabling motivation to be generated by localized glutamate disruptions in nucleus accumbens. *Journal of Neuroscience, 28*, 7184–7192.

Fawcett, J., Clark, D. C., Scheftner, W. A., & Gibbons, R. D. (1983). Assessing anhedonia in psychiatric patients: The Pleasure Scale. *Archives of General Psychiatry, 40*(1), 79–84.

Fawcett, J., Clark, D. C., Scheftner, W. A., & Hedeker, D. (1983). Differences between anhedonic and normally hedonic depressive states. *American Journal of Psychiatry, 140*(8), 1027–1030.

Feinstein, A., Roy, P., Lobaugh, N., Feinstein, K., O'Connor, P., & Black, S. (2004). Structural brain abnormalities in multiple sclerosis patients with major depression. *Neurology, 62*(4), 586–590.

Fellows, L. K., & Farah, M. J. (2005). Different underlying impairments in decision-making following ventromedial and dorsolateral frontal lobe damage in humans. *Cerebral Cortex, 15*(1), 58–63.

Fenn, D., & George, K. (1999). Post-stroke mania late in life involving the left hemisphere. *Australian and New Zealand Journal of Psychiatry, 33*(4), 598–600.

Fernandez-Duque, D., & Black, S. E. (2005). Impaired recognition of negative facial emotions in patients with frontotemporal dementia. *Neuropsychologia, 43*(11), 1673–1687.

Ferrier, D. (1878). The Goulstonian lecture on the localization of cerebral diseases. *British Medical Journal, 1*, 443–447.

Fertuck, E. A., Lenzenweger, M. F., & Clarkin, J. F. (2005). The association between attentional and executive controls in the expression of borderline personality disorder features: A preliminary study. *Psychopathology, 38*(2), 75–81.

Fibiger, H. C., & Phillips, A. G. (1988). Mesocorticolimbic dopamine systems and reward. *Annals of the New York Academy of Sciences, 537*, 206–215.

Finch, C. E., Seeman, T. E., Bengtson, V. L., & Schaie, K. W. (1999). Stress theories of aging. In V. L. Bengtson, D. Gans, N. M. Putney, & M. Silverstein (Eds.), *Handbook of theories of aging* (pp. 81–97). New York: Springer.

Fischer, A. R., & Good, G. E. (1997). Men and psychotherapy: An investigation of alexithymia, intimacy, and masculine gender roles. *Psychotherapy: Theory, Research, Practice, Training, 34*(2), 160–170.

Fischman, M. W., & Foltin, R. W. (1992). Self-administration of cocaine by humans: A laboratory perspective. In *Cocaine: Scientific and social dimensions* (CIBA Foundation Symposium, No. 166, pp. 165–173). Oxford, UK: Wiley.

Fischman, M. W., Sudakov, K. V., Ganten, D., & Nikolov, N. A. (1989). Measuring subjective effects in humans: Changes in moods and feeling states after drug administration. In *Emotions and behavior: A systems approach* (pp. 117–135). Amsterdam: Gordon & Breach.

Fish, B., & Kendler, K. S. (2005). Abnormal infant neurodevelopment predicts schizophrenia spectrum disorders. *Journal of Child and Adolescent Psychopharmacology, 15*(3), 348–361.

Fitzgerald, M., & Molyneux, G. (2004). Overlap between alexithymia and Asperger's syndrome. *American Journal of Psychiatry, 161*(11), 2134–2135.

Flachenecker, P., Rufer, A., Bihler, I., Hippel, C., Reiners, K., Toyka, K. V., et al. (2003). Fatigue in MS is related to sympathetic vasomotor dysfunction. *Neurology, 61*(6), 851–853.

Flory, J. D., Harvey, P. D., Mitropoulou, V., New, A. S., Silverman, J. M., Siever, L. J., et al. (2006). Dispositional impulsivity in normal and abnormal samples. *Journal of Psychiatry Research, 40*(5), 438–447.

Flykt, A. (2006). Preparedness for action: Responding to the snake in the grass. *American Journal of Psychology, 119*(1), 29–43.

Flykt, A., & Caldara, R. (2006). Tracking fear in snake and spider fearful participants during visual search: A multi-response domain study. *Cognition and Emotion, 20*(8), 1075–1091.

Fogarasi, A. S., Janszky, J. Z., & Tuxhorn, I. (2006). Autonomic symptoms during childhood partial epileptic seizures. *Epilepsia, 47*(3), 584–588.

Foisy, M.-L., Philippot, P., Verbanck, P., Pelc, I., Van Der Straten, G., & Kornreich, C. (2005). Emotional facial expression decoding impairment in persons dependent on multiple substances: Impact of a history of alcohol dependence. *Journal of Studies on Alcohol, 66*(5), 673–681.

Folkow, B. (1993). Physiological organization of neurohormonal responses to psychosocial stimuli: Implications for health and disease. *Annals of Behavioral Medicine, 15*, 226–234.

Fontana, A., & McLaughlin, M. (1998). Coping and appraisal of daily stressors predict heart rate and blood pressure levels in young women. *Behavioral Medicine, 24*(1), 5–16.

Ford, J. M., Pfefferbaum, A., Tinklenberg, J. R., & Kopell, B. S. (1982). Effects of perceptual and cognitive difficulty on P3 and RT in young and old adults. *Electroencephalography and Clinical Neurophysiology, 54*(3), 311–321.

Forgas, J. P. (1998). On being happy and mistaken: Mood effects on the fundamental attribution error. *Journal of Personality and Social Psychology, 75*(2), 318–331.

Forgas, J. P., & Cromer, M. (2004). On being sad and evasive: Affective influences on verbal communication strategies in conflict situations. *Journal of Experimental Social Psychology, 40*(4), 511–518.

Forgas, J. P., & East, R. (2008a). How real is that smile?: Mood effects on accepting or rejecting the veracity of emotional facial expressions. *Journal of Nonverbal Behavior, 32*(3), 157–170.

Forgas, J. P., & East, R. (2008b). On being happy and gullible: Mood effects on skepticism and the detection of deception. *Journal of Experimental Social Psychology, 44*(5), 1362–1367.

Forgas, J. P., Laham, S. M., & Vargas, P. T. (2005). Mood effects on eyewitness memory: Affective influences on susceptibility to misinformation. *Journal of Experimental Social Psychology, 41*(6), 574–588.

Forrest, B. J. (2004). The utility of math difficulties, internalized psychopathology, and visual–spatial deficits to identify children with the nonverbal learning disability syndrome: Evidence for a visualspatial disability. *Child Neuropsychology, 10*(2), 129–146.

Fossella, J., Posner, M. I., Fan, J., Swanson, J. M., & Pfaff, D. W. (2002). Attentional phenotypes for the analysis of higher mental functions. *Scientific World Journal, 2*, 217–223.

Frank, J. E., & Tomaz, C. (2000). Enhancement of declarative memory associated with emotional content in a Brazilian sample. *Brazilian Journal of Medical and Biological Research, 33*(12), 1483–1489.

Franken, I. H. A., & Muris, P. (2005a). Individual differences in decision-making. *Personality and Individual Differences, 39*(5), 991–998.

Franken, I. H. A., & Muris, P. (2005b). Individual differences in reward sensitivity are related to food craving and relative body weight in healthy women. *Appetite, 45*(2), 198–201.

Franken, I. H. A., Muris, P., & Rassin, E. (2005). Psychometric properties of the Dutch BIS/BAS scales. *Journal of Psychopathology and Behavioral Assessment, 27*(1), 25–30.

Franken, I. H. A., Rassin, E., & Muris, P. (2007). The assessment of anhedonia in clinical and non-clinical populations: Further validation of the Snaith–Hamilton Pleasure Scale (SHAPS). *Journal of Affective Disorders, 99*(1–3), 83–89.

Fredrikson, M., Furmark, T., Olsson, M. T., Fischer, H., Andersson, J., & Langstroem, B. (1998). Functional neuroanatomical correlates of electrodermal activity: A positron emission tomographic study. *Psychophysiology, 35*(2), 179–185.

Freeman, W., & Watts, J. W. (1939). An interpretation of the functions of the frontal lobe. *Yale Journal of Biology and Medicine, 11*, 527–539.

Freeman, W., & Watts, J. W. (1942a). Prefrontal lobotomy: The surgical relief of mental pain. *Bulletin of the New York Academy of Medicine, 18*, 794–812.

Freeman, W., & Watts, J. W. (1942b). *Psychosurgery.* Oxford, UK: Charles C. Thomas.

Freeman, W., & Watts, J. W. (1948). Psychosurgery. In E. A. Spiegel (Ed.), *Progress in neurology and psychiatry 1948* (pp. 409–420). Oxford, UK: Grune & Stratton.

Frey, S., Kostopoulos, P., & Petrides, M. (2000). Orbitofrontal involvement in the processing of unpleasant auditory information. *European Journal of Neuroscience, 12*(10), 3709–3712.

Frieboes, R.-M., Mueller, U., Murck, H., von Cramon, D. Y., Holsboer, F., & Steiger, A. (1999). Nocturnal hormone secretion and the sleep EEG in patients several months after traumatic brain injury. *Journal of Neuropsychiatry and Clinical Neurosciences, 11*(3), 354–360.

Friedman, N. P., Miyake, A., Young, S. E., Defries, J. C., Corley, R. P., & Hewitt, J. K.

(2008). Individual differences in executive functions are almost entirely genetic in origin. *Journal of Experimental Psychology: General, 137*(2), 201–225.

Fritsch, G., & Hitzig, E. (1870). Electric excitability of the cerebrum. *Archive fur Anatomie, Physiologie und Wissenschaftliche Medizine, 37*, 300–332.

Fuchs, R. A., Ramirez, D. R., & Bell, G. H. (2008). Nucleus accumbens shell and core involvement in drug context-induced reinstatement of cocaine seeking in rats. *Psychopharmacology, 200*(4), 545–556.

Fujiwara, E., Schwartz, M. L., Gao, F., Black, S. E., & Levine, B. (2008). Ventral frontal cortex functions and quantified MRI in traumatic brain injury. *Neuropsychologia, 46*(2), 461–474.

Fukunishi, I., Kawamura, N., Ishikawa, T., & Ago, Y. (1997). Mothers' low care in the development of alexithymia: A preliminary study in Japanese college students. *Psychological Reports, 80*(1), 143–146.

Fukunishi, I., & Tsurata, T. (2001). Alexithymic characteristics in children with refractory hematological diseases. *Psychosomatics: Journal of Consultation Liaison Psychiatry, 42*(3), 276–277.

Funayama, E. S., Grillon, C., Davis, M., & Phelps, E. A. (2001). A double dissociation in the affective modulation of startle in humans: Effects of unilateral temporal lobectomy. *Journal of Cognitive Neuroscience, 13*, 721–729.

Gafoor, R., & O'Keane, V. (2003). Three case reports of secondary mania: Evidence supporting a right frontotemporal locus. *European Psychiatry, 18*(1), 32–33.

Gainotti, G. (1972). Emotional behavior and hemispheric side of lesion. *Cortex, 8*, 41–45.

Gainotti, G. (2001). Components and levels of emotion disrupted in patients with unilateral brain damage. In G. Gainotti (Ed.), *Emotional behavior and its disorders* (2nd ed., pp. 161–179). New York: Elsevier.

Gallagher, E. N., & Vella-Brodrick, D. A. (2008). Social support and emotional intelligence as predictors of subjective well-being. *Personality and Individual Differences, 44*(7), 1551–1561.

Gallagher, H. L., & Frith, C. D. (2003). Functional imaging of "theory of mind." *Trends in Cognitive Sciences, 7*(2), 77–83.

Gallinat, J., Bajbouj, M., Sander, T., Schlattmann, P., Xu, K., Ferro, E. F., et al. (2003). Association of the G1947A COMT (Val(108/158)Met) gene polymorphism with prefrontal P300 during information processing. *Biological Psychiatry, 54*(1), 40–48.

Galvin, J. E., Malcom, H., Johnson, D., & Morris, J. C. (2007). Personality traits distinguishing dementia with Lewy bodies from Alzheimer's disease. *Neurology, 68*(22), 1895–1901.

Garcia, J. A. (1951). Theorie affective des hallucinations; recherches sur la fonction catathymique dans la genese des erreurs psychosensorielles [Affective theory of hallucinations; researches on the catathymic function in the genesis of psychosensory errors]. *Annales Medico-Psychologiques, 109*, 170–194.

Garcia-Sanchez, C., Estevez-Gonzalez, A., Suarez-Romero, E., & Junque, C. (1997). Right hemisphere dysfunction in subjects with attention-deficit disorder with and without hyperactivity. *Journal of Child Neurology, 12*(2), 107–115.

Gasbarri, A., Pompili, A., Arnone, B., d'Onofrio, A., Marchetti, A., Tavares, M. C., et al. (2005). Declarative memory retention and emotional stimuli: A study of an Italian sample. *Functional Neurology, 20*(4), 157–162.

Gaudreau, P., Sanchez, X., & Blondin, J.-P. (2006). Positive and negative affective states in a performance-related setting: Testing the factorial structure of the PANAS across two samples of French-Canadian participants. *European Journal of Psychological Assessment, 22*(4), 240–249.

Gaul, C., Jordan, B., Wustmann, T., & Preuss, U. W. (2007). Klüver–Bucy–syndrom beim menschen [Klüver–Bucy syndrome in humans]. *Der Nervenarzt, 78*(7), 821–824.

Gay, M. C., Vrignaud, P., Garitte, C., & Meunier, C. (2010). Predictors of depression in multiple sclerosis patients. *Acta Neurologica Scandinavica, 121*(3), 161–170.

Gellatly, I. R., & Meyer, J. P. (1992). The effects of goal difficulty on physiological arousal, cognition, and task performance. *Journal of Applied Psychology, 77*(5), 694–704.

Genovese, J. E. C., & Wallace, D. (2007). Reward sensitivity and substance abuse in middle school and high school students. *Journal of Genetic Psychology, 168*(4), 465–469.

George, M. S., Kellner, C. H., Bernstein, H., & Goust, J. M. (1994). A magnetic resonance imaging investigation into mood disorders in multiple sclerosis: A pilot study. *Journal of Nervous and Mental Disease, 182*(7), 410–412.

Gerardi-Caulton, G. (2000). Sensitivity to spatial conflict and the development of self-regulation in children 24–36 months of age. *Developmental Science, 3*(4), 397–404.

Germans, M. K., & Kring, A. M. (2000). Hedonic deficit in anhedonia: Support for the role of approach motivation. *Personality and Individual Differences, 28*(4), 659–672.

Gerrards-Hesse, A., Spies, K., & Hesse, F. W. (1994). Experimental inductions of emotional states and their effectiveness: A review. *British Journal of Psychology, 85*(1), 55–78.

Geuze, E., Vermetten, E., & Bremner, J. D. (2005). MR-based in vivo hippocampal volumetrics: 2. Findings in neuropsychiatric disorders. *Molecular Psychiatry, 10*(2), 160–184.

Ghigo, E., Masel, B., Aimaretti, G., Casanueva, F. F., Elovic, E., Stalla, G., et al. (2005). Consensus guidelines on screening for hypopituitarism following traumatic brain injury. *Brain Injury, 19*(9), 711–724.

Giancola, P. R., Martin, C. S., Tarter, R. E., & Pelham, W. E. (1996). Executive cognitive functioning and aggressive behavior in preadolescent boys at high risk for substance abuse/dependence. *Journal of Studies on Alcohol, 57*(4), 352–359.

Giancola, P. R., Moss, H. B., Martin, C. S., Kirisci, L., & Tarter, R. E. (1996). Executive cognitive functioning predicts reactive aggression in boys at high risk for substance abuse: A prospective study. *Alcoholism: Clinical and Experimental Research, 20*(4), 740–744.

Giardino, J., Gonzalez, A., Steiner, M., & Fleming, A. S. (2008). Effects of motherhood on physiological and subjective responses to infant cries in teenage mothers: A comparison with non-mothers and adult. *Hormones and Behavior, 53*(1), 149–158.

Gibson, E. L. (2006). Emotional influences on food choice: Sensory, physiological and psychological pathways. *Physiology and Behavior, 89*(1), 53–61.

Gillespie, C. F., & Nemeroff, C. B. (2007). Corticotropin-releasing factor and the psychobiology of early-life stress. *Current Directions in Psychological Science, 16*(2), 85–89.

Glascher, J., & Adolphs, R. (2003). Processing of the arousal of subliminal and supralimina emotional stimuli by the human amygdala. *Journal of Neuroscience, 23*, 10274–10282.

Glassman, J. N., Dryer, D., & McCartney, J. R. (1986). Complex partial status epilepticus presenting as gelastic seizures: A case report. *General Hospital Psychiatry, 8*, 61–64.

Gloor, P., & Aggleton, J. P. (1992). Role of the amygdala in temporal lobe epilepsy. In J. P. Aggleton (Ed.), *The amygdala: Neurobiological aspects of emotion, memory, and mental dysfunction* (pp. 505–538). New York: Wiley-Liss.

Goberman, A. M., Coelho, C. A., & Robb, M. P. (2005). Prosodic characteristics of parkinsonian speech: The effect of levodopa-based medication. *Journal of Medical Speech–Language Pathology, 13*(1), 51–68.

Goeders, N. E., Lane, J. D., & Smith, J. E. (1984). Self-administration of methionine enkephalin into the nucleus accumbens. *Pharmacology, Biochemistry, and Behavior, 20*(3), 451–455.

Goldin, P. R., McRae, K., Ramel, W., & Gross, J. J. (2008). The neural bases of emotion regulation: Reappraisal and suppression of negative emotion. *Biological Psychiatry, 63*(6), 577–586.

Goldstein, R. Z., Alia-Klein, N., Tomasi, D., Zhang, L., Cottone, L. A., Maloney, T., et al. (2007). Is decreased prefrontal cortical sensitivity to monetary reward associated with impaired motivation and self-control in cocaine addiction? *American Journal of Psychiatry, 164*(1), 43–51.

Goldstein, R. Z., Tomasi, D., Alia-Klein, N., Cottone, L. A., Zhang, L., Telang, F., et al. (2007). Subjective sensitivity to monetary gradients is associated with frontolimbic activation to reward in cocaine abusers. *Drug and Alcohol Dependence, 87*(2), 233–240.

Goltz, F. (1892). Der Hund ohne Grosshirn [Dog without cerebrum]. *Pfluger's Archive, 51*, 570–614.

Gomez, R., Cooper, A., & Gomez, A. (2005). An item response theory analysis of the carver and white (1994) BIS/BAS scales. *Personality and Individual Differences, 39*(6), 1093–1103.

Gordon, N. S. (2003). *The neural basis of joy and sadness: A functional magnetic resonance imaging study of the neuro-affective effects of music, laughter and crying.* Ann Arbor, MI: ProQuest Information & Learning.

Gorelick, P. B., & Ross, E. D. (1987). The aprosodias: Further functional–anatomical evidence for the organisation of affective language in the right hemisphere. *Journal of Neurology, Neurosurgery, and Psychiatry, 50*(5), 553–560.

Gornick, M. C., Addington, A., Shaw, P., Bobb, A. J., Sharp, W., Greenstein, D., et al. (2007). Association of the dopamine receptor D4 (DRD4) Gene 7-repeate allele with children with attention-deficit/hypereactivity disorder (ADHD): An update. *American Journal of Medical Genetics Part B, 144B*, 379–382.

Gorwood, P., Corruble, E., Falissard, B., & Goodwin, G. M. (2008). Toxic effects of depression on brain function: Impairment of delayed recall and the cumulative length of depressive disorder in a large sample of depressed outpatients. *American Journal of Psychiatry, 165*(6), 731–739.

Gosselin, N., Peretz, I., Johnsen, E., & Adolphs, R. (2007). Amygdala damage impairs emotion recognition from music. *Neuropsychologia, 45*(2), 236–244.

Gosselin, P., & Kirouac, G. (1995). Le decodage de prototypes emotionnels faciaux [The decoding of facial emotional prototypes]. *Canadian Journal of Experimental Psychology, 49*(3), 313–329.

Gottfried, J. A., & Dolan, R. J. (2004). Human orbitofrontal cortex mediates extinction learning while accessing conditioned representations of value. *Nature Neuroscience, 7*(10), 1144–1152.

Gottfried, J. A., O'Doherty, J., & Dolan, R. J. (2003). Encoding predictive reward value in human amygdala and orbitofrontal cortex. *Science, 301*, 1104–1107.

Gould, S. L., & Hyer, L. A. (2004). Dementia and behavioral disturbance: Does premorbid personality really matter? *Psychological Reports, 95*(3, Pt. 2), 1072–1078.

Goyal, R., Sameer, M., & Chandrasekaran, R. (2006). Mania secondary to right-sided stroke: Responsive to olanzapine. *General Hospital Psychiatry, 28*(3), 262–263.

Grabe, H. J., Moeller, B., Willert, C., Spitzer, C., Rizos, T., & Freyberger, H. J. (2004). Interhemispheric transfer in alexithymia: A transcallosal inhibition study. *Psychotherapy and Psychosomatics, 73*(2), 117–123.

Grabe, H. J., Ruhrmann, S., Ettelt, S., Mueller, A., Buhtz, F., Hochrein, A., et al. (2006). Alexithymia in obsessive–compulsive disorder: Results from a family study. *Psychotherapy and Psychosomatics, 75*(5), 312–318.

Grabenhorst, F., Rolls, E. T., Margot, C., da Silva, M. A., & Velazco, M. I. (2007). How pleasant and unpleasant stimuli combine in different brain regions: Odor mixtures. *Journal of Neuroscience, 27*(49), 13532–13540.

Graham, R., Devinsky, O., & LaBar, K. S. (2007). Quantifying deficits in the perception of fear and anger in morphed facial expressions after bilateral amygdala damage. *Neuropsychologia, 45*(1), 42–54.

Grassi, L., Rossi, E., Sabato, S., Cruciani, G., & Zambelli, M. (2004). Diagnostic criteria for psychosomatic research and psychosocial variables in breast cancer patients. *Psychosomatics: Journal of Consultation Liaison Psychiatry, 45*(6), 483–491.

Grattan, L. M., & Eslinger, P. J. (1989). Higher cognition and social behavior: Changes in cognitive flexibility and empathy after cerebral lesions. *Neuropsychology, 3*(3), 175–185.

Gray, H. M., & Tickle-Degnen, L. (2010). A meta-analysis of performance on emotion recognition tasks in Parkinson's disease. *Neuropsychology, 24*(2), 176–191.

Gray, J. A. (1970). The psychological basis of introversion–extraversion. *Behavior Research and Therapy, 26*, 67–70.

Gray, J. A. (1982). *The neuropsychology of anxiety*. New York: Oxford University Press.

Gray, J. A. (1987). *The psychology of fear and stress* (2nd ed.). Cambridge, UK: Cambridge University Press.

Gray, J. A., Gale, A., & Edwards, J. A. (1986). Anxiety, personality, and the brain. In A. Gale & J. A. Edwards (Eds.), *Physiological correlates of human behaviour: Vol. 3. Individual differences and psychopathology* (pp. 31–43). San Diego, CA: Academic Press.

Gray, J. A., van Goozen, S. H. M., Van de Poll, N. E., & Sergeant, J. A. (1994). Framework for a taxonomy of psychiatric disorder. In S. H. M. van Goozen, N. E. Van De Poll, & J. A. Sargeant (Eds), *Emotions: Essays on emotion theory* (pp. 29–59). Hillsdale, NJ: Erlbaum.

Grigsby, J., Kaye, K., Baxter, J., Shetterly, S. M., & Hamman, R. F. (1998). Executive cognitive abilities and functional status among community-dwelling older persons in the San Luis Valley Health and Aging Study. *Journal of the American Geriatrics Society, 46*(5), 590–596.

Grillon, C. (2008). Models and mechanisms of anxiety: Evidence from startle studies. *Psychopharmacology, 199*(3), 421–437.

Gross, J. J., & John, O. P. (2003). Individual differences in two emotion regulation processes: Implications for affect, relationships, and well-being. *Journal of Personality and Social Psychology, 85*(2), 348–362.

Gross, J. J., Richards, J. M., John, O. P., Snyder, D. K., Simpson, J., & Hughes, J. N. (2006). Emotion regulation in everyday life. In D. K. Snyder, J. A. Simpson, & J. N. Hughes (Eds.), *Emotion regulation in couples and families: Pathways to dysfunction and health* (pp. 13–35). Washington, DC: American Psychological Association.

Gross, J. J., & Thompson, R. A. (2007). Emotion regulation: Conceptual foundations. In J. J. Gross (Ed.), *Handbook of emotion regulation* (pp. 3–24). New York: Guilford Press.

Grossberg, S., Bullock, D., & Dranias, M. R. (2008). Neural dynamics underlying impaired autonomic and conditioned responses following amygdala and orbitofrontal lesions. *Behavioral Neuroscience, 122*(5), 1100–1125.

Gruber, S., Rathgeber, K., Braunig, P., & Gauggel, S. (2007). Stability and course of neuropsychological deficits in manic and depressed bipolar patients compared to patients with major depression. *Journal of Affective Disorders, 104*(1–3), 61–71.

Guang'an, L., Jinfang, L., & Lixin, C. (2004). Early comprehensive–intervention on post-stroke depression. *Chinese Mental Health Journal, 18*(1), 15–17.

Guendel, H., Lopez-Sala, A., Ceballos-Baumann, A. O., Deus, J., Cardoner, N., Marten-Mittag, B., et al. (2004). Alexithymia correlates with the size of the right anterior cingulate. *Psychosomatic Medicine, 66*(1), 132–140.

Guilbaud, O., Loas, G., Corcos, M., Speranza, M., Stephan, P., Perez-Diaz, F., et al. (2002). L'alexithymie dans les conduites de dependance et chez le sujet sain: Valeur en populatino francaise et francophone [Alexithymie in addictive behaviors and in healthy subjects: Results of a study in French speaking subjects]. *Annales Medico-Psychologiques, 160*(1), 77–85.

Gunal, D. I., Afsar, N., Tanridag, T., & Aktan, S. (2002). Autonomic dysfunction in multiple sclerosis: Correlation with disease-related parameters. *European Neurology, 48*(1), 1–5.

Gunning-Dixon, F. M., Gur, R. C., Perkins, A. C., Schroeder, L., Turner, T., Turetsky, B. I., et al. (2003). Aged related differences in brain activation during emotional face processing. *Neurobiology of Aging, 24*(2), 285–295.

Gurrera, R. J., O'Donnell, B. F., Nestor, P. G., Gainski, J., & McCarley, R. W. (2001). The P3 auditory event-related brain potential indexes major personality traits. *Biological Psychiatry, 49*(11), 922–929.

Guttman, H., & Laporte, L. (2002). Alexithymia, empathy, and psychological symptoms in a family context. *Comprehensive Psychiatry, 43*(6), 448–455.

Guyton, A. C., & Hall, J. E. (2005). *Textbook of medical physiology* (11th ed.). San Francisco: Elsevier.

Haaland, K. Y. (2006). Left hemisphere dominance for movement. *Clinical Neuropsychologist, 20*(4), 609–622.

Haas, B. W., Mills, D., Yam, A., Hoeft, F., Bellugi, U., & Reiss, A. (2009). Genetic influences on sociability: Heightened amygdala reactivity and event-related responses to positive social stimuli in Williams syndrome. *Journal of Neuroscience, 29*(4), 1132–1139.

Haas, B. W., Omura, K., Amin, Z., Constable, R. T., & Canli, T. (2006). Functional connectivity with the anterior cingulate is associated with extraversion during the emotional Stroop task. *Social Neuroscience, 1*(1), 16–24.

Haas, B. W., Omura, K., Constable, R. T., & Canli, T. (2007). Emotional conflict and neuroticism: Personality-dependent activation in the amygdala and subgenual anterior cingulate. *Behavioral Neuroscience, 121*(2), 249–256.

Habib, M., Daquin, G. R., Pelletier, J., Montreuil, M., Robichon, F., Zaidel, E., et al. (2003). Alexithymia as a consequence of impaired callosal function: Evidence from multiple sclerosis patients and normal individuals. In E. Zaidel & M. Iacoboni (Eds.), *The parallel brain: The cognitive neuroscience of the corpus callosum* (pp. 415–422). Cambridge, MA: MIT Press.

Hadjikhani, N., & de Gelder, B. (2003). Seeing fearful body expressions activates the fusiform cortex and amygdala. *Current Biology, 13*(24), 2201–2205.

Haga, S. M., Kraft, P. l., & Corby, E.-K. (2009). Emotion regulation: Antecedents and well-being outcomes of cognitive reappraisal and expressive suppression in cross-cultural samples. *Journal of Happiness Studies, 10*(3), 271–291.

Hagan, C. C., Hoeft, F., Mackey, A., Mobbs, D., & Reiss, A. L. (2008). Aberrant neural function during emotion attribution in female subjects with fragile X syndrome. *Journal of the American Academy of Child and Adolescent Psychiatry, 47*(12), 1443–1454.

Hagemann, D., Naumann, E., Becker, G., Maier, S., & Bartussek, D. (1998). Frontal brain asymmetry and affective style: A conceptual replication. *Psychophysiology, 35*(4), 372–388.

Hagerman, P. J., & Hagerman, R. J. (2004). Fragile X–associated tremor/ataxia syndrome (FXTAS). *Mental Retardation and Developmental Disabilities Research Reviews, 10*(1), 25–30.

Hagerman, R., Leehey, M., Heinrichs, W., Tassone, F., Wilson, R., Hills, J., et al. (2001). Intention tremor, parkinsonism, and generalized brain atrophy in male carriers of fragile X. *Neurology, 57*(1), 127–130.

Haller, J. F. (1986). Decline of bloodletting: A study in 19th century ratiocinations. *Southern Medical Journal, 79*, 469–475.

Hama, S., Yamashita, H., Shigenobu, M., Watanabe, A., Kurisu, K., Yamawaki, S., et al. (2007). Post-stroke affective or apathetic depression and lesion location: Left frontal lobe and bilateral basal ganglia. *European Archives of Psychiatry and Clinical Neuroscience, 257*(3), 149–152.

Hamann, S. B., Ely, T. D., Grafton, S. T., & Kilts, C. D. (1999). Amygdala activity related to enhanced memory for pleasant and aversive stimuli. *Nature: Neuroscience, 2*, 289–293.

Hamann, S. B., & Mao, H. (2002). Positive and negative emotional verbal stimuli elicit activity in the left amygdala. *NeuroReport, 13*(1), 15–19.

Hamberg, K., & Lee, J. W. (2005). Biology, gender and behaviour: A critical discussion of the biological models used for explaining cognitive and behavioural gender differences. In A. H. Eagly, A. E. Beall, & R. J. Sternberg (Eds.), *Psychology of gender identity* (2nd ed., pp. 127–144). Hauppauge, NY: Nova Biomedical Books.

Hamm, A. O., Schupp, H. T., & Weike, A. I. (2003). Motivational organization of emotions: Autonomic changes, cortical responses, and reflex modulation. In R. J. Davidson, K. R. Scherer, & H. H. Goldsmith (Eds.), *Handbook of affective sciences* (pp. 187–211). New York: Oxford University Press.

Handel, S. F., Ovitt, L., Spiro, J. R., & Rao, V. (2007). Affective disorder and personality change in a patient with traumatic brain injury. *Psychosomatics: Journal of Consultation Liaison Psychiatry, 48*(1), 67–70.

Hankinson, R. J. (1991). Greek medical models of mind. In S. Everson (Ed.), *Psychology* (pp. 194–217). New York: Cambridge University Press.

Harden, C. L. (2002). Depression and anxiety in epilepsy patients. *Epilepsy and Behavior, 3*(3), 296.

Hariri, A. R., Drabant, E. M., Munoz, K. E., Kolachana, B. S., Mattay, V. S., Egan, M. F., et al. (2005). A susceptibility gene for affective disorders and the response of the human amygdala. *Archives of General Psychiatry, 62(2)*, 146–152.

Hariri, A. R., Mattay, V. S., Tessitore, A., Kolachana, B., Fera, F., Goldman, D., et al. (2002). Serotonin transporter genetic variation and the response of the human amygdala. *Science, 297*, 400–403.

Harkins, P. W., & Riese, W. (1963). *Galen on the passions and errors of the soul.* Columbus: Ohio State University Press.

Harlow, J. M. (1848). Passage of an iron rod through the head. *Boston Medical and Surgical Journal, 20*, 389–393.

Harlow, J. M. (1868). Recovery from the passage of an iron bar through the head. *Publications of the Massachusetts Medical Society, 2*, 327–347.

Harrington, D. L., & Haaland, K. Y. (1991). Hemispheric specialization for motor sequencing: Abnormalities in levels of programming. *Neuropsychologia, 29*(2), 147–163.

Harris, G. T., Rice, M. E., & Cormier, C. A. (1991). Psychopathy and violent recidivism. *Law and Human Behavior, 15*(6), 625–637.

Harvey, P. O., Pruessner, J., Czechowska, Y., & Lepage, M. (2007). Individual differences in trait anhedonia: A structural and functional magnetic resonance imaging study in non-clinical subjects. *Molecular Psychiatry, 12*(8), 767–775.

Harwood, D. G., Barker, W. W., Ownby, R. L., & Duara, R. (1999). Prevalence and correlates of Capgras syndrome in Alzheimer's disease. *International Journal of Geriatric Psychiatry, 14*(6), 415–420.

Hasler, G., Fromm, S., Alvarez, R. P., Luckenbaugh, D. A., Drevets, W. C., & Grillon, C. (2007). Cerebral blood flow in immediate and sustained anxiety. *Journal of Neuroscience, 27*(23), 6313–6319.

Hastings, M. E., Tangney, J. P., & Stuewig, J. (2008). Psychopathy and identification of facial expressions of emotion. *Personality and Individual Differences, 44*(7), 1474–1483.

Hatfield, E., Rapson, R. L., Greco, M., & Stenner, P. (2008). Emotional contagion. In M. Greco & P. Stenner (Eds.), *Emotions: A social science reader* (pp. 443–448). New York: Routledge/Taylor & Francis.

Hawkley, L. C., & Cacioppo, J. T. (2003). Loneliness and pathways to disease. *Brain, Behavior, and Immunity, 17*(Suppl. 1), S98–S105.

Hayano, F., Nakamura, M., Asami, T., Uehara, K., Yoshida, T., Roppongi, T., et al. (2009). Smaller amygdala is associated with anxiety in patients with panic disorder. *Psychiatry and Clinical Neurosciences, 63*(3), 266–276.

Hayes, C. J., Stevenson, R. J., & Coltheart, M. (2007). Disgust and Huntington's disease. *Neuropsychologia, 45*(6), 1135–1151.

Heaton, K. W. (2006). Fails, fits, and fatalities from emotion in Shakespeare's characters: Survey of the canon. *British Medical Journal, 333*, 1335–1338.

Heaton, R. K., Chelune, G. J., Talley, J. L., Kay, G. G., & Curtiss, G. (1993). *Wisconsin Card Sorting Test Manual: Revised and Expanded.* Odessa, FL: Psychological Assessment Resources.

Heck, E. T., & Bryer, J. B. (1986). Superior sorting and categorizing ability in a case of bilateral frontal atrophy: An exception to the rule. *Journal of Clinical and Experimental Neuropsychology, 8*(3), 313–316.

Heilman, K. M., Bowers, D., Speedie, L., & Coslett, H. B. (1984). Comprehension of affective and nonaffective prosody. *Neurology, 34*(7), 917–921.

Heilman, K. M., Leon, S. A., & Rosenbek, J. C. (2004). Affective aprosodia from a medial frontal stroke. *Brain and Language, 89*(3), 411–416.

Heilman, K. M., & Zaidel, D. W. (1994). Emotion and the brain: A distributed modular network mediating emotional experience. In D. W. Zaidel (Ed.), *Neuropsychology* (pp. 139–158). San Diego, CA: Academic Press.

Heilman, R. M., Crisan, L. G., Houser, D., Miclea, M., & Miu, A. C. (2010). Emotion regulation and decision making under risk and uncertainty. *Emotion, 10*(2), 257–265.

Heim, C., Mletzko, T., Purselle, D., Nemeroff, C. B., & Musselman, D. L. (2008). The dexamethasone/corticotropin-releasing factor test in men with major depression: Role of childhood trauma. *Biological Psychiatry, 63*(4), 398–405.

Heim, C., Newport, D. J., Mletzko, T., Nemeroff, C. B., & Miller, A. H. (2008). The link between childhood trauma and depression: Insights from HPA axis studies in humans. *Psychoneuroendocrinology, 33*(6), 693–710.

Heims, H. C., Critchley, H. D., Dolan, R., Mathias, C. J., & Cipolotti, L. (2004). Social and motivational functioning is not critically dependent on feedback of autonomic responses: Neuropsychological evidence from patients with pure autonomic failure. *Neuropsychologia, 42*(14), 1979–1988.

Heinaman, R. (1997). *Plato: Methaphysics and epistemology.* New York: Routledge.

Heine, V. M., Maslam, S., Zareno, J., Joels, M., & Lucassen, P. J. (2004). Suppressed proliferation and apoptotic changes in the rat dentate gyrus after acute and chronic stress are reversible. *European Journal of Neuroscience, 19*(1), 131–144.

Heinz, A., & Smolka, M. N. (2006). The effects of catechol-O-methyltransferase genotype on brain activation elicited by affective stimuli and cognitive tasks. *Reviews in the Neurosciences, 17*(3), 359–367.

Hennenlotter, A., Schroeder, U., Erhard, P., Haslinger, B., Stahl, R., Weindl, A., et al. (2004). Neural correlates associated with impaired disgust processing in presymptomatic Huntington's disease. *Brain: A Journal of Neurology, 127*(6), 1446–1453.

Henriques, J. B., & Davidson, R. J. (1990). Regional brain electrical asymmetries discriminate between previously depressed and healthy control subjects. *Journal of Abnormal Psychology, 99*(1), 22–31.

Henriques, J. B., & Davidson, R. J. (1991). Left frontal hypoactivation in depression. *Journal of Abnormal Psychology, 100*(4), 535–545.

Henry, J. D., Phillips, L. H., Crawford, J. R., Theodorou, G., & Summers, F. (2006). Cognitive and psychosocial correlates of alexithymia following traumatic brain injury. *Neuropsychologia, 44*(1), 62–72.

Henry, J. D., Phillips, L. H., Maylor, E. A., Hosie, J., Milne, A. B., & Meyer, C. (2006). A new conceptualization of alexithymia in the general adult population: Implications for research involving older adults. *Journal of Psychosomatic Research, 60*(5), 535–543.

Henry, J. D., Ruffman, T., McDonald, S., O'Leary, M.-A. P., Phillips, L. H., Brodaty, H., et al. (2008). Recognition of disgust is selectively preserved in Alzheimer's disease. *Neuropsychologia, 46*(5), 1363–1370.

Herbert, B. M., & Pollatos, O. (2008). Interozeptive sensitivitaet, gefuehle und verhaltensregulation [Interoceptive sensitivity, feelings and behavioral control]. *Zeitschrift fuer Neuropsychologie, 19*(3), 125–137.

Hermann, B. P., Seidenberg, M., Haltiner, A., & Wyler, A. R. (1991). Mood state in unilateral temporal lobe epilepsy. *Biological Psychiatry, 30*(12), 1205–1218.

Hernandez, N., Metzger, A., Magne, R., Bonnet-Brilhault, F., Roux, S., Barthelemy, C., et al. (2009). Exploration of core features of a human face by healthy and autistic adults analyzed by visual scanning. *Neuropsychologia, 47*(4), 1004–1012.

Herry, C., Bach, D. R., Esposito, F., Di Salle, F., Perrig, W. J., Scheffler, K., et al. (2007). Processing of temporal unpredictability in human and animal amygdala. *Journal of Neuroscience, 27*(22), 5958–5966.

Herve, H. F., Hayes, P. J., & Hare, R. D. (2003). Psychopathy and sensitivity to the emotional polarity of metaphorical statements. *Personality and Individual Differences, 35*(7), 1497–1507.

Hess, W. R., & Akert, K. (1955). Experimental data on role of hypothalamus in mechanism of emotional behavior. *Archives of Neurology and Psychiatry (Chicago), 73*, 127–129.

Hessl, D., Rivera, S., Koldewyn, K., Cordeiro, L., Adams, J., Tassone, F., et al. (2007). Amygdala dysfunction in men with the fragile X premutation. *Brain: A Journal of Neurology, 130*(2), 404–416.

Hessl, D., Rivera, S. M., & Reiss, A. L. (2004). The neuroanatomy and neuroendocrinology of fragile X syndrome. *Mental Retardation and Developmental Disabilities Research Reviews, 10*(1), 17–24.

Heubeck, B. G., Wilkinson, R. B., & Cologon, J. (1998). A second look at Carver and White's (1994) BIS/BAS scales. *Personality and Individual Differences, 25*(4), 785–800.

Heym, N., Ferguson, E., & Lawrence, C. (2008). An evaluation of the relationship between Gray's revised RST and Eysenck's pen: Distinguishing BIS and FFFS in Carver and White's BIS/BAS scales. *Personality and Individual Differences, 45*(8), 709–715.

Hierons, R., Janota, I., & Corsellis, J. A. (1978). The late effects of necrotizing encephalitis of the temporal lobes and limbic areas: A clinico-pathological study of 10 cases. *Psychological Medicine, 8*(1), 21–42.

Hintikka, J., Honkalampi, K., Lehtonen, J., & Viinamaeki, H. (2001). Are alexithymia and depression distinct or overlapping constructs?: A study in a general population. *Comprehensive Psychiatry, 42*(3), 234–239.

Hiott, D. W., & Labbate, L. (2002). Anxiety disorders associated with traumatic brain injuries. *NeuroRehabilitation, 17*(4), 345–355.

Hoefer, M., Allison, S. C., Schauer, G. F., Neuhaus, J. M., Hall, J., Dang, J. N., et al. (2008). Fear conditioning in frontotemporal lobar degeneration and Alzheimer's disease. *Brain: A Journal of Neurology, 131*(6), 1646–1657.

Hoelzel, B. K., Ott, U., Gard, T., Hempel, H., Weygandt, M., Morgen, K., et al. (2008). Investigation of mindfulness meditation practitioners with voxel-based morphometry. *Social Cognitive and Affective Neuroscience, 3*(1), 55–61.

Hoeschl, C., & Hajek, T. (2001). Hippocampal damage mediated by corticosteroids: A neuropsychiatric research challenge. *European Archives of Psychiatry and Clinical Neuroscience, 251*(8), II81–II88.

Hoffman, J. L. (1949). Clinical observations concerning schizophrenic patients treated by prefrontal leukotomy. *New England Journal of Medicine, 241*, 233–236.

Holland, D. C., Dollinger, S. J., Holland, C. J., & MacDonald, D. A. (1995). The relationship between psychometric intelligence and the five-factor model of personality in a rehabilitation sample. *Journal of Clinical Psychology, 51*(1), 79–88.

Holroyd, C. B., Baker, T. E., Kerns, K. A., & Mueller, U. (2008). Electrophysiological evidence of atypical motivation and reward processing in children with attention-deficit hyperactivity disorder. *Neuropsychologia, 46*(8), 2234–2242.

Honer, W. G., Hurwitz, T., Li, D. K., Palmer, M., & Paty, D. W. (1987). Temporal lobe involvement in multiple sclerosis patients with psychiatric disorders. *Archives of Neurology, 44*(2), 187–190.

Honkalampi, K., Hintikka, J., Laukkanen, E., Lehtonen, J., & Viinamaki, H. (2001). Alexithymia and depression: A prospective study of patients with major depressive disorder. *Psychosomatics: Journal of Consultation Liaison Psychiatry, 42*(3), 229–234.

Honkalampi, K., Koivumaa-Honkanen, H., Lehto, S. M., Hintikka, J., Haatainen, K., Rissanen, T., et al. (2010). Is alexithymia a risk factor for major depression, personality disorder, or alcohol use disorders?: A prospective population-based study. *Journal of Psychosomatic Research, 68*(3), 269–273.

Hook, J. N., Giordani, B., Schteingart, D. E., Guire, K., Giles, J., Ryan, K., et al. (2007). Patterns of cognitive change over time and relationship to age following successful treatment of Cushing's disease. *Journal of the International Neuropsychological Society, 13*(1), 21–29.

Hooker, C. I., Verosky, S. C., Germine, L. T., Knight, R. T., & D'Esposito, M. (2010). Neural activity during social signal perception correlates with self-reported empathy. *Brain Research, 1308*, 100–113.

Hopf, H. C., Fitzek, C., Marx, J., Urban, P. P., & Thoemke, F. (2000). Emotional facial paresis of pontine origin. *Neurology, 54*, 1217.

Hopf, H. C., Mueller-Forell, W., & Hopf, N. J. (1992). Localization of emotional and volitional facial paresis. *Neurology, 42*, 195–201.

Hoptman, M. J., & Davidson, R. J. (1998). Baseline EEG asymmetries and performance on neuropsychological tasks. *Neuropsychologia, 36*(12), 1343–1353.

Horan, W. P., Reise, S. P., Subotnik, K. L., Ventura, J., & Nuechterlein, K. H. (2008). The validity of Psychosis Proneness Scales as vulnerability indicators in recent-onset schizophrenia patients. *Schizophrenia Research, 100*(1–3), 224–236.

Horn, L. J. (1988). Pharmacologic interventions in neuroendocrine disorders following traumatic brain injury: II. Hypothalamic–pituitary disorders. *Journal of Head Trauma Rehabilitation, 3*(3), 86–90.

Hornak, J., Bramham, J., Rolls, E. T., Morris, R. G., O'Doherty, J., Bullock, P. R., et al. (2003). Changes in emotion after circumscribed surgical lesions of the orbitofrontal and cingulate cortices. *Brain: A Journal of Neurology, 126*(7), 1691–1712.

Horner, M. D., Selassie, A. W., Lineberry, L., Ferguson, P. L., & Labbate, L. A. (2008). Predictors of psychological symptoms 1 year after traumatic brain injury: A population-based, epidemiological study. *Journal of Head Trauma Rehabilitation, 23*(2), 74–83.

Howland, E. W., & Newman, J. P. (1993). *The effect of incentives on Wisconsin Card Sorting Task performance in psychopaths.* Unpublished manuscript.

Hubbard, K., & Trauner, D. A. (2007). Intonation and emotion in autistic spectrum disorders. *Journal of Psycholinguistic Research, 36*(2), 159–173.

Huebner, T., Vloet, T. D., Marx, I., Konrad, K., Fink, G. R., Herpertz, S. C., et al. (2008). Morphometric brain abnormalities in boys with conduct disorder. *Journal of the American Academy of Child and Adolescent Psychiatry, 47*(5), 540–547.

Hugdahl, K. (1996). Brain laterality: Beyond the basics. *European Psychologist, 1*(3), 206–220.

Hughes, S. L., Case, H. S., Stuempfle, K. J., & Evans, D. S. (2003). Personality profiles of Iditasport ultra-marathon participants. *Journal of Applied Sport Psychology, 15*(3), 256–261.

Hull, C. L. (1943). *Principles of behavior.* New York: Appleton Century.

Humphreys, K., Minshew, N., Leonard, G. L., & Behrmanna, M. (2007). A fine-grained analysis of facial expression processing in high-functioning adults with autism. *Neuropsychologia, 45*(4), 685–695.

Husain, M. M. (2005). Emotional lability (pseudobulbar affect) in general psychiatry: An introduction. *American Journal of Geriatric Pharmacotherapy, 3*, 3–3.

Iannaccone, S., & Ferini-Strambi, L. (1996). Pharmacologic treatment of emotional lability. *Clinical Neuropharmacology, 19*(6), 532–535.

Infrasca, R. (1997). Alexithymia, neurovegetative arousal and neuroticism: An experimental study. *Psychotherapy and Psychosomatics, 66*(5), 276–280.

Irwin, M. (2002). Effects of sleep and sleep loss on immunity and cytokines. *Brain, Behavior, and Immunity, 16*, 503–512.

Isenschmid, R., & Krehl, L. (1912). Ueber den Einfluss des Gehirns auf die Warmeregulation [About the influence of the brain on temperature regulation]. *Archive fuer Experimentell Pathologie und Pharmakologie, 70*, 109–134.

Ito, R., Robbins, T. W., McNaughton, B. L., & Everitt, B. J. (2006). Selective excitotoxic lesions of the hippocampus and basolateral amygdala have dissociable effects on appetitive cue and place conditioning based on path integration in a novel Y-maze procedure. *European Journal of Neuroscience, 23*(11), 3071–3080.

Izard, C. E. (1971). *The face of emotion.* East Norwalk, CT: Appleton-Century-Crofts.

Izquierdo, A., & Murray, E. A. (2004). Combined unilateral lesions of the amygdala and orbital prefrontal cortex impair affective processing in rhesus monkeys. *Journal of Neurophysiology, 91*(5), 2023–2039.

Izquierdo, A., Suda, R. K., & Murray, E. A. (2005). Comparison of the effects of bilateral orbital prefrontal cortex lesions and amygdala lesions on emotional responses in rhesus monkeys. *Journal of Neuroscience, 25*(37), 8534–8542.

Jaeger, J., Borod, J. C., & Peselow, E. (1986). Facial expression of positive and negative emotions in patients with unipolar depression. *Journal of Affective Disorders, 11*(1), 43–50.

Jaenig, W. (2003). The autonomic nervous system and its coordination by the brain. In R. J. Davidson, K. R. Scherer, & H. H. Goldsmith (Eds.), *Handbook of affective sciences* (pp. 135–186). New York: Oxford University Press.

James, W. (1884). What is an emotion? *Mind, 9*, 188–205.

James, W. (1890). *The principles of psychology.* New York: Holt.

Jamieson, J., Flood, K., & Lavoie, N. (1994). Physical fitness and heart rate recovery from stress. *Canadian Journal of Behavioural Science/Revue Canadienne des Sciences du Comportement, 26*(4), 566–577.

Jang, K. L., Wolf, H., & Larstone, R. (2006). What is the role of personality in psychopathology?: A view from behavior genetics. In R. F. Krueger & J. L. Tackett (Eds.), *Personality and psychopathology* (pp. 153–173). New York: Guilford Press.

Janszky, J., Fogarasi, A., Magalova, V., Tuxhorn, I., & Ebner, A. (2005). Hyperorality in epileptic seizures: Periictal incomplete Kluever–Bucy syndrome. *Epilepsia, 46*(8), 1235–1240.

Jefferson, G. (1949). René Descartes on the localisation of the soul. *Irish Journal of Medical Science, 285*(Ser. 6), 691–706.

Jin, Y., Mai, C., & Ding, K. (2001). A study of alexithymia of hemodialysis patients. *Chinese Journal of Clinical Psychology, 9*(3), 226–227.

Jing, L., & Jiamei, L. (2007). Impacts of different approaches of emotion regulation on memory. *Acta Psychologica Sinica, 39*(6), 1084–1092.

John, O. P., & Gross, J. J. (2004). Healthy and unhealthy emotion regulation: Personality processes, individual differences, and life span development. *Journal of Personality, 72*(6), 1301–1333.

Johns, M., Inzlicht, M., & Schmader, T. (2008). Stereotype threat and executive resource depletion: Examining the influence of emotion regulation. *Journal of Experimental Psychology: General, 137*(4), 691–705.

Johnson, E. O., Roth, T., & Breslau, N. (2006). The association of insomnia with anxiety disorders and depression: Exploration of the direction of risk. *Journal of Psychiatric Research, 40*, 700–708.

Johnson, S. C., Pinkston, J. B., Bigler, E. D., & Blatter, D. D. (1996). Corpus callosum morphology in normal controls and traumatic brain injury: Sex differences, mechanisms of injury, and neuropsychological correlates. *Neuropsychology, 10*(3), 408–415.

Johnstone, T., van Reekum, C. M., Oakes, T. R., & Davidson, R. J. (2006). The voice of emotion: An FMRI study of neural responses to angry and happy vocal expressions. *Social Cognitive and Affective Neuroscience, 1*(3), 242–249.

Jonsdottir, S., Bouma, A., Sergeant, J. A., & Scherder, E. J. A. (2006). Relationships between neuropsychological measures of executive function and behavioral measures of ADHD symptoms and comorbid behavior. *Archives of Clinical Neuropsychology, 21*(5), 383–394.

Jorge, R. E., Robinson, R. G., Arndt, S., & Starkstein, S. (2003). Mortality and poststroke depression: A placebo-controlled trial of antidepressants. *American Journal of Psychiatry, 160*(10), 1823–1829.

Jorge, R. E., Robinson, R. G., Starkstein, S. E., & Arndt, S. V. (1993). Secondary mania following traumatic brain injury. *American Journal of Psychiatry, 150*(6), 916–921.

Jorge, R. E., Robinson, R. G., Tateno, A., Narushima, K., Acion, L., Moser, D., et al. (2004). Repetitive transcranial magnetic stimulation as treatment of poststroke depression: A preliminary study. *Biological Psychiatry, 55*(4), 398–405.

Jorm, A. F., Christensen, H., Henderson, A. S., Jacomb, P. A., Korten, A. E., & Rodgers, B. (1999). Using the BIS/BAS scales to measure behavioural inhibition and behavioural activation: Factor structure, validity, and norms in a large community sample. *Personality and Individual Differences, 26*(1), 49–58.

Josephs, K. A. (2007). Capgras syndrome and its relationship to neurodegenerative disease. *Archives of Neurology, 64*(12), 1762–1766.

Kagan, J. (1988). The meanings of personality predicates. *American Psychologist, 43*(8), 614–620.

Kales, H. C., Maixner, D. F., & Mellow, A. M. (2005). Cerebrovascular disease and late-life depression. *American Journal of Geriatric Psychiatry, 13*(2), 88–98.

Kalin, N. H., Shelton, S. E., & Davidson, R. J. (2004). The role of the central nucleus of the amygdala in mediating fear and anxiety in the primate. *Journal of Neuroscience, 24*(24), 5506–5515.

Kalisch, R., Wiech, K., Herrmann, K., & Dolan, R. J. (2006). Neural correlates of self-distraction from anxiety and a process model of cognitive emotion regulation. *Journal of Cognitive Neuroscience, 18*(8), 1266–1276.

Kan, Y., Kawamura, M., Hasegawa, Y., Mochizuki, S., & Nakamura, K. (2002). Recognition of emotion from facial, prosodic and written verbal stimuli in Parkinson's disease. *Cortex, 38*(4), 623–630.

Kapoor, A., Kostaki, A., Janus, C., & Matthews, S. G. (2009). The effects of prenatal stress on learning in adult offspring is dependent on the timing of the stressor. *Behavioural Brain Research, 197*(1), 144–149.

Kappas, A. (2006). Appraisals are direct, immediate, intuitive, and unwitting ... and some are reflective. *Cognition and Emotion, 20*(7), 952–975.

Karlsson, H., Naaanen, P., & Stenman, H. (2008). Cortical activation in alexithymia as a response to emotional stimuli. *British Journal of Psychiatry, 192*(1), 32–38.

Karow, C. M., Marquardt, T. P., & Marshall, R. C. (2001). Affective processing in left and right hemisphere brain-damaged subjects with and without subcortical involvement. *Aphasiology, 15*(8), 715–729.

Kasari, C., Freeman, S. F. N., & Hughes, M. A. (2001). Emotion recognition by children with Down syndrome. *American Journal on Mental Retardation, 106*(1), 59–72.

Kauhanen, J., Julkunen, J., & Salonen, J. T. (1991). Alexithymia and perceived symptoms: Criterion validity of the Toronto Alexithymia Scale. *Psychotherapy and Psychosomatics, 56*(4), 247–252.

Kauhanen, J., Kaplan, G. A., Cohen, R. D., & Julkunen, J. (1996). Alexithymia and risk of death in middle-aged men. *Journal of Psychosomatic Research, 41*(6), 541–549.

Kawashima, R., Yamada, K., Kinomura, S., Yamaguchi, T., Matsui, H., Yoshioka, S., et al. (1993). Regional cerebral blood flow changes of cortical motor areas and prefrontal areas in humans related to ipsilateral and contralateral hand movement. *Brain Research, 623*(1), 33–40.

Kawashima, S., Nakazawa, T., Kishiro, M., Seki, N., Hihara, H., & Ogura, K. (1999). A case of frontotemporal dementia with paraphilia. *Seishin Igaku (Clinical Psychiatry), 41*(4), 413–416.

Kawata, A. K. (2006). *Measurement invariance of the Positive and Negative Affect Schedule (PANAS) in a community sample of older people.* Ann Arbor, MI: ProQuest Information & Learning.

Kazui, H., Mori, E., Hashimoto, M., Hirono, N., Imamura, T., Tanimukai, S., et al. (2000). Impact of emotion on memory: Controlled study of the influence of emotionally charged material on declarative memory in Alzheimer's disease. *British Journal of Psychiatry, 177*, 343–347.

Keane, J., Calder, A. J., Hodges, J. R., & Young, A. W. (2002). Face and emotion processing in frontal variant frontotemporal dementia. *Neuropsychologia, 40*(6), 655–665.

Keightley, M. L., Chiew, K. S., Winocur, G., & Grady, C. L. (2007). Age-related differences in brain activity underlying identification of emotional expressions in faces. *Social Cognitive and Affective Neuroscience, 2*(4), 292–302.

Keillor, J. M., Barrett, A. M., Crucian, G. P., Kortenkamp, S., & Heilman, K. M. (2002). Emotional experience and perception in the absence of facial feedback. *Journal of the International Neuropsychological Society, 8*(1), 130–135.

Keilp, J. G., Sackeim, H. A., & Mann, J. J. (2005). Correlates of trait impulsiveness in performance measures and neuropsychological tests. *Psychiatry Research, 135*(3), 191–201.

Keller, J., Buckley, T. M., Schatzberg, A. F., Roose, S. P., & Sackeim, H. A. (2004). Hypothalamic–pituitary–adrenal axis activity in mood and cognition in the elderly: Implications for symptoms and outcomes. In S. P. Roose & H. A. Sackeim (Eds.), *Late-life depression* (pp. 157–166). New York: Oxford University Press.

Keltner, D., & Buswell, B. N. (1997). Embarrassment: Its distinct form and appeasement functions. *Psychological Bulletin, 122*(3), 250–270.

Kendall-Tackett, K. (Ed.). (2007). *The psychoneuroimmunology of chronic disease: Exploring the links between inflammation, stress, and illness.* Washington, DC: American Psychological Association.

Kent, J. M., Coplan, J. D., Mawlawi, O., Martinez, J. M., Browne, S. T., Slifstein, M., et al. (2005). Prediction of panic response to a respiratory stimulant by reduced orbitofrontal cerebral blood flow in panic disorder. *American Journal of Psychiatry, 162*(7), 1379–1381.

Kesler, S. R., Garrett, A., Bender, B., Yankowitz, J., Zeng, S. M., & Reiss, A. L. (2004). Amygdala and hippocampal volumes in Turner syndrome: A high-resolution MRI study of X-monosomy. *Neuropsychologia, 42*(14), 1971–1978.

Kessler, R. C., Berglund, P., Demler, O., Jin, R., Koretz, D., Meriknagas, K. R., et al. (2003). The epidemiology of major depressive disorder. *Journal of the American Medical Association, 289*, 3095–3105.

Kessler, R. C., Sonnega, A., Bromet, E., & Hughes, M. (1995). Posttraumatic stress disorder in the National Comorbidity Survey. *Archives of General Psychiatry, 52*(12), 1048–1060.

Khalfa, S. P., Guye, M., Peretz, I., Chapon, F. D. R., Girard, N., Chauvel, P., et al. (2008). Evidence of lateralized anteromedial temporal structure involvement in musical emotion processing. *Neuropsychologia, 46*(10), 2485–2493.

Khan-Bourne, N., & Brown, R. G. (2003). Cognitive behaviour therapy for the treatment of depression in individuals with brain injury. *Neuropsychological Rehabilitation, 13*(1), 89–107.

Kiehl, K. A., Bates, A. T., Laurens, K. R., Hare, R. D., & Liddle, P. F. (2006). Brain potentials implicate temporal lobe abnormalities in criminal psychopaths. *Journal of Abnormal Psychology, 115*(3), 443–453.

Kile, S. J., Ellis, W. G., Olichney, J. M., Farias, S., & DeCarli, C. (2009). Alzheimer abnormalities of the amygdala with Kluever–Bucy syndrome symptoms: An amygdaloid variant of Alzheimer disease. *Archives of Neurology, 66*(1), 125–129.

Kim, J. J., Haller, J., Sulyok, K., Csermely, P., & Korcsmaros, T. (2007). Glucocorticoid hyper- and hypofunction: Stress effects on cognition and aggression. In P. Csermely & T. Korcsmáros (Eds.), *Stress responses in biology and medicine: Stress of life in molecules, organisms, and psychosocial communities* (pp. 291–303). Malden, MA: Blackwell.

Kim, J. S., Choi, E. A., Kwon, S. U., & Seo, Y. S. (2002). Inability to control anger or aggression after stroke. *Neurology, 58*, 1106–1108.

Kim, J. S., & Choi-Kwon, S. (2000). Poststroke depression and emotional incontinence: Correlation with lesion location. *Neurology, 54*(9), 1805–1810.

Kim, S.-E., Kim, J.-W., Kim, J.-J., Jeong, B. S., Choi, E. A., Jeong, Y.-G., et al. (2007). The neural mechanism of imagining facial affective expression. *Brain Research, 1145*, 128–137.

King, C. R., Knutson, K. I., Rathouz, P. J., Sidney, S., Liu, K., & Lauderdale, D. S. (2008). *Journal of the American Medical Association, 300*(24), 2859–2866.

Kinney, D. K., Munir, K. M., Crowley, D. J., & Miller, A. M. (2008). Prenatal stress and risk for autism. *Neuroscience and Biobehavioral Reviews, 32*(8), 1519–1532.

Kinsbourne, M. (1978). *Asymmetrical function of the brain.* Oxford, UK: Cambridge University Press.

Kippin, T. E., Sotiropoulos, V., Badih, J., & Pfaus, J. G. (2004). Opposing roles of the nucleus accumbens and anterior lateral hypothalamic area in the control of sexual behaviour in the male rat. *European Journal of Neuroscience, 19*(3), 698–704.

Kipps, C. M., Nestor, P. J., Acosta-Cabronero, J., Arnold, R., & Hodges, J. R. (2009). Understanding social dysfunction in the behavioural variant of frontotemporal dementia: The role of emotion and sarcasm processing. *Brain: A Journal of Neurology, 132*(3), 592–603.

Kirsch, L. G., & Becker, J. V. (2007). Emotional deficits in psychopathy and sexual sadism: Implications for violent and sadistic behavior. *Clinical Psychology Review, 27*(8), 904–922.

Kirschbaum, C., Klauer, T., Filipp, S.-H., & Hellhammer, D. H. (1995). Sex-specific effects of social support on cortisol and subjective responses to acute pychological stress. *Psychosomatic Medicine, 57*(1), 23–31.

Kirschbaum, C., Pruessner, J. C., Stone, A. A., & Federenko, I. (1995). Persistent high cortisol responses to repeated psychological stress in a subpopulation of healthy men. *Psychosomatic Medicine, 57*(5), 468–474.

Kirsch-Darrow, L., Fernandez, H. F., Marsiske, M., Okun, M. S., & Bowers, D. (2006). Dissociating apathy and depression in Parkinson's disease. *Neurology, 67*(1), 33–38.

Kleen, J. K., Sitomer, M. T., Killeen, P. R., & Conrad, C. D. (2006). Chronic stress impairs spatial memory and motivation for reward without disrupting motor ability and motivation to explore. *Behavioral Neuroscience, 120*(4), 842–851.

Kleinginna, P. R., & Kleinginna, A. M. (1985). Cognition and affect: A reply to Lazarus and Zajonc. *American Psychologist, 40*(4), 470–471.

Kluger, B. M., & Heilman, K. M. (2007). Dysfunctional facial emotional expression and comprehension in a patient with corticobasal degeneration. *Neurocase, 13*(3), 165–168.

Klüver, H., & Bucy, P. C. (1937). "Psychic blindness" and other symptoms following bilateral temporal lobectomy in rhesus monkeys. *American Journal of Physiology, 119*, 352–353.

Klüver, H., & Bucy, P. C. (1938). An analysis of certain effects of bilateral temporal lobectomy in the rhesus monkey, with special reference to "psychic blindness." *Journal of Psychology, 5*, 33–54.

Klüver, H., & Bucy, P. C. (1939). Preliminary analysis of functions of the temporal lobes in monkeys. *Archives of Neurology and Psychiatry (Chicago), 42*, 979–1000.

Knott, J. (1911). Phrenology and its founder: The claims of Franz Joseph Gall on the homage of scientific posterity. *New York Medical Journal, 93*, 305–310, 372–376, 419–423, 470–473.

Knutson, B., Adams, C. M., Fong, G. W., & Hommer, D. (2001). Anticipation of increasing monetary reward selectively recruits nucleus accumbens. *Journal of Neuroscience, 21*(16), RC159.

Knutson, B., Fong, G. W., Adams, C. M., Varner, J. L., & Hommer, D. (2001). Dissociation of reward anticipation and outcome with event-related fMRI. *NeuroReport, 12*(17), 3683–3687.

Knuuttila, S. (2004). *Emotions in ancient and medieval philosophy.* Oxford, UK: Clarendon Press.

Knyazev, G. G., Slobodskaya, H. R., & Wilson, G. D. (2004). Comparison of the construct validity of the Gray–Wilson Personality Questionnaire and the BIS/BAS scales. *Personality and Individual Differences, 37*(8), 1565–1582.

Kochanska, G., Aksan, N., Penney, S. J., & Doobay, A. F. (2007). Early positive emotionality as a heterogeneous trait: Implications for children's self-regulation. *Journal of Personality and Social Psychology, 93*(6), 1054–1066.

Kodounis, A., Stamboulis, E., Constantinidis, T. S., & Liolios, A. (2005). Measurement of autonomic dysregulation in multiple sclerosis. *Acta Neurologica Scandinavica, 112*(6), 403–408.

Koehler, P. J., & Jagella, C. (2002). Constantin von Monakow (1853–1930). *Journal of Neurology, 249*, 115–116.

Konrad, K., Gauggel, S., Manz, A., & Schoell, M. (2000). Lack of inhibition: A motivational deficit in children with attention deficit/hyperactivity disorder and children with traumatic brain injury. *Child Neuropsychology, 6*(4), 286–296.

Koponen, S., Taiminen, T., Honkalampi, K., Joukamaa, M., Viinamaki, H., Kurki, T., et al. (2005). Alexithymia after traumatic brain injury: Its relation to magnetic resonance imaging findings and psychiatric disorders. *Psychosomatic Medicine, 67*(5), 807–812.

Kornreich, C., Blairy, S., Philippot, P., Dan, B., Foisy, M.-L., Hess, U., et al. (2001). Impaired emotional facial expression recognition in alcoholism compared with obsessive–compulsive disorder and normal controls. *Psychiatry Research, 102*(3), 235–248.

Koskinen, S., & Alaranta, H. (2008). Traumatic brain injury in Finland 1991–2005: A nationwide register study of hospitalized and fatal TBI. *Brain Injury, 22*(3), 205–214.

Kosson, D. S., Suchy, Y., Mayer, A. R., & Libby, J. (2002). Facial affect recognition in criminal psychopaths. *Emotion, 2*(4), 398–411.

Kramer, J. H., Quitania, L., Dean, D., Neuhaus, J., Rosen, H. J., Halabi, C., et al. (2007). Magnetic resonance imaging correlates of set shifting. *Journal of the International Neuropsychological Society, 13*(3), 386–392.

Krantz, D. S., & Manuck, S. B. (1984). Acute physiologic reactivity and risk of cardiovascular disease: A review and methodologic critique. *Psychological Bulletin, 96*, 435–464.

Kremen, W. S., Eisen, S. A., Tsuang, M. T., & Lyons, M. J. (2007). Is the Wisconsin Card Sorting Test a useful neurocognitive endophenotype? *American Journal of Medical Genetics and Part B: Neuropsychiatric Genetics, 144B*(4), 403–406.

Kring, A. M., Persons, J. B., & Thomas, C. (2007). Changes in affect during treatment for depression and anxiety. *Behaviour Research and Therapy, 45*(8), 1753–1764.

Kronholm, E., Partonen, T., Salminen, J. K., Mattila, A. K., & Joukamaa, M. (2007). Alexithymia, depression and sleep disturbance symptoms. *Psychotherapy and Psychosomatics, 77*(1), 63–65.

LaBar, K. S., Crupain, M. J., Voyvodic, J. T., & McCarthy, G. (2003). Dynamic perception of facial affect and identity in the human brain. *Cerebral Cortex, 13*(10), 1023–1033.

Ladavas, E., Cimatti, D., del Pesce, M., & Tuozzi, G. (1993). Emotional evaluation with and without conscious stimulus identification: Evidence from a split-brain patient. *Cognition and Emotion, 7*(1), 95–114.

Lafora, G. R. (1940). Sobre el hambre y la anorexia de origen cerebral [On hunger and anorexia of cerebral origin]. *Archivos de Neurologia y Psiquiatria de Mexico, 3*, 633–667.

Lamb, R. J., Preston, K. L., Schindler, C. W., & Meisch, R. A. (1991). The reinforcing and subjective effects of morphine in post-addicts: A dose–response study. *Journal of Pharmacology and Experimental Therapeutics, 259*(3), 1165–1173.

Lambert, K. G. (2003). The life and career of Paul MacLean: A journey toward neurobiological and social harmony. *Physiology and Behavior, 79*, 343–349.

Landry, S. H., Swank, P., Stuebing, K., Prasad, M., & Ewing-Cobbs, L. (2004). Social competence in young children with inflicted traumatic brain injury. *Developmental Neuropsychology, 26*(3), 707–733.

Lane, R. D. (1996). Impaired verbal and nonverbal emotion recognition in alexithymia. *Psychosomatic Medicine, 58*(6), 581–581.

Lane, R. D., Reiman, E. M., Ahern, G. L., & Thayer, J. F. (2001). Activity in medial prefrontal cortex correlates with vagal component of heart rate variability during emotion. *Brain and Cognition, 47*, 97–100.

Lane-Brown, A. T., & Tate, R. L. (2009). Measuring apathy after traumatic brain injury: Psychometric properties of the Apathy Evaluation Scale and the Frontal Systems Behavior Scale. *Brain Injury, 23*(13–14), 999–1007.

Lang, P. J. (1994). The varieties of emotional experience: A meditation on James–Lange theory. *Psychological Review, 101*(2), 211–221.

Lange, C. G. (1922). The emotions. In C. G. Lange & W. James (Eds.), *The emotions* (Vol. 1, pp. 33–90). Baltimore: Williams & Wilkins.

Lange, T., Perras, B., Fehm, H. L., & Born, J. (2003). Sleep enhances the human antibody response to hepatitis A vaccination. *Psychosomatic Medicine, 65*, 831–835.

Larsen, J. K., Brand, N., Bermond, B., & Hijman, R. (2003). Cognitive and emotional characteristics of alexithymia: A review of neurobiological studies. *Journal of Psychosomatic Research, 54*(6), 533–541.

Larson, M. J., Kelly, K. G., Stigge-Kaufman, D. A., Schmalfuss, I. M., & Perlstein, W. M. (2007). Reward context sensitivity impairment following severe TBI: An event-related potential investigation. *Journal of the International Neuropsychological Society, 13*(4), 615–625.

LaRusso, L. (1978). Sensitivity of paranoid patients to nonverbal cues. *Journal of Abnormal Psychology, 87*(5), 463–471.

Lattner, S., Meyer, M. E., & Friederici, A. D. (2005). Voice perception: Sex, pitch, and the right hemisphere. *Human Brain Mapping, 24*(1), 11–20.

Lautin, A. (2001). *The limbic brain*. New York: Kluwer Academic/Plenum Press.

Lavenu, I., & Pasquier, F. (2004). Perception of emotion on faces in frontotemporal dementia and Alzheimer's disease: A longitudinal study. *Dementia and Geriatric Cognitive Disorders, 19*(1), 37–41.

Lavretsky, H., Zheng, L., Weiner, M. W., Mungas, D., Reed, B., Kramer, J. H., et al. (2008). The MRI brain correlates of depressed mood, anhedonia, apathy, and anergia in older adults with and without cognitive impairment or dementia. *International Journal of Geriatric Psychiatry, 23*(10), 1040–1050.

Lawrence, A. D., Goerendt, I. K., & Brooks, D. J. (2007). Impaired recognition of facial expressions of anger in Parkinson's disease patients acutely withdrawn from dopamine replacement therapy. *Neuropsychologia, 45*(1), 65–74.

Lawrence, K., Campbell, R., Swettenham, J., Terstegge, J., Akers, R., Coleman, M., et al. (2003). Interpreting gaze in Turner syndrome: Impaired sensitivity to intention and emotion, but preservation of social cueing. *Neuropsychologia, 41*(8), 894–905.

Lawrence, K., Kuntsi, J., Coleman, M., Campbell, R., & Skuse, D. (2003). Face and emotion recognition deficits in Turner syndrome: A possible role for X-linked genes in amygdala development. *Neuropsychology, 17*(1), 39–49.

Lawrence, N. S., Jollant, F., O'Daly, O., Zelaya, F., & Phillips, M. L. (2009). Distinct roles of prefrontal cortical subregions in the Iowa Gambling Task. *Cerebral Cortex, 19*(5), 1134–1143.

Lazarus, R. S. (1982). Thoughts on the relations between emotion and cognition. *American Psychologist, 37*(9), 1019–1024.

Lazarus, R. S. (1999). *Stress and emotion: A new synthesis*. New York: Springer.

Lazarus, R. S., & Folkman, S. (1984). *Stress, appraisal, and coping*. New York: Springer.

Lazarus, R. S., & Lazarus, B. N. (1994). *Passions and reasons: Making sense of our emotions*. New York: Oxford University Press.

Lazzaro, I., Gordon, E., Li, W., Lim, C. L., Plahn, M., Whitmont, S., et al. (1999). Simultaneous EEG and EDA measures in adolescent attention deficit hyperactivity disorder. *International Journal of Psychophysiology, 34*(2), 123–134.

Le, H.-N., Berenbaum, H., & Raghavan, C. (2002). Culture and alexithymia: Mean levels, correlates, and the role of parental socialization of emotions. *Emotion, 2*(4), 341–360.

Lebert, F., Pasquier, F., & Petit, H. (1995). Personality traits and frontal lobe dementia. *International Journal of Geriatric Psychiatry, 10*(12), 1047–1049.

Lebre, A. A. T., Mendes, M. F., Tilbery, C. P., Almeida, A. L., & Neto, A. S. (2007). Relacao entre fadiga e disturbios autonomicos na esclerose multipla [Relation between fatigue and autonomic disturbances in multiple sclerosis]. *Arquivos de Neuro-Psiquiatria, 65*(3-A), 663–668.

Lechowski, L., Benoit, M., Chassagne, P., Vedel, I., Tortrat, D., Teillet, L., et al. (2009). Persistent apathy in Alzheimer's disease as an independent factor of rapid functional decline: The REAL longitudinal cohort study. *International Journal of Geriatric Psychiatry, 24*(4), 341–346.

LeDoux, J. (1996). *The emotional brain: The mysterious underpinnings of emotional life*. New York: Touchstone.

Lee, A. C. K., Tang, S. W., Yu, G. K. K., & Cheung, R. T. F. (2007). Incidence and predictors of depression after stroke (DAS). *International Journal of Psychiatry in Clinical Practice, 11*(3), 200–206.

Lee, B. K., Glass, T. A., McAtee, M. J., Wand, G. S., Bandeen-Roche, K., Bolla, K. I., et al. (2007). Associations of salivary cortisol with cognitive function in the Baltimore memory study. *Archives of General Psychiatry, 64*, 810–818.

Lee, G. P., Meador, K. J., Loring, D. W., Allision, J. D., Brown, W. S., Paul, L. K., et al. (2004). Neural substrates of emotion as revealed by functional magnetic resonance imaging. *Cognitive and Behavioral Neurology, 17*(1), 9–17.

Lee, P. R., Brady, D. L., Shapiro, R. A., Dorsa, D. M., & Koenig, J. I. (2007). Prenatal stress generates deficits in rat social behavior: Reversal by oxytocin. *Brain Research, 1156*, 152–167.

Lee, T. M. C., Liu, H. L., Chan, C. C. H., Fang, S. Y., & Gao, J. H. (2005). Neural activities associated with emotion recognition observed in men and women. *Molecular Psychiatry, 10*(5), 450–455.

Lee, T.-W., Josephs, O., Dolan, R. J., & Critchley, H. D. (2006). Imitating expressions: Emotion-specific neural substrates in facial mimicry. *Social Cognitive and Affective Neuroscience, 1*(2), 122–135.

Lee, Y., Kim, Y.-T., Seo, E., Park, O., Jeong, S.-H., Kim, S. H., et al. (2007). Dissociation of emotional decision-making from cognitive decision-making in chronic schizophrenia. *Psychiatry Research, 152*(2/3), 113–120.

Leentjens, A. F. G., Wielaert, S. M., van Harskamp, F., & Wilmink, F. (1998). Disturbances of affective prosody in patients with schizophrenia: A cross sectional study. *Journal of Neurology, Neurosurgery, and Psychiatry, 64*(3), 375–378.

Lenzi, G. L., Altieri, M., & Maestrini, I. (2008). Post-stroke depression. *Revue Neurologique, 164*(10), 837–840.

Leone, L., Pierro, A., & Mannetti, L. (2002). Validita della versione Italiana delle Scale BIS/BAS di Carver e White (1994): Generalizzabilita della struttura e relazioni con costrutti affini [Validity of the Italian version of the BIS/BAS Scale of Carver and White (1994): Generalizability of structure and relationships of related constructs]. *Giornale Italiano di Psicologia, 29*(2), 413–434.

Leterme, A., Brun, L., Dittmar, A., & Robin, O. (2008). Autonomic nervous system responses to sweet taste: Evidence for habituation rather than pleasure. *Physiology and Behavior, 93*(4), 994–999.

Levenson, R. W. (2003). Autonomic specificity and emotion. In R. J. Davidson, K. R. Scherer, & H. H. Goldsmith (Eds.), *Handbook of affective sciences* (pp. 212–224). New York: Oxford University Press.

Levenson, R. W., Ekman, P., Heider, K., & Friesen, W. V. (1992). Emotion and autonomic nervous system activity in the Minangkabau of West Sumatra. *Journal of Personality and Social Psychology, 62*, 972–988.

Leventhal, A. M., Chasson, G. S., Tapia, E., Miller, E. K., & Pettit, J. W. (2006). Measuring hedonic capacity in depression: A psychometric analysis of three anhedonia scales. *Journal of Clinical Psychology, 62*(12), 1545–1558.

Levison, P. K., & Flynn, J. P. (1965). The objects attacked by cats during stimulation of the hypothalamus. *Animal Behaviour, 13*(2), 217–220.

Lewis, M. B., Sherwood, S., Moselhy, H., & Ellis, H. D. (2001). Autonomic responses to familiar faces without autonomic responses to familiar voices: Evidence for voice-specific Capgras delusion. *Cognitive Neuropsychiatry, 6*(3), 217–228.

Lezak, M. D., Howieson, D. B., & Loring, D. W. (2004). *Neuropsychological assessment.* Oxford, UK: Oxford University Press.

Li, C.-S. R., Huang, C.-Y., Lin, W.-Y., & Sun, C.-W. V. (2007). Gender differences in punishment and reward sensitivity in a sample of Taiwanese college students. *Personality and Individual Differences, 43*(3), 475–483.

Li, Y.-Z., Zhang, Y., Jiang, Y., Li, H., Mi, S., Yi, G.-J., et al. (2008). The Chinese version of the BIS/BAS Scale: Reliability and validity. *Chinese Mental Health Journal, 22*(8), 613–616.

Libby, P. (2002). Inflammation in atherosclerosis. *Nature, 420*, 868–874.

Liberzon, I., Phan, K. L., Decker, L. R., & Taylor, S. F. (2003). Extended amygdala and emotional salience: A PET activation study of positive and negative affect. *Neuropsychopharmacology, 28*(4), 726–733.

Lichtenstein, P. E. (1950). Studies of anxiety: II. The effects of lobotomy on a feeding inhibition in dogs. *Journal of Comparative and Physiological Psychology, 43*(6), 419–427.

Lieberman, M. D., Eisenberger, N. I., Crockett, M. J., Tom, S. M., Pfeifer, J. H., & Way, B. M. (2007). Putting feelings into words: Affect labeling disrupts amygdala activity in response to affective stimuli. *Psychological Science, 18*(5), 421–428.

Lieberman, M. D., & Rosenthal, R. (2001). Why introverts can't always tell who likes them: Multitasking and nonverbal decoding. *Journal of Personality and Social Psychology, 80*(2), 294–310.

Liebermann, D., Giesbrecht, G. F., & Maller, U. (2007). Cognitive and emotional aspects of self-regulation in preschoolers. *Cognitive Development, 22*(4), 511–529.

Lilly, R., Cummings, J. L., Benson, D. F., & Frankel, M. (1983). The human Klüver–Bucy syndrome. *Neurology, 33*(9), 1141–1145.

Lin, C.-H., Chiu, Y.-C., Cheng, C.-M., & Hsieh, J.-C. (2008). Brain maps of Iowa Gambling Task. *BMC Neuroscience, 9*, 72.

Lind, K., Edman, A., Sjogren, M., Wallin, A., & Karlsson, I. (2002). Relationship between depressive symptomatology and the subcortical brain syndrome in dementia. *International Journal of Geriatric Psychiatry, 17*(8), 744–778.

Lindsley, D. B., & Stevens, S. S. (1951). Emotion. In S. S. Stevens (Ed.), *Handbook of experimental psychology* (pp. 473–516). Oxford, UK: Wiley.

Links, K. A., Chow, T. W., Binns, M., Freedman, M., Stuss, D. T., Scott, C. J. M., et al. (2009). Apathy is not associated with basal ganglia atrophy in frontotemporal dementia. *American Journal of Geriatric Psychiatry, 17*(9), 819–821.

Lipp, A., Sandroni, P., Ahlskog, J. E., Fealey, R. D., Kimpinski, K., Iodice, V., et al. (2009). Prospective differentiation of multiple system atrophy from Parkinson's disease, with and without autonomic failure. *Archives of Neurology, 66*(6), 742–750.

Liston, C., McEwen, B. S., & Casey, B. J. (2009). Psychosocial stress reversibly disrupts prefrontal processing and attentional control. *Proceedings of the National Academy of Sciences of the United States of America, 106*(3), 912–917.

Liston, C., Miller, M. M., Goldwater, D. S., Radley, J. J., Rocher, A. B., Hof, P. R., et al. (2006). Stress-induced alterations in prefrontal cortical dendritic morphology predict selective impairments in perceptual attentional set-shifting. *Journal of Neuroscience, 26*(30), 7870–7874.

Loas, G., & Boyer, P. (1993). Relationships between anhedonia and depressive symptoms in major depressive disorder. *European Psychiatry, 8*(1), 51–52.

Loas, G., Boyer, P., Fremaux, D., & Gayant, C. (1995). L'Echelle de Plaisir–Deplaisir Physique (EPD-P): Etude de validation chez 295 sujets [The Physical Pleasure–Displeasure Scale (P-PDS): A validation study among 295 subjects]. *European Review of Applied Psychology/Revue Europeenne de Psychologie Appliquee, 45*(3), 193–202.

Loas, G., Noisette, C., Legrand, A., & Boyer, P. (2000). Is anhedonia a specific dimension in chronic schizophrenia? *Schizophrenia Bulletin, 26*(2), 495–506.

Loas, G., Perot, J. M., Hardy, P., & Jouvent, R. (1994). Physical anhedonia and subtypes of major depressive disorder. *European Psychiatry, 9*(6), 304–306.

LoBue, V., & DeLoache, J. S. (2008). Detecting the snake in the grass: Attention to fear-relevant stimuli by adults and young children. *Psychological Science, 19*(3), 284–289.

Loesel, F., & Schmucker, M. (2004). Psychopathy, risk taking, and attention: A differentiated test of the somatic marker hypothesis. *Journal of Abnormal Psychology, 113*(4), 522–529.

Loewy, A. D., & Holstege, G. (1991). Forebrain nuclei involved in autonomic control. In G. Holstege (Ed.), *Role of the forebrain in sensation and behavior* (pp. 253–268). Amsterdam: Elsevier Science.

Loiseau, P., Cohadon, F., & Cohadon, S. (1971). Gelastic epilepsy: A review and report of five cases. *Epilepsia, 12*, 313–323.

Lopez-Meza, E., Corona-Vazquez, T., Ruano-Calderon, L. A., & Ranirez-Bermudez, J. (2005). Severe impulsiveness as the primary manifestation of multiple sclerosis in a young female. *Psychiatry and Clinical Neurosciences, 59*(6), 739–742.

Lough, S., Kipps, C. M., Treise, C., Watson, P., Blair, J. R., & Hodges, J. R. (2006). Social reasoning, emotion and empathy in frontotemporal dementia. *Neuropsychologia, 44*(6), 950–958.

Lucassen, P. J., Bosch, O. J., Jousma, E., Kroemer, S. A., Andrew, R., Seckl, J. R., et al. (2009). Prenatal stress reduces postnatal neurogenesis in rats selectively bred for high, but not low, anxiety: Possible key role of placental 11 beta-hydroxysteroid dehydrogenase type 2. *European Journal of Neuroscience, 29*(1), 97–103.

Lueken, U., Seidl, U., Schwarz, M., Voelker, L., Naumann, D., Mattes, K., et al. (2006). Die Apathy Evaluation Scale: Erste Ergebnisse zu den psychometrischen Eigenschaften einer deutschsprachigen Uebersetzung der Skala [Psychometric properties of a German version of the Apathy Evaluation Scale]. *Fortschritte der Neurologie, Psychiatrie, 74*(12), 714–722.

Lueken, U., Seidl, U., Voelker, L., Schweiger, E., Kruse, A., & Schroeder, J. (2007). Development of a short version of the Apathy Evaluation Scale specifically adapted for demented nursing home residents. *American Journal of Geriatric Psychiatry, 15*(5), 376–385.

Luminet, O., Bagby, R. M., Wagner, H., Taylor, G. J., & Parker, J. D. A. (1999). Relation between alexithymia and the five-factor model of personality: A facet-level analysis. *Journal of Personality Assessment, 73*(3), 345–358.

Luminet, O., Rime, B., Bagby, R. M., & Taylor, G. J. (2004). A multimodal investigation of emotional responding in alexithymia. *Cognition and Emotion, 18*(6), 741–766.

Luminet, O., Vermeulen, N., Demaret, C., Taylor, G. J., & Bagby, R. M. (2006). Alexithymia and levels of processing: Evidence for an overall deficit in remembering emotion words. *Journal of Research in Personality, 40*(5), 713–733.

Lumley, M. A., Beyer, J., Radcliffe, A., Vingerhoets, A., Nyklicek, I., & Denollet, J. (2008). Alexithymia and physical health problems: A critique of potential pathways and a research agenda. In A Vingerhoets, I. Nyklicek, & J. Denollet (Eds.), *Emotion regulation: Conceptual and clinical issues* (pp. 43–68). New York: Springer Science+Business Media.

Lumme, V., Aalto, S., Ilonen, T., Nagren, K., & Hietala, J. (2007). Dopamine D2/D3 receptor binding in the anterior cingulate cortex and executive functioning. *Psychiatry Research, 156*(1), 69–74.

Lunazzi de Jubany, H. (2000). Investigacion de variables en el constructo Alexitimia en 550 casos [On alexithymia construct variables in 550 cases]. *Revista Iberoamericana de Diagnostico y Evaluacion Psicologica, 10*(2), 101–119.

Lupien, S. J., Fiocco, A., Wan, N., Maheu, F., Lord, C., Schramek, T., et al. (2005). Stress hormones and human memory function across the lifespan. *Psychoneuroendocrinology, 30*, 225–242.

Lupien, S. J., Meaney, M. J., Wang, E., & Snyder, D. S. (1998). Stress, glucocorticoids, and hippocampal aging in rat and human. In E. Wang & D. S. Snyder (Eds.), *Handbook of the aging brain* (pp. 19–50). San Diego, CA: Academic Press.

Luu, P., Collins, P., & Tucker, D. M. (2000). Mood, personality, and self-monitoring:

Negative affect and emotionality in relation to frontal lobe mechanisms of error monitoring. *Journal of Experimental Psychology, 129*(1), 43–60.

Mabuchi, N., Hirayama, M., Koike, Y., Watanabe, H., Ito, H., Kobayashi, R., et al. (2005). Progression and prognosis in pure autonomic failure (PAF): Comparison with multiple system atrophy. *Journal of Neurology, Neurosurgery, and Psychiatry, 76*(7), 947–952.

MacCoon, D. G., Wallace, J. F., & Newman, J. P. (2004). Self-regulation: Context-appropriate balanced attention. In R. F. Baumeister & K. D. Vohs (Eds.), *Handbook of self-regulation: Research, theory, and applications* (pp. 422–446). New York: Guilford Press.

Macdonnell, M. F., & Flynn, J. P. (1964). Attack elicited by stimulation of the thalamus of rats. *Science, 144*, 1249–1250.

MacLean, P. (1949). Psychosomatic disease and the "visceral brain." Recent developments bearing on the Papez theory of emotion. *Psychosomatic Medicine, 11*, 338–352.

MacLean, P. (1952). Some psychiatric implications of physiological studies on the frontotemporal portions of the limbic system (visceral brain), electroencephalography: The basal and temporal regions. *Yale Journal of Biological Medicine, 22*, 407–418.

MacLean, P. (1990). *The triune brain in evloution: Role in paleocerebral function.* New York: Plenum Press.

Macmillan, M. (2008). Phineas Gage: Unravelling the myth [Electronic version]. *The Psychologist, 21*, 828–831. Retrieved from *www.thepsychologist.org.uk.*

MacMillan, S., Szeszko, P. R., Moore, G. J., Madden, R., Lorch, E., Ivey, J., et al. (2003). Increased amygdala: Hippocampal volume ratios associated with severity of anxiety in pediatric major depression. *Journal of Child and Adolescent Psychopharmacology, 13*(1), 65–73.

MacPherson, S. E., Phillips, L. H., Della Sala, S., & Cantagallo, A. (2008). Iowa Gambling Task impairment is not specific to ventromedial prefrontal lesions. *Clinical Neuropsychologist, 23*(3), 510–522.

Magai, C., Cohen, C. I., Culver, C., Gomberg, D., & Malatesta, C. (1997). Relation between premorbid personality and patterns of emotion expression in mid- to late-stage dementia. *International Journal of Geriatric Psychiatry, 12*(11), 1092–1099.

Magar, E. C. E., Phillips, L. H., & Hosie, J. A. (2008). Self-regulation and risk-taking. *Personality and Individual Differences, 45*(2), 153–159.

Maggi, R., Tavola, T., & Gala, C. (1996). Psychobiological responses to stress in ageing. *New Trends in Experimental and Clinical Psychiatry, 12*(3), 179–188.

Maheu, F. S., Mazzone, L., Merke, D. P., Keil, M. F., Stratakis, C. A., Pine, D. S., et al. (2008). Altered amygdala and hippocampus function in adolescents with hypercortisolemia: A functional magnetic resonance imaging study of Cushing syndrome. *Development and Psychopathology, 20*(4), 1177–1189.

Mahler, S. V., Smith, K. S., & Berridge, K. C. (2007). Endocannabinoid hedonic hotspot for sensory pleasure: Anandamide in nucleus accumbens shell enhances "liking" of a sweet reward. *Neuropsychopharmacology, 32*(11), 2267–2278.

Maia, T. V., & McClelland, J. L. (2005). The somatic marker hypothesis: Still many questions but no answers. *Trends in Cognitive Sciences, 9*(4), 162–164.

Malberg, J. E., & Duman, R. S. (2003). Cell proliferation in adult hippocampus is decreased by inescapable stress: Reversal by fluoxetine treatment. *Neuropsychopharmacology, 28*(9), 1562–1571.

Manes, F., Paradiso, S., & Robinson, R. G. (1999). Neuropsychiatric effects of insular stroke. *Journal of Nervous and Mental Disease, 187*(12), 707–712.

Manes, F., Sahakian, B., Clark, L., Rogers, R., Antoun, N., Aitken, M., et al. (2002). Decision-making processes following damage to the prefrontal cortex. *Brain: A Journal of Neurology, 125*(3), 624–639.

Mangelli, L., Semprini, F., Sirri, L., Fava, G., & Sonino, N. (2006). Use of the diagnostic criteria for psychosomatic research (DCPR) in a community sample. *Psychosomatics: Journal of Consultation Liaison Psychiatry, 47*(2), 143–146.

Mann, L. S., Wise, T. N., Trinidad, A., & Kohanski, R. E. (1994). Alexithymia, affect recognition, and the five-factor model of personality in normal subjects. *Psychological Reports, 74*(2), 563–567.

Mantani, T., Okamoto, Y., Shirao, N., Okada, G., & Yamawaki, S. (2005). Reduced activation of posterior cingulate cortex during imagery in subjects with high degrees of alexithymia: A functional magnetic resonance imaging study. *Biological Psychiatry, 57*(9), 982–990.

Manuck, S. B., Flory, J. D., Ferrell, R. E., Dent, K. M., Mann, J. J., & Muldoon, M. F. (1999). Aggression and anger-related traits associated with a polymorphism of the tryptophan hydroxylase gene. *Biological Psychiatry, 45*(5), 603–614.

Marchesi, C., Brusamonti, E., & Maggini, C. (2000). Are alexithymia, depression, and anxiety distinct constructs in affective disorders? *Journal of Psychosomatic Research, 49*(1), 43–49.

Maren, S., & Hobin, J. A. (2007). Hippocampal regulation of context-dependent neuronal activity in the lateral amygdala. *Learning and Memory, 14*(4), 318–324.

Marin, R. S., Biedrzycki, R. C., & Firinciogullari, S. (1991). Reliability and validity of the Apathy Evaluation Scale. *Psychiatry Research, 38*(2), 143–162.

Marin, R. S., & Chakravorty, S. (2005). Disorders of diminished motivation. In J. M. Silver, T. W. McAllister, & S. C. Yudofsky (Eds.), *Textbook of traumatic brain injury* (pp. 337–352). Arlington, VA: American Psychiatric Publishing.

Marin, R. S., Firinciogullari, S., & Biedrzycki, R. C. (1993). The sources of convergence between measures of apathy and depression. *Journal of Affective Disorders, 28*(2), 117–124.

Marin, R. S., & Wilkosz, P. A. (2005). Disorders of diminished motivation. *Journal of Head Trauma Rehabilitation, 20*(4), 377–388.

Markowitsch, H. J., Vandekerckhove, M. M. P., Lanfermann, H., & Russ, M. O. (2003). Engagement of lateral and medial prefrontal areas in the ecphory of sad and happy autobiographical memories. *Cortex, 39*(4), 643–665.

Marschark, M., Richtsmeier, L. M., Richardson, J. T. E., Crovitz, H. F., & Henry, J. (2000). Intellectual and emotional functioning in college students following mild traumatic brain injury in childhood and adolescence. *Journal of Head Trauma Rehabilitation, 15*(6), 1227–1245.

Marsh, A. A., Finger, E. C., Mitchell, D. G. V., Reid, M. E., Sims, C., Kosson, D. S., et al. (2008). Reduced amygdala response to fearful expressions in children and adolescents with callous-unemotional traits and disruptive behavior disorders. *American Journal of Psychiatry, 165*(6), 712–720.

Marshall, G. A., Monserratt, L., Harwood, D., Mandelkern, M., Cummings, J. L., & Sultzer, D. L. (2007). Positron emission tomography metabolic correlates of apathy in Alzheimer's disease. *Archives of Neurology, 64*(7), 1015–1020.

Martel, M. M. (2009). Research review: A new perspective on attention-deficit hyperactivity disorder: Emotion dysregulation and trait models. *Journal of Child Psychology and Psychiatry, 50*(9), 1042–1051.

Martin, L. E., & Potts, G. F. (2009). Impulsivity in decision-making: An event-related potential investigation. *Personality and Individual Differences, 46*(3), 303–308.

Martinez, M. F., Flores, J. C., de las Heras, S. P., Lekumberri, A. M., Menocal, M. G., & Imirizaldu, J. J. Z. (2008). Prevalence of neuropsychiatric symptoms in elderly patients with dementia in Mungialde County (Basque country, Spain). *Dementia and Geriatric Cognitive Disorders, 25*(2), 103–108.

Marumo, K., Takizawa, R., Kawakubo, Y., Onitsuka, T., & Kasai, K. (2009). Gender difference in right lateral prefrontal hemodynamic response while viewing fearful faces: A multi-channel near-infrared spectroscopy. *Neuroscience Research, 63*(2), 89–94.

Mashour, G. A., Walker, E. E., & Martuza, R. L. (2005). Psychosurgery: Past, present, and future. *Brain Research Reviews, 48*(3), 409–419.

Massimo, L., Powers, C., Moore, P., Vesely, L., Avants, B., Gee, J., et al. (2009). Neuroanatomy of apathy and disinhibition in frontotemporal lobar degeneration. *Dementia and Geriatric Cognitive Disorders, 27*(1), 96–104.

Mast, B. T., Yochim, B., MacNeill, S. E., & Lichtenberg, P. A. (2004). Risk factors for geriatric depression: The importance of executive functioning within the vascular depression hypothesis. *Journals of Gerontology: Series A: Biological Sciences and Medical Sciences, 12*, 1290–1294.

Masunami, T., Okazaki, S., & Maekawa, H. (2009). Decision-making patterns and sensitivity to reward and punishment in children with attention-deficit hyperactivity disorder. *International Journal of Psychophysiology, 72*(3), 283–288.

Mataix-Cols, D., An, S. K., Lawrence, N. S., Caseras, X., Speckens, A., Giampietro, V., et al. (2008). Individual differences in disgust sensitivity modulate neural responses to aversive/disgusting stimuli. *European Journal of Neuroscience, 27*(11), 3050–3058.

Matheson, E., & Jahoda, A. (2005). Emotional understanding in aggressive and nonaggressive individuals with mild or moderate mental retardation. *American Journal on Mental Retardation, 110*(1), 57–67.

Mathiesen, B. B., Farster, P. L. V., & Svendsen, H. A. (2004). Affect regulation and loss of initiative in a case of orbitofrontal injury. *Neuro-Psychoanalysis, 6*(1), 47–62.

Matthys, W., Van Goozen, S. H. M., Snoek, H., & Van Engeland, H. (2004). Response perseveration and sensitivity to reward and punishment in boys with oppositional defiant disorder. *European Child and Adolescent Psychiatry, 13*(6), 362–364.

Mattila, A. K., Kronholm, E., Jula, A., Salminen, J. K., Koivisto, A.-M., Mielonen, R.-L., et al. (2008). Alexithymia and somatization in general population. *Psychosomatic Medicine, 70*(6), 716–722.

Mattila, A. K., Saarni, S. I., Salminen, J. K., Huhtala, H., Sintonen, H., & Joukamaa, M. (2009). Alexithymia and health-related quality of life in a general population. *Psychosomatics: Journal of Consultation Liaison Psychiatry, 50*(1), 59–68.

Mattox, S. T., Valle-Inclan, F., & Hackley, S. A. (2006). Psychophysiological evidence for impaired reward anticipation in Parkinson's disease. *Clinical Neurophysiology, 117*(10), 2144–2153.

Max, J. E., Robertson, B. A. M., & Lansing, A. E. (2001). The phenomenology of personality change due to traumatic brain injury in children and adolescents. *Journal of Neuropsychiatry and Clinical Neurosciences, 13*(2), 161–170.

Mazzeo, S. E., Mitchell, K. S., & Williams, L. J. (2008). Anxiety, alexithymia, and depression as mediators of the association between childhood abuse and eating disordered behavior in African American and European American women. *Psychology of Women Quarterly, 32*(3), 267–280.

Mazzola, F., Seigal, A., MacAskill, A., Corden, B., Lawrence, K., & Skuse, D. H. (2006). Eye tracking and fear recognition deficits in Turner syndrome. *Social Neuroscience, 1*(3), 259–269.

McCauley, E., Kay, T., Ito, J., & Treder, R. (1987). The Turner syndrome: Cognitive deficits, affective discrimination, and behavior problems. *Child Development, 58*(2), 464–473.

McCauley, S. R., McDaniel, M. A., Pedroza, C., Chapman, S. B., & Levin, H. S. (2009). Incentive effects on event-based prospective memory performance in children and adolescents with traumatic brain injury. *Neuropsychology, 23*(2), 201–209.

McClendon, R., & Kadis, L. B. (1994). Shame and early decisions: Theory and clinical implications. *Transactional Analysis Journal, 24*(2), 130–138.

McClure, E. B., Monk, C. S., Nelson, E. E., Parrish, J. M., Adler, A., Blair, R. J. R., et al. (2007). Abnormal attention modulation of fear circuit function in pediatric generalized anxiety disorder. *Archives of General Psychiatry, 64*(1), 97–106.

McCown, W. G., Johnson, J. L., & Austin, S. H. (1986). Inability of delinquents to recognize facial affects. *Journal of Social Behavior and Personality, 1*(4), 489–496.

McCown, W. G., Johnson, J. L., & Austin, S. H. (1988). Patterns of facial affect recognition errors in delinquent adolescent males. *Journal of Social Behavior and Personality, 3*(3), 215–224.

McCrae, R. R. (1987). Creativity, divergent thinking, and Openness to Experience. *Journal of Personality and Social Psychology, 52*(6), 1258–1265.

McDermott, L. M., & Ebmeier, K. P. (2009). A meta-analysis of depression severity and cognitive function. *Journal of Affective Disorders, 119*(1–3), 1–8.

McDonald, S., Flanagan, S., & Rollins, J. (2002). *The Awareness of Social Interference Test (TASIT)*. San Antonio, TX: Pearson.

McDougall, J. (1982). Alexithymia: A psychoanalytic viewpoint. *Psychotherapy and Psychosomatics, 38*(1), 81–90.

McElroy, T., & Dowd, K. (2007). Susceptibility to anchoring effects: How openness-to-experience influences responses to anchoring cues. *Judgment and Decision Making, 2*(1), 48–53.

McEwen, B. S. (1999). Stress and hippocampal plasticity. *Annual Review of Neuroscience, 22*, 105–122.

McEwen, B. S. (2005). Stressed or stressed out: What is the difference? *Journal of Psychiatry and Neuroscience, 30*(5), 315–318.

McEwen, B. S. (2007). Physiology and neurobiology of stress and adaptation: Central role of the brain. *Physiological Reviews, 87*, 873–904.

McEwen, B. S., Angulo, J., Cameron, H., & Chao, H. M. (1992). Paradoxical effects of adrenal steroids on the brain: Protection versus degeneration. *Biological Psychiatry, 31*(2), 177–199.

McEwen, B. S., & Lasley, E. N. (2003). Allostatic load: When protection gives way to damage. *Advances in Mind–Body Medicine, 19*(1), 28–33.

McEwen, B. S., Magarinos, A. M., & Gorman, J. M. (2004). Does stress damage the brain? In J. M. Gorman (Ed.), *Fear and anxiety: The benefits of translational research* (pp. 23–45). Arlington, VA: American Psychiatric Publishing.

Mecklinger, A., von Cramon, D. Y., Springer, A., & Matthes-von Cramon, G. (1999).

Executive control functions in task switching: Evidence from brain injured patients. *Journal of Clinical and Experimental Neuropsychology, 21*, 606–619.

Melis, C., & van Boxtel, A. (2007). Autonomic physiological response patterns related to intelligence. *Intelligence, 35*(5), 471–487.

Melnick, S. M., & Hinshaw, S. P. (2000). Emotion regulation and parenting in AD/HD and comparison boys: Linkages with social behaviors and peer preference. *Journal of Abnormal Child Psychology, 28*(1), 73–86.

Mendez, M. F., Chow, T., Ringman, J., Twitchell, G., & Hinkin, C. H. (2000). Pedophilia and temporal lobe disturbances. *Journal of Neuropsychiatry and Clinical Neurosciences, 12*(1), 71–76.

Mendez, M. F., & Foti, D. J. (1997). Lethal hyperoral behaviour from the Klüver–Bucy syndrome. *Journal of Neurology, Neurosurgery, and Psychiatry, 62*(3), 293–294.

Mendez, M. F., Lauterbach, E. C., & Sampson, S. M. (2008). An evidence-based review of the psychopathology of frontotemporal dementia: A report of the ANPA committee on research. *Journal of Neuropsychiatry and Clinical Neurosciences, 20*(2), 130–149.

Mendez, M. F., & Perryman, K. M. (2002). Neuropsychiatric features of frontotemporal dementia: Evaluation of consensus criteria and review. *Journal of Neuropsychiatry and Clinical Neurosciences, 14*(4), 424–429.

Mendez, M. F., & Shapira, J. S. (2009). Altered emotional morality in frontotemporal dementia. *Cognitive Neuropsychiatry, 14*(3), 165–179.

Merkelbach, S., Koenig, J., & Sittinger, H. (2003). Personality traits in multiple sclerosis (MS) patients with and without fatigue experience. *Acta Neurologica Scandinavica, 107*(3), 195–201.

Merriam–Webster. (2004). *The Merriam–Webster dictionary* (11th ed.). Springfield, MA: Author.

Meyer, T. D., Barton, S., Baur, M., & Jordan, G. (2010). Vulnerability factors for bipolar disorders as predictors of attributions in ability-based and chance-based tests. *Journal of Individual Differences, 31*(1), 29–37.

Meyer-Lindenberg, A., Buckholtz, J. W., Kolachana, B., Hariri, A. R., Pezawas, L., Blasi, G., et al. (2006). Neural mechanisms of genetic risk for impulsivity and violence in humans. *Proceedings of the National Academy of Sciences of the United States of America, 103*(16), 6269–6274.

Miao, Y. K. (2003). Mania associated with multiple sclerosis. *Hong Kong Journal of Psychiatry, 13*(1), 34–38.

Michaud, K., Forget, H., & Cohen, H. (2009). Chronic glucocorticoid hypersecretion in Cushing's syndrome exacerbates cognitive aging. *Brain and Cognition, 71*(1), 1–8.

Milad, M. R., Rauch, S. L., Schoenbaum, G., Gottfried, J. A., Murray, E. A., & Ramus, S. J. (2007). The role of the orbitofrontal cortex in anxiety disorders. In G. Schoenbaum, J. Gottfried, E. A. Murray, & S. Ramus (Eds.), *Linking affect to action: Critical contributions of the orbitofrontal cortex* (pp. 546–561). Malden, MA: Blackwell.

Milders, M., Ietswaart, M., Crawford, J. R., & Currie, D. (2008). Social behavior following traumatic brain injury and its association with emotion recognition, understanding of intentions, and cognitive flexibility. *Journal of the International Neuropsychological Society, 14*(2), 318–326.

Miles, L., Johnston, L., Fletcher-Flinn, C. M., & Haberman, G. M. (2006). Not all smiles are created equal: Perceiver sensitivity to the differences between posed and genuine smiles. In C. M. Fletcher-Flinn (Ed.), *Cognition and language: Perspectives from New Zealand* (pp. 51–64). Bowen Hills, Queensland, Australia: Australian Academic Press.

Milham, M. P., Nugent, A. C., Drevets, W. C., Dickstein, D. P., Leibenluft, E., Ernst, M., et al. (2005). Selective reduction in amygdala volume in pediatric anxiety disorders: A voxel-based morphometry investigation. *Biological Psychiatry, 57*(9), 961–966.

Miller, A., & Panitch, H. (2007). Therapeutic use of dextromethorphan: Key learnings from treatment of pseudobulbar affect. *Journal of the Neurological Sciences, 259*(1–2), 67–73.

Mingote, S., Font, L., Farrar, A. M., Vontell, R., Worden, L. T., Stopper, C. M., et al. (2008). Nucleus accumbens adenosine A-sub(2A) receptors regulate exertion of effort by acting on the ventral striatopallidal pathway. *Journal of Neuroscience, 28*, 9037–9046.

Mitchell, A. J. (1995). The contribution of hypercortisolaemia to the cognitive decline of geriatric depression. *International Journal of Geriatric Psychiatry, 10*(5), 401–409.

Mitchell, D. G. V., Fine, C., Richell, R. A., Newman, C., Lumsden, J., Blair, K. S., et al. (2006). Instrumental learning and relearning in individuals with psychopathy and in patients with lesions involving the amygdala or orbitofrontal cortex. *Neuropsychology, 20*(3), 280–289.

Mitchell, J. T., Kimbrel, N. A., Hundt, N. E., Cobb, A. R., Nelson-Gray, R. O., & Lootens, C. M. (2007). An analysis of reinforcement sensitivity theory and the five-factor model. *European Journal of Personality, 21*(7), 869–887.

Mittal, V. A., & Walker, E. F. (2007). Movement abnormalities predict conversion to Axis I psychosis among prodromal adolescents. *Journal of Abnormal Psychology, 116*(4), 796–803.

Mitterschiffthaler, M. T., Fu, C. H. Y., Dalton, J. A., Andrew, C. M., & Williams, S. C. R. (2007). A functional MRI study of happy and sad affective states induced by classical music. *Human Brain Mapping, 28*(11), 1150–1162.

Mizoguchi, K., Ishige, A., Takeda, S., Aburada, M., & Tabira, T. (2004). Endogenous glucocorticoids are essential for maintaining prefrontal cortical cognitive function. *Journal of Neuroscience, 24*(24), 5492–5499.

Mizoguchi, K., Shoji, H., Ikeda, R., Tanaka, Y., & Tabira, T. (2008). Persistent depressive state after chronic stress in rats is accompanied by HPA axis dysregulation and reduced prefrontal dopaminergic neurotransmission. *Pharmacology, Biochemistry, and Behavior, 91*(1), 170–175.

Moayeri, S. E., Cahill, L., Jin, Y., & Potkin, S. G. (2000). Relative sparing of emotionally influenced memory in Alzheimer's disease. *NeuroReport, 11*(4), 653–655.

Moffitt, T. E. (2005). The new look of behavioral genetics in developmental psychopathology: Gene–environment interplay in antisocial behaviors. *Psychological Bulletin, 131*(4), 533–554.

Mohr, D. C., & Pelletier, D. (2006). A temporal framework for understanding the effects of stressful life events on inflammation in patients with multiple sclerosis. *Brain, Behavior, and Immunity, 20*(1), 27–36.

Moller, A., Wiedemann, G., Rohde, U., Backmund, H., & Sonntag, A. (1994). Correlates of cognitive impairment and depressive mood disorder in multiple sclerosis. *Acta Neurolgica Scandinavica, 89*, 117–121.

Mondelli, V., Dazzan, P., Gabilondo, A., Tournikioti, K., Walshe, M., Marshall, N., et al. (2008). Pituitary volume in unaffected relatives of patients with schizophrenia and bipolar disorder. *Psychoneuroendocrinology, 33*(7), 1004–1012.

Moniz, E. (1937). Psycho-chirurgie [Psychosurgery]. *Nervenarzt, 10*, 113–118.

Monnot, M., Lovallo, W. R., Nixon, S. J., & Ross, E. (2002). Neurological basis of deficits in affective prosody comprehension among alcoholics and fetal alcohol-exposed adults. *Journal of Neuropsychiatry and Clinical Neuroscience, 14*(3), 321–328.

Monnot, M., Nixon, S., Lovallo, W., & Ross, E. (2001). Altered emotional perception in alcoholics: Deficits in affective prosody comprehension. *Alcoholism: Clinical and Experimental Research, 25*(3), 362–369.

Montaron, M. F., Drapeau, E., Dupret, D., Kitchener, P., Aurousseau, C., Moal, M. L., et al. (2006). Lifelong corticosterone level determines age-related decline in neurogenesis and memory. *Neurobiology of Aging, 27*(4), 645–654.

Montreys, C. R., & Borod, J. C. (1998). A preliminary evaluation of emotional experience and expression following unilateral braiin damage. *International Journal of Neuroscience, 96*(3), 269–283.

Moore, E. L., Terryberry-Spohr, L., & Hope, D. A. (2006). Mild traumatic brain injury and anxiety sequelae: A review of the literature. *Brain Injury, 20*(2), 117–132.

Moore, S. A., Zoellner, L. A., & Mollenholt, N. (2008). Are expressive suppression and cognitive reappraisal associated with stress-related symptoms? *Behaviour Research and Therapy, 46*(9), 993–1000.

Moriguchi, Y., Decety, J., Ohnishi, T., Maeda, M., Mori, T., Nemoto, K., et al. (2007). Empathy and judging other's pain: An fMRI study of alexithymia. *Cerebral Cortex, 17*(9), 2223–2234.

Morris, J. S., de Gelder, B., Weiskrantz, L., & Dolan, R. J. (2001). Differential extrageniculostriate and amygdala responses to presentation of emotional faces in a cortically blind field. *Brain: A Journal of Neurology, 124*(6), 1241–1252.

Morrison, V., Pollard, B., Johnston, M., & MacWalter, R. (2005). Anxiety and depression 3 years following stroke: Demographic, clinical, and psychological predictors. *Journal of Psychosomatic Research, 59*(4), 209–213.

Morton, B. E., & Rafto, S. E. (2006). Corpus callosum size is linked to dichotic deafness and hemisphericity, not sex or handedness. *Brain and Cognition, 62*(1), 1–8.

Mosely, J. V., & Linden, W. (2006). Predicting blood pressure and heart rate change with cardiovascular reactivity and recovery: Results from a 3-year and 10-year follow-up. *Psychosomatic Medicine, 68*, 833–843.

Moses, S. N., Houck, J. M., Martin, T., Hanlon, F. M., Ryan, J. D., Thoma, R. J., et al. (2007). Dynamic neural activity recorded from human amygdala during fear conditioning using magnetoencephalography. *Brain Research Bulletin, 71*(5), 452–460.

Mueller, E. M., Nguyen, J., Ray, W. J., & Borkovec, T. D. (2010). Future-oriented decision-making in generalized anxiety disorder is evident across different versions of the Iowa Gambling Task. *Journal of Behavior Therapy and Experimental Psychiatry, 41*(2), 165–171.

Mueller, J. M., & Wytykowska, A. M. (2005). Psychometric properties and validation of a Polish adaptation of Carver and White's BIS/BAS scales. *Personality and Individual Differences, 39*(4), 795–805.

Muller, J., Buhner, M., & Ellgring, H. (2003). Relationship and differential validity of alexithymia and depression: A comparison of the Toronto Alexithymia and Self-Rating Depression Scales. *Psychopathology, 36*(2), 71–77.

Mullin, B. C., & Hinshaw, S. P. (2007). Emotion regulation and externalizing disorders in children and adolescents. In J. J. Gross (Ed.), *Handbook of emotion regulation* (pp. 523–541). New York: Guilford Press.

Munson, J., Dawson, G., Abbott, R., Faja, S., Webb, S. J., Friedman, S. D., et al. (2006). Amygdalar volume and behavioral development in autism. *Archives of General Psychiatry, 63*(6), 686–693.

Munver, R., & Volfson, I. A. (2007). Adrenal insufficiency: Diagnosis and management. *Current Urology Reports, 7*, 80–85.

Murayama, J., Kashiwagi, T., Kashiwagi, A., & Mimura, M. (2004). Impaired pitch production and preserved rhythm production in a right brain-damaged patient with amusia. *Brain and Cognition, 56*(1), 36–42.

Murphy, F. C., Nimmo-Smith, I., & Lawrence, A. D. (2003). Functional neuroanatomy of emotions: A meta-analysis. *Cognitive, Affective, and Behavioral Neuroscience, 3*(3), 207–233.

Myers, L. B., Burns, J. W., Derakshan, N., Elfant, E., Eysenck, M. W., Phipps, S., et al. (2008). Current issues in repressive coping and health. In A. Vingerhoets, I. Nyklicek, & J. Denollet (Eds.), *Emotion regulation: Conceptual and clinical issues* (pp. 69–86). New York: Springer Science+Business Media.

Myhill, P. C., Sillars, B. A., Starkstein, S., Annus, T., & Yeap, B. B. (2008). Reduction in salivary cortisol concentration correlates with resolution of psychosis in Cushing's syndrome. *Journal of Neuropsychiatry and Clinical Neurosciences, 20*(1), 113–115.

Naccache, L., Gaillard, R. l., Adam, C., Hasboun, D., Clemenceau, S. P., Baulac, M., et al. (2005). A direct intracranial record of emotions evoked by subliminal words. *Proceedings of the National Academy of Sciences of the United States of America, 102*(21), 7713–7717.

Nagaratnam, N., Wong, K.-K., & Patel, I. (2006). Secondary mania of vascular origin in elderly patients: A report of two clinical cases. *Archives of Gerontology and Geriatrics, 43*(2), 223–232.

Nakhutina, L., Borod, J. C., & Zgaljardic, D. J. (2006). Posed prosodic emotional expression in unilateral stroke patients: Recovery, lesion location, and emotional perception. *Archives of Clinical Neuropsychology, 21*(1), 1–13.

Nakimuli-Mpungu, E., Musisi, S., Mpungu, S. K., & Katabira, E. (2006). Primary mania versus HIV-related secondary mania in Uganda. *American Journal of Psychiatry, 163*(8), 1349–1354.

Narashima, K., Kosier, J. T., & Robinson, R. G. (2003). A reappraisal of poststroke depression, intra- and inter-hemispheric lesion location using meta-analysis. *Journal of Neuropsychiatry and Clinical Neurosciences, 15*(4), 422–430.

Narushima, K., & Robinson, R. G. (2003). The effect of early versus late antidepressant treatment on physical impairment associated with poststroke depression: Is there a time-related therapeutic window? *Journal of Nervous and Mental Disease, 191*(10), 645–652.

Nauta, W. J. H. (1946). Hypothalamic regulation of sleep in rats: An experimental study. *Journal of Neurophysiology, 9*, 285–316.

Newman, J. P., MacCoon, D. G., Vaughn, L. J., & Sadeh, N. (2005). Validating a distinction between primary and secondary psychopathy with measures of Gray's BIS and BAS constructs. *Journal of Abnormal Psychology, 114*(2), 319–323.

Newman, J. P., Patterson, C. M., Howland, E. W., & Nichols, S. L. (1990). Passive avoidance in psychopaths: The effects of reward. *Personality and Individual Differences, 11*(11), 1101–1114.

Newman, J. P., & Schmitt, W. A. (1998). Passive avoidance in psychopathic offenders: A replication and extension. *Journal of Abnormal Psychology, 107*(3), 527–532.

Ng, D. M., & Jeffrey, R. W. (2003). Relationships between perceived stress and health behaviors in a sample of working adults. *Health Psychology, 22*, 638–642.

Nicholl, C. R., Lincoln, N. B., Muncaster, K., & Thomas, S. (2002). Cognitions and post-stroke depression. *British Journal of Clinical Psychology, 41*(3), 221–231.

Nichols, H. (1896). Review of fear. *Psychological Review, 3*(4), 445–447.

Nichols, N. R., Zieba, M., & Bye, N. (2001). Do glucocorticoids contribute to brain aging? *Brain Research Reviews, 37*(1), 273–286.

Nicholson, C. (2006). Thinking it over: fMRI and psychological science [Electronic version]. *The APS Observer, 19*. Retrieved from *www.psychologicalscience.org/observer.*

Niedenthal, P. M. (2007). Embodying emotion. *Science, 316*, 1002–1005.

Niedenthal, P. M., Winkielman, P., Mondillon, L., & Vermeulen, N. (2009). Embodiment of emotion concepts. *Journal of Personality and Social Psychology, 96*(6), 1120–1136.

Niedermaier, N., Bohrer, E., Schulte, K., Schlattmann, P., & Heuser, I. (2004). Prevention and treatment of poststroke depression with mirtazapine in patients with acute stroke. *Journal of Clinical Psychiatry, 65*(12), 1619–1623.

Nielson, K. A., Langenecker, S. A., & Garavan, H. (2002). Differences in the functional neuroanatomy of inhibitory control across the adult life span. *Psychology and Aging, 17*, 56–71.

Nigg, J. T., John, O. P., Blaskey, L. G., Huang-Pollock, C. L., Willcutt, E. G., Hinshaw, S. P., et al. (2002). Big five dimensions and ADHD symptoms: Links between personality traits and clinical symptoms. *Journal of Personality and Social Psychology, 83*(2), 451–469.

Nigg, J. T., Wong, M. M., Martel, M. M., Jester, J. M., Puttler, L. I., Glass, J. M., et al. (2006). Poor response inhibition as a predictor of problem drinking and illicit drug use in adolescents at risk for alcoholism and other substance use disorders. *Journal of the American Academy of Child and Adolescent Psychiatry, 45*(4), 468–475.

Niijima, A. (1991). Effects of taste stimulation on the efferent activity of the autonomic nerves in the rat. *Brain Research Bulletin, 26*(1), 165–167.

Nilsson, J. P., Soderstrom, M., Karlsson, A. U., Lekander, M., Akerstedt, T., Erixon, N., et al. (2005). Less effective executive functioning after one night's sleep deprivation. *Journal of Sleep Research, 14*(1), 1–6.

Nishida, T., Kudo, T., Inoue, Y., Nakamura, F., Yoshimura, M., Matsuda, K., et al. (2006). Postictal mania versus postictal psychosis: Differences in clinical features, epileptogenic zone, and brain functional changes during postictal period. *Epilepsia, 47*(12), 2104–2114.

Nobel Lectures, Physiology or Medicine 1942–1962. (1964). Amsterdam: Elsevier.

Noble, E. P. (1968). The effects of physiological doses of corticosteroid on catecholamine metabolism in man. *Journal of Psychiatric Research, 6*(2), 159–167.

Nordby, G., Ekeberg, O., Knardahl, S., & Os, I. (1995). A double-blind study of psychosocial factors in 40-year-old women with essential hypertension. *Psychotherapy and Psychosomatics, 63*(3), 142–150.

Nowak, L. G., & Bullier, J. (1997). The timing of information transfer in the visual system. In K. S. Rockland, J. H. Kaas, & A. Peters (Eds.), *Cerebral cortex: Extrastriate cortex in primates* (pp. 205–241). New York: Springer.

Ochsner, K. N., Bunge, S. A., Gross, J. J., & Gabrieli, J. D. E. (2002). Rethinking feelings: An fMRI study of the cognitive regulation of emotion. *Journal of Cognitive Neuroscience, 14*(8), 1215–1229.

Ochsner, K. N., & Gross, J. J. (2007). The neural architecture of emotion regulation. In J. J. Gross (Ed.), *Handbook of emotion regulation* (pp. 87–109). New York: Guilford Press.

Ochsner, K. N., & Gross, J. J. (2008). Cognitive emotion regulation: Insights from social cognitive and affective neuroscience. *Current Directions in Psychological Science, 17*(2), 153–158.

O'Connell, R. G., Bellgrove, M. A., Dockree, P. M., Lau, A., Fitzgerald, M., & Robertson, I. H. (2008). Self-alert training: Volitional modulation of autonomic arousal improves sustained attention. *Neuropsychologia, 46*(5), 1379–1390.

O'Connell, R. G., Bellgrove, M. A., Dockree, P. M., Lau, A., Hester, R., Garavan, H., et al. (2009). The neural correlates of deficient error awareness in attention-deficit hyperactivity disorder (ADHD). *Neuropsychologia, 47*(4), 1149–1159.

O'Dwyer, A. M., & Orrell, M. W. (1994). Stress, ageing and dementia. *International Review of Psychiatry, 6*(1), 73–83.

O'Hara, R., Schroeder, C. M., Mahadevan, R., Lindley, S., Weiner, M., Noda, A., et al. (2007). Serotonin transporter polymorphism, memory and hippocampal volume in the elderly: Association and interaction with cortisol. *Molecular Psychiatry, 12*(6), 544–555.

Ohayon, M. M., & Roth, T. (2003). Place of chronic insomnia in the course of depressive and anxiety disorders. *Journal of Psychiatric Research, 37*, 9–15.

Ohira, H., Nomura, M., Ichikawa, N., Isowa, T., Iidaka, T., Sato, A., et al. (2006). Association of neural and physiological responses during voluntary emotion suppression.. *NeuroImage, 29*, 721–733.

Ohman, A. (2002). Automaticity and the amygdala: Nonconscious responses to emotional faces. *Current Directions in Psychological Science, 11*(2), 62–66.

Ohman, A. (2005). The role of the amygdala in human fear: Automatic detection of threat. *Psychoneuroendocrinology, 30*(10), 953–958.

Ohman, A., Flykt, A., & Esteves, F. (2001). Emotion drives attention: Detecting the snake in the grass. *Journal of Experimental Psychology: General, 130*(3), 466–478.

Ohman, A., & Mineka, S. (2001). Fears, phobias, and preparedness: Toward an evolved module of fear and fear learning. *Psycholgical Review, 108*, 483–522.

Ohmura, Y., Yamaguchi, T., Futami, Y., Izumi, T., Yoshida, T., Yoshioka, M., et al. (2009). Corticotropin releasing factor enhances attentional function as assessed by the five-choice serial reaction time task in rats. *Behavioural Brain Research, 198*(2), 429–433.

O'Jile, J. R., Ryan, L. M., Parks-Levy, J., Betz, B., & Gouvier, W. D. (2004). Sensation seeking and risk behaviors in young adults with and without a history of head injury. *Applied Neuropsychology, 11*(2), 107–112.

Okuda, M., Harada, H., Mizutani, H., & Hamanaka, T. (1998). Pica in demented patients. *Seishin Igaku (Clinical Psychiatry), 40*(10), 1103–1105.

Olley, A., Malhi, G., & Sachdev, P. (2007). Memory and executive functioning in obsessive–compulsive disorder: A selective review. *Journal of Affective Disorders, 104*(1–3), 15–23.

Olson, I. R., Plotzker, A., & Ezzyat, Y. (2007). The enigmatic temporal pole: A review of findings on social and emotional processing. *Brain: A Journal of Neurology, 130*(7), 1718–1731.

Oppenheimer, S. M. (1992). Cardiovascular effects of human insular cortex stimulation. *Cardiology, 42*, 1727–1732.

Orbelo, D. M., Grim, M. A., Talbott, R. E., & Ross, E. D. (2005). Impaired comprehension of affective prosody in elderly subjects is not predicted by age-related hearing loss or age-related cognitive decline. *Journal of Geriatric Psychiatry and Neurology, 18*(1), 25–32.

Osaka, M., Komori, M., Morishita, M., & Osaka, N. (2007). Neural bases of focusing attention in working memory: An fMRI study based on group differences. *Cognitive, Affective, and Behavioral Neuroscience, 7*(2), 130–139.

O'Sullivan, S. S., Massey, L. A., Williams, D. R., Silveira-Moriyama, L., Kempster, P. A., Holton, J. L., et al. (2008). Clinical outcomes of progressive supranuclear palsy and multiple system atrophy. *Brain: A Journal of Neurology, 131*(5), 1362–1372.

Oyebode, F., Edelstyn, N. M. J., Patel, A., & Riddoch, M. J. (1996). Capgras syndrome in vascular dementia: Recognition memory and visual processing. *International Journal of Geriatric Psychiatry, 11*(1), 71–73.

Ozdemir, O., & Hachinski, V. (2008). Brain lateralization and sudden death: Its role in the neurogenic heart syndrome. *Journal of the Neurological Sciences, 268*(1), 6–11.

Ozonoff, S. (1995). Reliability and validity of the Wisconsin Card Sorting Test in studies of autism. *Neuropsychology, 9*(4), 491–500.

Pacak, K., Armando, I., Kvetnansky, R., Palkovits, M., Goldstein, D. S., Kopin, I. J., et al. (1992). Stress-induced changes in norepinephrine, dihydroxyphenylglycol, and 3,4-dihydroxyphenylacetic acid levels in the hypothalamic paraventricular nucleus of conscious rats. In R. Kvetnansky (Ed.), *Stress: Neuroendocrine and molecular approaches* (Vols. 1 & 2, pp. 93–98). Philadelphia: Gordon & Breach Science.

Paelecke-Habermann, Y., Pohl, J., & Leplow, B. (2005). Attention and executive functions in remitted major depression patients. *Journal of Affective Disorders, 89*(1–3), 125–135.

Pajouhi, M., Shaban, N. K. Z., & Mohajeri, T. M. R. (2007). Evaluation and prevention of diabetic neuropathy. *Tehran University Medical Journal, 65*(3), 1–6.

Palmiter, R. D. (2007). Is dopamine a physiologically relevant mediator of feeding behavior? *Trends in Neurosciences, 30*(8), 375–381.

Panzer, A., Viljoen, M., & Roos, J. L. (2007). The neurobiological basis of fear: A concise review. *South African Psychiatry Review, 10*(2), 71–75.

Paolucci, S. (2008). Epidemiology and treatment of post-stroke depression. *Neuropsychiatric Disease and Treatment, 4*, 145–154.

Papagno, C., & Vallar, G. (2002). Anosognosia for left hemiplegia: Banbinski's (1914) cases. In C. Code, E. Joanette, A. R. Lecours, & C.-W. Wallesch (Eds.), *Classic cases in neuropsychology: II. Brain damage, behaviour, and cognition* (pp. 171–189). Hove, UK: Psychology Press.

Papez, J. W. (1937). A proposed mechanism of emotion. *Archives of Neurology and Psychiatry, 79*, 217–224.

Paradiso, S., Vaidya, J. G., McCormick, L. M., Jones, A., & Robinson, R. G. (2008). Aging and alexithymia: Association with reduced right rostral cingulate volume. *American Journal of Geriatric Psychiatry, 16*(9), 760–769.

Pariante, C. M. (2006). The glucocorticoid receptor: Part of the solution or part of the problem? *Journal of Psychopharmacology, 20*(4), 79–84.

Pariante, C. M., & Lightman, S. L. (2008). The HPA axis in major depression: Classical theories and new developments. *Trends in Neurosciences, 31*(9), 464–468.

Parker, J. D. A., Bagby, R. M., Taylor, G. J., & Endler, N. S. (1993). Factorial validity of the 20-item Toronto Alexithymia Scale. *European Journal of Personality, 7*(4), 221–232.

Parker, J. D. A., Keefer, K. V., Taylor, G. J., & Bagby, R. M. (2008). Latent structure of the alexithymia construct: A taxometric investigation. *Psychological Assessment, 20*(4), 385–396.

Parker, J. D. A., Taylor, G. J., & Bagby, R. M. (1998). Alexithymia: Relationship with ego defense and coping styles. *Comprehensive Psychiatry, 39*(2), 91–98.

Parker, J. D. A., Taylor, G. J., & Bagby, R. M. (2003). The 20-item Toronto Alexithymia Scale III: Reliability and factorial validity in a community population. *Journal of Psychosomatic Research, 55*(3), 269–275.

Parker, K. J., Buckmaster, C. L., Sundlass, K., Schatzberg, A. F., Lyons, D. M., & McEwen, B. S. (2006). Maternal mediation, stress inoculation, and the development of neuroendocrine stress resistance in primates. *Proceedings of the National Academy of Sciences of the United States of America, 103*(8), 3000–3005.

Parker, P. D., Prkachin, K. M., & Prkachin, G. C. (2005). Processing of facial expressions of negative emotion in alexithymia: The influence of temporal constraint. *Journal of Personality, 73*(4), 1087–1107.

Patten, S. B., Beck, C. A., Williams, J. V. A., Barbui, C., & Metz, L. M. (2003). Major depression in multiple sclerosis: A population-based perspective. *Neurology, 61*(11), 1524–1527.

Patten, S. B., Svenson, L., & Metz, L. M. (2005). Descriptive epidemiology of affective disorders in multiple sclerosis. *CNS Specrums, 10*, 365–382.

Paul, L. K., Lautzenhiser, A., Brown, W. S., Hart, A., Neumann, D., Spezio, M., et al. (2006). Emotional arousal in agenesis of the corpus callosum. *International Journal of Psychophysiology, 61*(1), 47–56.

Pearce, J. M. S. (2004). A note on gelastic epilepsy. *European Neurology, 52*, 172–174.

Pearson. (2009). *Advanced clinical solutions for the WAIS-IV/WMS-IV*. San Antonio, TX: Author.

Pecina, S., & Berridge, K. C. (2005). Hedonic hot spot in nucleus accumbens shell: Where do mu-opioids cause increased hedonic impact of sweetness? *Journal of Neuroscience, 25*, 11777–11786.

Pedersen, K. F., Alves, G., Aarsland, D., & Larsen, J. P. (2009). Occurrence and risk factors for apathy in Parkinson's disease: A 4-year prospective longitudinal study. *Journal of Neurology, Neurosurgery, and Psychiatry, 80*(11), 1279–1282.

Pell, M. D. (1998). Recognition of prosody following unilateral brain lesion: Influence of functional and structural attributes of prosodic contours. *Neuropsychologia, 36*(8), 701–715.

Pell, M. D., & Leonard, C. L. (2005). Facial expression decoding in early Parkinson's disease. *Cognitive Brain Research, 23*(2), 327–340.

Pelletier, M., Bouthillier, A., Levesque, J., Carrier, S., Breault, C., Paquette, V., et al.

(2003). Separate neural circuits for primary emotions?: Brain activity during self-induced sadness and happiness in professional actors. *NeuroReport, 14*(8), 1111–1116.

Persinger, M. A. (1993). Personality changes following brain injury as a grief response to the loss of sense of self: Phenomenological themes as indices of local lability and neurocognitive structuring as psychotherapy. *Psychological Reports, 72*(3), 1059–1068.

Pessoa, L. (2009). How do emotion and motivation direct executive control? *Trends in Cognitive Sciences, 13*(4), 160–166.

Petrovic, P., Pleger, B., Seymour, B., Kloeppel, S., Martino, B. D., Critchley, H., et al. (2008). Blocking central opiate function modulates hedonic impact and anterior cingulate response to rewards and losses. *Journal of Neuroscience, 28*(42), 10509–10516.

Pezawas, L., Meyer-Lindenberg, A., Drabant, E. M., Verchinski, B. A., Munoz, K. E., Kolachana, B. S., et al. (2005). 5-HTTLPR polymorphism impacts human cingulate–amygdala interactions: A genetic susceptibility mechanism for depression. *Nature Neuroscience, 8*(6), 828–834.

Phan, K. L., Fitzgerald, D. A., Nathan, P. J., Moore, G. J., Uhde, T. W., & Tancer, M. E. (2005). Neural substrates for voluntary suppression of negative affect: A functional magnetic resonance imaging study. *Biological Psychiatry, 57*(3), 210–219.

Phan, K. L., Orlichenko, A., Boyd, E., Angstadt, M., Coccaro, E. F., Liberzon, I., et al. (2009). Preliminary evidence of white matter abnormality in the uncinate fasciculus in generalized social anxiety disorder. *Biological Psychiatry, 66*(7), 691–694.

Phelps, E. A. (2004). Human emotion and memory: Interactions of the amygdala and hippocampal complex. *Current Opinion in Neurobiology, 14*(2), 198–202.

Phelps, E. A., Fiske, S. T., Kazdin, A. E., & Schacter, D. L. (2006). Emotion and cognition: Insights from studies of the human amygdala. In S. T. Fiske, A. E. Kazdin, & D. L. Schacter (Eds.), *Annual review of psychology* (Vol 57, pp. 27–53). Palo Alto, CA: Annual Reviews.

Phelps, E. A., LaBar, K. S., Anderson, A. K., O'Connor, K. J., Fulbright, R. K., & Spencer, D. D. (1998). Specifying the contributions of the human amygdala to emotional memory: A case study. *Neurocase, 4*(6), 527–540.

Philippot, P., Kornreich, C., Blairy, S., Den Dulk, A., Le Bon, O., Streel, E., et al. (1999). Alcoholics' deficits in the decoding of emotional facial expression. *Alcoholism: Clinical and Experimental Research, 23*(6), 1031–1038.

Phillips, L. H., Saldias, A., McCarrey, A., Henry, J. D., Scott, C., Summers, F., et al. (2009). Attentional lapses, emotional regulation and quality of life in multiple sclerosis. *British Journal of Clinical Psychology, 48*(1), 101–106.

Phillips, L. J., McGorry, P. D., Garner, B., Thompson, K. N., Pantelis, C., Wood, S. J., et al. (2006). Stress, the hippocampus and the hypothalamic–pituitary–adrenal axis: Implications for the development of psychotic disorders. *Australian and New Zealand Journal of Psychiatry, 40*(9), 725–741.

Pick, L. H. (2002). *Lexical expression of emotion in cortical stroke patients: Intra- and interhemispheric effects.* Ann Arbor, MI: ProQuest Information & Learning.

Pieper, S., & Brosschot, J. F. (2005). Prolonged stress-related cardiovascular activation: Is there any? *Annals of Behavioral Medicine, 30*(2), 91–103.

Pier, M. P., Hulstijn, W., & Sabbe, B. G. C. (2004). Differential patterns of psychomotor functioning in unmedicated melancholic and nonmelancholic depressed patients. *Journal of Psychiatric Research, 38*(4), 425–435.

Pietrzak, R. H., Maruff, P., Mayes, L. C., Roman, S. A., Sosa, J. A., & Snyder, P. J. (2008). An examination of the construct validity and factor structure of the Groton Maze Learning Test, a new measure of spatial working memory, learning efficiency, and error monitoring. *Archives of Clinical Neuropsychology, 23*(4), 433–445.

Pizzagalli, D. A., Sherwood, R. J., Henriques, J. B., & Davidson, R. J. (2005). Frontal brain asymmetry and reward responsiveness: A source-localization study. *Psychological Science, 16*(10), 805–813.

Platel, H., Price, C., Baron, J.-C., Wise, R., Lambert, J., Frackowiak, R. S. J., et al. (1997). The structural components of music perception: A functional anatomical study. *Brain: A Journal of Neurology, 120*(2), 229–243.

Pluck, G. C., & Brown, R. G. (2002). Apathy in Parkinson's disease. *Journal of Neurology, Neurosurgery, and Psychiatry, 73*(6), 636–642.

Plutchik, R. (1985). On emotion: The chicken-and-egg problem revisited. *Motivation and Emotion, 9*(2), 197–200.

Pol, H. E. H., Schnack, H. G., Posthuma, D., Mandl, R. C. W., Baare, W. F., van Oel, C., et al. (2006). Genetic contributions to human brain morphology and intelligence. *Journal of Neuroscience, 26*(40), 10235–10242.

Polich, J., & Kok, A. (1995). Cognitive and biological determinants of P300: An integrative review. *Biological Psychology, 41*(2), 103–146.

Pollatos, O., Gramann, K., & Schandry, R. (2007). Neural systems connecting interoceptive awareness and feelings. *Human Brain Mapping, 28*(1), 9–18.

Pollatos, O., Kirsch, W., & Schandry, R. (2005a). Brain structures involved in interoceptive awareness and cardioafferent signal processing: A dipole source localization study. *Human Brain Mapping, 26*(1), 54–64.

Pollatos, O., Kirsch, W., & Schandry, R. (2005b). On the relationship between interoceptive awareness, emotional experience, and brain processes. *Cognitive Brain Research, 25*(3), 948–962.

Pollatos, O., Schandry, R., Auer, D. P., & Kaufmann, C. (2007). Brain structures mediating cardiovascular arousal and interoceptive awareness. *Brain Research, 1141*, 178–187.

Pomerantz, J. M. (2008). Early antidepressant treatment is effective for post-stroke depression. *Drug Benefit Trends, 20*(3), 115–116.

Porges, S. W. (2007). The polyvagal perspective. *Biological Psychology, 74*, 116–143.

Posner, M. I., Rothbart, M. K., & Sheese, B. E. (2007). Attention genes. *Developmental Science, 10*(1), 24–29.

Posner, M. I., Rothbart, M. K., Vizueta, N., Levy, K. N., Evans, D. E., Thomas, K. M., et al. (2002). Attentional mechanisms of borderline personality disorder. *Proceedings of the National Academy of Sciences, 99*(25), 16366–16370.

Pourtois, G., de Gelder, B., Bol, A., & Crommelick, M. (2005). Perception of facial expressions and voiced and of their combination in the human brain. *Cortex, 41*, 9–59.

Poythress, N. G., Skeem, J. L., Weir, J., Lilienfeld, S. O., Douglas, K. S., Edens, J. F., et al. (2008). Psychometric properties of Carver and White's (1994) BIS/BAS scales in a large sample of offenders. *Personality and Individual Differences, 45*(8), 732–737.

Premack, D., & Woodruff, G. (1978). Does the chimpanzee have a theory of mind? *Behavioral and Brain Sciences, 1*(4), 515–526.

Premkumar, P., Fannon, D., Kuipers, E., Simmons, A., Frangou, S., & Kumari, V.

(2008). Emotional decision-making and its dissociable components in schizophrenia and schizoaffective disorder: A behavioural and MRI investigation. *Neuropsychologia, 46*(7), 2002–2012.

Preston, S. D., Bechara, A., Damasio, H., Grabowski, T. J., Stansfield, R. B., Mehta, S., et al. (2007). The neural substrates of cognitive empathy. *Social Neuroscience, 2*(3), 254–275.

Pribram, K. H. (1967). The new neurology and the biology of emotion: A structural approach. *American Psychologist, 22*(10), 830–838.

Pribram, K. H., & Bagshaw, M. (1953). Further analysis of the temporal lobe syndrome utilizing fronto-temporal ablations in monkeys. *Journal of Comparative and Physiological Psychology, 99*, 347–375.

Prigatano, G. P., Wethe, J. V., Gray, J. A., Wang, N., Chung, S., Ng, Y.-T., et al. (2008). Intellectual functioning in presurgical patients with hypothalamic hamartoma and refractory epilepsy. *Epilepsy and Behavior, 13*(1), 149–155.

Pruessner, J. C., Lord, C., Meaney, M., Lupien, S., Yehuda, R., & McEwen, B. (2004). Effects of self-esteem on age-related changes in cognition and the regulation of the hypothalamic–pituitary–adrenal axis. In R. Yehuda & B. S. McEwen (Eds.), *Biobehavioral stress response: Protective and damaging effects* (pp. 186–190). New York: New York Academy of Sciences.

Psychological Corporation (1997). *WAIS-III and WMS-III technical manual.* San Antonio, TX: Author.

Puccetti, R. (1969). The sensation of pleasure. *British Journal for the Philosophy of Science, 20*(3), 239–245.

Pujol, J. S., Bello, J., Deus, J., Cardoner, N. S., Marta-Vilalta, J. L., & Capdevila, A. (2000). Beck Depression Inventory factors related to demyelinating lesions of the left arcuate fasciculus region. *Psychiatry Research: Neuroimaging, 99*(3), 151–159.

Pujol, J. S., Bello, J., Deus, J., Marta-Vilalta, J. L., & Capdevila, A. (1997). Lesions in the left arcuate fasciculus region and depressive symptoms in multiple sclerosis. *Neurology, 49*(4), 1105–1110.

Pushkar, D., Basevitz, P., Arbuckle, T., Nohara-LeClair, M., Lapidus, S., & Peled, M. (2000). Social behavior and off-target verbosity in elderly people. *Psychology and Aging, 15*(2), 361–374.

Putman, P., Hermans, E. J., & van Honk, J. (2007). Exogenous cortisol shifts a motivated bias from fear to anger in spatial working memory for facial expressions. *Psychoneuroendocrinology, 32*(1), 14–21.

Putnam, K. M., Pizzagalli, D. A., Gooding, D. C., Kalin, N. H., & Davidson, R. J. (2008). Neural activity and diurnal variation of cortisol: Evidence from brain electrical tomography analysis and relevance to anhedonia. *Psychophysiology, 45*(6), 886–895.

Quigg, M., & Barbaro, N. M. (2008). Stereotactic radiosurgery for treatment of epilepsy. *Archives of Neurology, 65*(2), 177–183.

Quiske, A., Frings, L., Wagner, K., Unterrainer, J., & Schulze-Bonhage, A. (2006). Cognitive functions in juvenile and adult patients with gelastic epilepsy due to hypothalamic hamartoma. *Epilepsia, 47*(1), 153–158.

Rabe, S., Zoellner, T., Beauducel, A., Maercker, A., & Karl, A. (2008). Changes in brain electrical activity after cognitive behavioral therapy for posttraumatic stress disorder in patients injured in motor vehicle accidents. *Psychosomatic Medicine, 70*(1), 13–19.

Rader, N., & Hughes, E. (2005). The influence of affective state on the performance of a block design task in 6- and 7-year-old children. *Cognition and Emotion, 19*(1), 143–150.

Radice-Neumann, D., Zupan, B., Babbage, D. R., & Willer, B. (2007). Overview of impaired facial affect recognition in persons with traumatic brain injury. *Brain Injury, 21*(8), 807–816.

Radley, J. J., Rocher, A. B., Miller, M., Janssen, W. G. M., Listen, C., Hof, P. R., et al. (2006). Repeated stress induces dendritic spine loss in the rat medial prefrontal cortex. *Cerebral Cortex, 16*(3), 313–320.

Raftery, J. N., & Bizer, G. Y. (2009). Negative feedback and performance: The moderating effect of emotion regulation. *Personality and Individual Differences, 47*(5), 481–486.

Rankin, K. P., Baldwin, E., Pace-Savitsky, C., Kramer, J. H., & Miller, B. L. (2005). Self awareness and personality change in dementia. *Journal of Neurology, Neurosurgery, and Psychiatry, 76*(5), 632–639.

Rankin, K. P., Kramer, J. H., & Miller, B. L. (2005). Patterns of cognitive and emotional empathy in frontotemporal lobar degeneration. *Cognitive and Behavioral Neurology, 18*(1), 28–36.

Rao, V., Spiro, J. R., Schretlen, D. J., & Cascella, N. G. (2007). Apathy syndrome after traumatic brain injury compared with deficits in schizophrenia. *Psychosomatics: Journal of Consultation Liaison Psychiatry, 48*(3), 217–222.

Rauch, S. L., Savage, C. R., Alpert, N. M., Fischman, A. J., & Jenike, M. A. (1997). The functional neuroanatomy of anxiety: A study of three disorders using positron emission tomography and symptom provocation. *Biological Psychiatry, 42*(6), 446–452.

Ravnkilde, B., Videbech, P., Rosenberg, R., Gjedde, A., & Gade, A. (2002). Putative tests of frontal lobe function: A PET-study of brain activation during Stroop's test and verbal fluency. *Journal of Clinical and Experimental Neuropsychology, 24*(4), 534–547.

Ray, R. D., Ochsner, K. N., Cooper, J. C., Robertson, E. R., Gabrieli, J. D. E., & Gross, J. J. (2005). Individual differences in trait rumination and the neural systems supporting cognitive reappraisal. *Cognitive, Affective, and Behavioral Neuroscience, 5*(2), 156–168.

Raymond, J. D., Shapiro, K. L., & Arnell, K. M. (1992). Temporary suppression of visual procesing in a RSVP task: An attention blink? *Journal of Experimental Psychology, 18*, 849–860.

Ready, R. E., Ott, B. R., & Grace, J. (2007). Factor structure of patient and caregiver ratings on the Dementia Quality of Life instrument. *Aging, Neuropsychology, and Cognition, 14*(2), 144–154.

Reiman, E. M., Lane, R. D., Ahern, G. L., Schwartz, G. E., Davidson, R. J., Friston, K. J., et al. (1997). Neuroanatomical correlates of externally and internally generated human emotions. *American Journal of Psychiatry, 154*, 918–925.

Reiss, S. (2000). Human individuality, happiness, and flow. *American Psychologist, 55*(10), 1161–1162.

Reiss, S. (2004). Multifaceted nature of intrinsic motivation: The theory of 16 basic desires. *Review of General Psychology, 8*(3), 179–193.

Reuter, M., Ott, U., Vaitl, D., & Hennig, J. (2007). Impaired executive control is associated with a variation in the promoter region of the tryptophan hydroxylase 2 gene. *Journal of Cognitive Neuroscience, 19*(3), 401–408.

Rey, V., Cereda, C., & Michel, P. (2008). Recurrent asystolia in right middle cerebral artery infarct with predominant insular involvement. *Journal of Neurology, Neurosurgery, and Psychiatry, 79*(6), 618–618.

Reynolds, B., Ortengren, A., Richards, J. B., & de Wit, H. (2006). Dimensions of impulsive behaviors: Personality and behavioral measures. *Personality and Individual Differences, 40*(2), 305–315.

Reynolds, S. M., & Berridge, K. C. (2002). Positive and negative motivation in nucleus accumbens shell: Bivalent rostrocaudal gradients for GABA-elicited eating, taste "liking"/"disliking" reactions, place preference/avoidance, and fear. *Journal of Neuroscience, 22*(16), 7308–7320.

Richards, J. M., & Gross, J. J. (2000). Emotion regulation and memory: The cognitive costs of keeping one's cool. *Journal of Personality and Social Psychology, 79*(3), 410–424.

Richards, J. M., & Gross, J. J. (2006). Personality and emotional memory: How regulating emotion impairs memory for emotional events. *Journal of Research in Personality, 40*(5), 631–651.

Richter, J., Moeller, B., Spitzer, C., Letzel, S., Bartols, S., Barnow, S., et al. (2006). Transcallosal inhibition in patients with and without alexithymia. *Neuropsychobiology, 53*(2), 101–107.

Ridout, N., Thom, C., & Wallis, D. J. (2010). Emotion recognition and alexithymia in females with non-clinical disordered eating. *Eating Behaviors, 11*(1), 1–5.

Rieger, M., Pirke, K.-M., Buske-Kirschbaum, A., Wurmser, H., Papousek, M., Hellhammer, D. H., et al. (2004). Influence of stress during pregnancy on HPA activity and neonatal behavior. In R. Yehuda & B. S. McEwen (Eds.), *Biobehavioral stress response: Protective and damaging effects* (pp. 228–230). New York: New York Academy of Sciences.

Rinn, W. E. (2007). Emotional facial expression in Parkinson's disease: A response to Bowers (2006). *Journal of the International Neuropsychological Society, 13*(4), 721–722.

Ritchie, K., & Lovestone, S. (2002). The dementias. *Lancet, 360*, 1767–1769.

Robbins, T. W., & Arnsten, A. F. T. (2009). The neuropsychopharmacology of fronto-executive function: Monoaminergic modulation. *Annual Review of Neuroscience, 32*, 267–287.

Robbins, T. W., & Everitt, B. (2007). A role of mesencephalic dopamine in activation: A commentary on Berridge. *Psychopharmacology, 191*, 433–437.

Robert, P. H., Berr, C., Volteau, M., Bertogliati-Fileau, C., Benoit, M., Guerin, O., et al. (2008). Importance of lack of interest in patients with mild cognitive impairment. *American Journal of Geriatric Psychiatry, 16*(9), 770–776.

Roberts, B. W., Walton, K. E., & Bogg, T. (2005). Conscientiousness and health across the life course. *Review of General Psychology, 9*(2), 156–168.

Robertson, D. (2008). The pathophysiology and diagnosis of orthostatic hypotension. *Clinical Autonomic Research, 18*, 2–7.

Robertsson, B., Blennow, K., Brane, G., Edman, A., Karlsson, I., Wallin, A., et al. (2001). Hyperactivity in the hypothalamic–pituitary–adrenal axis in demented patients with delirium. *International Clinical Psychopharmacology, 16*(1), 39–47.

Robin, A. A. (1958). A controlled study of the effects of leucotomy. *Journal of Neurology, Neurosurgery, and Psychiatry, 21*, 262–269.

Robin, A. A. (1959). The value of leucotomy in relation to diagnosis. *Journal of Neurology, Neurosurgery, and Psychiatry, 22*, 132–136.

Robins, R. W., Fraley, R. C., Roberts, B. W., & Trzesniewksi, K. H. (2001). A longitudinal study of personality change in young adulthood. *Journal of Personality, 64*(4), 618–640.

Robinson, R. G. (1983). Mood changes in stroke patients: Relationship to lesion location. *Comprehensive Psychiatry, 24*(6), 555–566.

Robinson, R. G. (1985a). Mood disorders in left-handed stroke patients. *American Journal of Psychiatry, 142*(12), 1424–1429.

Robinson, R. G. (1985b). A two-year longitudinal study of poststroke mood disorders: In-hospital prognostic factors associated with six-month outcome. *Journal of Nervous and Mental Disease, 173*(4), 221–226.

Robinson, R. G. (1997). Neuropsychiatric consequences of stroke. *Annual Review of Medicine, 48*, 217–229.

Robinson, R. G., Boston, J. D., Starkstein, S. E., & Price, T. R. (1988). Comparison of mania and depression after brain injury: Causal factors. *American Journal of Psychiatry, 145*(2), 172–178.

Robinson, R. G., Jorge, R. E., Moser, D. J., Acion, L., Solodkin, A., Small, S. L., et al. (2008). Escitalopram and problem-solving therapy for prevention of poststroke depression: A randomized control trial. *Journal of the American Medical Association, 299*(20), 2391–2400.

Robinson, R. G., Parikh, R. M., Lipsey, J. R., & Starkstein, S. E. (1993). Pathological laughing and crying following stroke: Validation of a measurement scale and a double-blind treatment study. *American Journal of Psychiatry, 150*(2), 286–293.

Robinson, S., Sandstrom, S. M., Denenberg, V. H., & Palmiter, R. D. (2005). Distinguishing whether dopamine regulates liking, wanting, and/or learning about rewards. *Behavioral Neuroscience, 119*(1), 5–15.

Robinson, T. E., & Berridge, K. C. (2000). The psychology and neurobiology of addiction: An incentive-sensitization view. *Addiction, 95*, S91–S117.

Robles, R., & Paez, F. (2003). El estudio sabre la traducción al español y las propiedades psicomótricas de las Escalas de Afecto Positivo y Negativo (PANAS) [Study of Spanish translation and Psychometric Properties of the Positive and Negative Affect Scales (PANAS)]. *Salud Mental, 26*(1), 69–75.

Rockwell, E., Choure, J., Galasko, D., Olichney, J., & Jeste, D. V. (2000). Psychopathology at initial diagnosis in dementia with Lewy bodies versus Alzheimer disease: Comparison of matched groups with autopsy-confirmed diagnoses. *International Journal of Geriatric Psychiatry, 15*(9), 819–823.

Rodriguez-Jimenez, R., Cubillo, A., Jimenez-Arriero, M. A., Ponce, G., Aragues-Figuero, M., & Palomo, T. (2006). Executive dysfunction in adults with attention deficit hyperactivity disorder. *Revista de Neurologia, 43*(11), 678–684.

Roelofs, K., van Peer, J., Berretty, E., Spinhoven, P., Elzinga, B. M., & de Jong, P. (2009). Hypothalamus–pituitary–adrenal axis hyperresponsiveness is associated with increased social avoidance behavior in social phobia. *Biological Psychiatry, 65*(4), 336–343.

Roffman, J. L., Marci, C. D., Glick, D. M., Dougherty, D. D., & Rauch, S. L. (2005). Neuroimaging and the functional neuroanatomy of psychotherapy. *Psychological Medicine, 35*(10), 1385–1398.

Rogers, J. M., & Read, C. A. (2007). Psychiatric comorbidity following traumatic brain injury. *Brain Injury, 21*(13), 1321–1333.

Rogers, R. D., Sahakian, B. J., Hodges, J. R., Polkey, C. E., Kennard, C., & Robbins,

T. W. (1998). Dissociating executive mechanisms of task control following frontal lobe damage and Parkinson's disease. *Brain, 121*, 815–842.

Rogstad, J. E., & Rogers, R. (2008). Gender differences in contributions of emotion to psychopathy and antisocial personality disorder. *Clinical Psychology Review, 28*(8), 1472–1484.

Roitman, M. F., Wheeler, R. A., Wightman, R. M., & Carelli, R. M. (2008). Real-time chemical responses in the nucleus accumbens differentiate rewarding and aversive stimuli. *Nature Neuroscience, 11*(12), 1376–1377.

Rolls, E. T. (2004). The functions of the orbitofrontal cortex. *Brain and Cognition, 55*(1), 11–29.

Rolls, E. T., Kringelbach, M. L., & de Araujo, I. E. T. (2003). Different representations of pleasant and unpleasant odours in the human brain. *European Journal of Neuroscience, 18*(3), 695–703.

Rolls, E. T., O'Doherty, J., Kringelbach, M. L., Francis, S., Bowtell, R., & McGlone, F. (2003). Representations of pleasant and painful touch in the human orbitofrontal and cingulate cortices. *Cerebral Cortex, 13*(3), 308–317.

Rosen, H. J., & Cummings, J. (2007). A real reason for patients with pseudobulbar affect to smile. *Annals of Neurology, 61*(2), 92–96.

Rosen, H. J., Pace-Savitsky, K., Perry, R. J., Kramer, J. H., Miller, B. L., & Levenson, R. W. (2004). Recognition of emotion in the frontal and temporal variants of frontotemporal dementia. *Dementia and Geriatric Cognitive Disorders, 17*(4), 277–281.

Ross, E. D. (1981). The aprosodias: Functional–anatomic organization of the affective components of language in the right hemisphere. *Archives of Neurology, 38*, 561–569.

Ross, E. D. (1984). Right hemisphere's role in language, affective behavior and emotion. *Trends in Neurosciences, 7*(9), 342–346.

Ross, E. D., & Mesulam, M. M. (2000). Affective prosody and the aprosodias. In M.-M. Mesulam (Ed.), *Principles of behavioral and cognitive neurology* (2nd ed., pp. 316–331). New York: Oxford University Press.

Ross, E. D., & Monnot, M. (2008). Neurology of affective prosody and its functional–anatomic organization in right hemisphere. *Brain and Language, 104*(1), 51–74.

Ross, E. D., Thompson, R. D., & Yenkosky, J. (1997). Lateralization of affective prosody in brain and the callosal integration of hemispheric language functions. *Brain and Language, 56*(1), 27–54.

Roth, R. M., Flashman, L. A., Saykin, A. J., McAllister, T. W., & Vidaver, R. (2004). Apathy in schizophrenia: Reduced frontal lobe volume and neuropsychological deficits. *American Journal of Psychiatry, 161*(1), 157–159.

Rothbart, M. K. (2007). Temperament, development, and personality. *Current Directions in Psychological Science, 16*(4), 207–212.

Rothbart, M. K., Ahadi, S. A., & Evans, D. E. (2000). Temperament and personality: Origins and outcomes. *Journal of Personality and Social Psychology, 78*(1), 122–135.

Rothbart, M. K., Ahadi, S. A., Hershey, K. L., & Fisher, P. (2001). Investigations of temperament at three to seven years: The Children's Behavior Questionnaire. *Child Development, 72*(5), 1394–1408.

Rothbart, M. K., Ellis, L. K., & Posner, M. I. (2004). Temperament and self-regulation. In R. F. Baumeister & K. D. Vohs (Eds.), *Handbook of self-regulation* (pp. 357–370). New York: Guilford Press.

Rothbart, M. K., Ellis, L. K., Rueda, M. R., & Posner, M. I. (2003). Developing mechanisms of temperamental effortful control. *Journal of Personality, 71*(6), 1113–1143.

Rothbart, M. K., & Sheese, B. E. (2007). Temperament and emotion regulation. In J. J. Gross (Ed.), *Handbook of emotion regulation* (pp. 331–350). New York: Guilford Press.

Rothman, M. S., Arciniegas, D. B., Filley, C. M., & Wierman, M. E. (2007). The neuroendocrine effects of traumatic brain injury. *Journal of Neuropsychiatry and Clinical Neurosciences, 19*(4), 363–372.

Rousmans, S., Robin, O., Dittmar, A., & Vernet-Maury, E. (2000). Autonomic nervous system responsess associated with primary tastes. *Chemical Senses, 25*(6), 709–718.

Royall, D. R., Chiodo, L. K., Mouton, C., & Polk, M. J. (2007). Cognitive predictors of mortality in elderly retirees: Results from the Freedom House Study. *American Journal of Geriatric Psychiatry, 15*(3), 243–251.

Royall, D. R., Palmer, R., Chiodo, L. K., & Polk, M. J. (2005). Executive control mediates memory's association with change in instrumental activities of daily living: The Freedom House Study. *Journal of the American Geriatrics Society, 53*(1), 11–17.

Rubinsztein, J. S., Michael, A., Paykel, E. S., & Sahakian, B. J. (2000). Cognitive impairment in remission in bipolar affective disorder. *Psychological Medicine, 30*(5), 1025–1036.

Ruff, R. (2005). Two decades of advances in understanding of mild traumatic brain injury. *Journal of Head Trauma Rehabilitation, 20*(1), 5–18.

Rushworth, M. F., Johansen-Berg, H., Gobel, S. M., & Devlin, J. T. (2003). The left parietal and premotor cortices: Motor attention and selection. *NeuroImage, 20*(Suppl. 1), S89–S100.

Ryan, M. C. M., Sharifi, N., Condren, R., & Thakore, J. H. (2004). Evidence of basal pituitary–adrenal overactivity in first episode, drug naive patients with schizophrenia. *Psychoneuroendocrinology, 29*(8), 1065–1070.

Rylander, G. S., Fulton, J. F., Aring, C. D., & Wortis, S. B. (1949). Personality analysis before and after frontal lobotomy. In J. F. Fulton, C. D. Aring, & S. B. Wortis (Eds.), *The frontal lobes* (Vol. 27, pp. 691–705). Oxford, UK: Williams & Wilkins.

Ryle, G. (1967). Plato. In P. Edwards (Ed.), *Encyclopedia of philosophy* (pp. 314–333). New York: Macmillan.

Saarijarvi, S., Salminen, J. K., Tamminen, T., & Aarela, E. (1993). Alexithymia in psychiatric consultation-liasion patients. *General Hospital Psychiatry, 15*(5), 330–330.

Saarijarvi, S., Salminen, J. K., & Toikka, T. B. (2001). Alexithymia and depression: A 1-year follow-up study in outpatients with major depression. *Journal of Psychosomatic Research, 51*(6), 729–733.

Saarijarvi, S., Salminen, J. K., & Toikka, T. B. (2006). Temporal stability of alexithymia over a five-year period in outpatients with major depression. *Psychotherapy and Psychosomatics, 75*(2), 107–112.

Sachs, G., Steger-Wuchse, D., Kryspin-Exner, I., Gur, R. C., & Katschnig, H. (2004). Facial affect recognition deficits and cognition in schizophrenia. *Schizophrenia Research, 68*(1), 27–35.

Sackeim, H. A., & Roose, S. P. (2004). Structural and functional brain imaging in late-life depression. In S. P. Roose & H. A. Sackeim (Eds.), *Late-life depression* (pp. 129–147). New York: Oxford University Press.

Sagduyu, K. (2002). Association of mild traumatic brain injury with bipolar disorder. *Journal of Clinical Psychiatry, 63*(7), 594–594.

Salamone, J. D., Correa, M., Farrar, A., & Mingote, S. M. (2007). Effort-related functions of nucleus accumbens dopamine and associated forebrain circuits. *Psychopharmacology, 191*(3), 461–482.

Salamone, J. D., Cousins, M. S., & Snyder, B. J. (1997). Behavioral functions of nucleus accumbens dopamine: Empirical and conceptual problems with the anhedonia hypothesis. *Neuroscience and Biobehavioral Reviews, 21*(3), 341–359.

Salminen, J. K., Saarijarvi, S., Aarela, E., Toikka, T., & Kauhanen, J. (1999). Prevalence of alexithymia and its association with sociodemographic variables in the general population of Finland. *Journal of Psychosomatic Research, 46*(1), 75–82.

Salzman, C. D., Paton, J. J., Belova, M. A., Morrison, S. E., Schoenbaum, G., Gottfried, J. A., et al. (2007). Flexible neural representations of value in the primate brain. In G. Schoenbaum, J. Gottfried, E. A. Murry, & S. Ramus (Eds.), *Linking affect to action: Critical contributions of the orbitofrontal cortex* (pp. 336–354). Malden, MA: Blackwell.

Sambataro, F., Dimalta, S., Di Giorgio, A., Taurisano, P., Blasi, G., Scarabino, T., et al. (2006). Preferential responses in amygdala and insula during presentation of facial contempt and disgust. *European Journal of Neuroscience, 24*(8), 2355–2362.

Sanchez, M. M., Ladd, C. O., & Plotsky, P. M. (2001). Early adverse experience as a developmental risk factor for later psychopathology: Evidence from rodent and primate models. *Development and Psychopathology, 13*(3), 419–449.

Sanders, R. D., & Mathews, T. A. (1994). Hypergraphia and secondary mania in temporal lobe epilepsy: Case reports and literature review. *Neuropsychiatry, Neuropsychology, and Behavioral Neurology, 7*(2), 114–117.

Sandin, B. (2003). Escalas PANAS de afecto positivo y negativo para ninos y adolescentes (PANASN) [The PANAS scales of positive and negative affect for children and adolscents (PANASN)]. *Revista de Psicopatologia y Psicologia Clinica, 8*(2), 173–182.

Santesso, D. L., Reker, D. L., Schmidt, L. A., & Segalowitz, S. J. (2006). Frontal electroencephalogram activation asymmetry, emotional intelligence, and externalizing behaviors in 10-year-old children. *Child Psychiatry and Human Development, 36*(3), 311–328.

Sarchiapone, M., Carli, V., Camardese, G., Cuomo, C., Di Giuda, D., Calcagni, M.-L., et al. (2006). Dopamine transporter binding in depressed patients with anhedonia. *Psychiatry Research: Neuroimaging, 147*(2), 243–248.

Sato, W., Kubota, Y., Okada, T., Murai, T., Yoshikawa, S., & Sengoku, A. (2002). Seeing happy emotion in fearful and angry faces: Qualitative analysis of facial expression recognition in a bilateral amygdala-damaged patient. *Cortex, 38*(5), 727–742.

Saxena, S., Gorbis, E., O'Neill, J., Baker, S. K., Mandelkern, M. A., Maidment, K. M., et al. (2009). Rapid effects of brief intensive cognitive-behavioral therapy on brain glucose metabolism in obsessive–compulsive disorder. *Molecular Psychiatry, 14*(2), 197–205.

Schachter, S., & Singer, J. (1962). Cognitive, social, and physiological determinants of emotional state. *Psychological Review, 69*(5), 379–399.

Schaefer, A., Schienle, A., & Vaitl, D. (2005). Stimulus type and design influence hemodynamic responses towards visual disgust and fear elicitors. *International Journal of Psychophysiology, 57*(1), 53–59.

Schaefer, R., Popp, K., Jergens, S., Lindenberg, R., Franz, M., & Seitz, R. J. (2007). Alexithymia-like disorder in right anterior cingulate infarction. *Neurocase, 13*(3), 201–208.

Schaefer, S. M. (2007). *Neural and dispositional correlates of components of affective style: Individual differences in perceiving, appraising, and regulating emotion.* Ann Arbor, MI: ProQuest Information & Learning.

Scheff, T. J. (1985). The primacy of affect. *American Psychologist, 40*(7), 849–850.

Schenkel, L. S., Pavuluri, M. N., Herbener, E. S., Harral, E. M., & Sweency, J. A. (2007). Facial emotion processing in acutely ill and euthymic patients with pediatric bipolar disorder. *Journal of the American Academy of Child and Adolescent Psychiatry, 46*(8), 1070–1079.

Scherer, K. R., & Peper, M. (2001). Psychological theories of emotion and neuropsychological research. In G. Gainotti (Ed.), *Handbook of neuropsychololology: Vol. 5. Emotional behavior and its disorders* (pp. 17–48). New York: Elsevier.

Schinka, J. A., Busch, R. M., & Robichaux-Keene, N. (2004). A meta-analysis of the association between the serotonin transporter gene polymorphism (*5-HTTLPR*) and trait anxiety. *Molecular Psychiatry, 9*(2), 197–202.

Schmahmann, J. D. (2001). The cerebrocerebellar system: Anatomic substrates of the cerebellar contribution to cognition and emotion. *International Review of Psychiatry, 13*(4), 247–260.

Schmeichel, B. J. (2007). Attention control, memory updating, and emotion regulation temporarily reduce the capacity for executive control. *Journal of Experimental Psychology: General, 136*(2), 241–255.

Schmeichel, B. J., Volokhov, R. N., & Demaree, H. A. (2008). Working memory capacity and the self-regulation of emotional expression and experience. *Journal of Personality and Social Psychology, 95*(6), 1526–1540.

Schmitter, A. M. (2006). 17th and 18th century theories of emotions. In E. M. Zalta (Ed.), *Stanford encyclopedia of philosophy*. Available at *plato.stanford.edu/archives/sum2006/entries/emotions-17th18th*.

Schmitz, A., Kirsch, P., Reuter, M., Alexander, N., Kozyra, E., Kuepper, Y., et al. (2009). The 5-HT1A C(–1019)G polymorphism, personality and electrodermal reactivity in a reward/punishment paradigm. *International Journal of Neuropsychopharmacology, 12*(3), 383–392.

Schneider, H. J. R., Kreitschmann-Andermahr, I., Ghigo, E., Agha, A., & Stalla, G. N. K. (2007). Hypothalamopituitary dysfunction following traumatic brain injury and aneurysmal subarachnoid hemorrhage: A systematic review. *Journal of the American Medical Association, 298*(12), 1429–1438.

Schneider, T. R., Lyons, J. B., & Williams, M. (2005). Emotional intelligence and autonomic self-perception: Emotional abilities are related to visceral acuity. *Personality and Individual Differences, 39*(5), 853–861.

Schneiderman, J. S., Buchsbaum, M. S., Haznedar, M. M., Hazlett, E. A., Brickman, A. M., Shihabuddin, L., et al. (2007). Diffusion tensor anisotropy in adolescents and adults. *Neuropsychobiology, 55*(2), 96–111.

Schneirla, T. C., & Jones, M. R. (1959). An evolutionary and developmental theory of biphasic processes underlying approach and withdrawal. In M. R. Jones (Ed.), *Nebraska Symposium on Motivation, 1959* (pp. 1–42). Lincoln: University of Nebraska Press.

Scholten, M. R. M., Aleman, A., & Kahn, R. S. (2008). The processing of emotional prosody and semantics in schizophrenia: Relationship to gender and IQ. *Psychological Medicine, 38*(6), 887–898.

Schommer, N. C., Hellhammer, D. H., & Kirschbaum, C. (2003). Dissociation between reactivity of the hypothalamus–pituitary–adrenal axis and the sympathetic–adrenal–medullary system to repeated psychosocial stress. *Psychosomatic Medicine, 65*(3), 450–460.

Schroeder, U., Hennenlotte, A., Erhard, P., Haslinger, B., Stahl, R., Lange, K. W., et al. (2004). Functional neuroanatomy of perceiving surprised faces. *Human Brain Mapping, 23*(4), 181–187.

Schulkin, J. (2004). *Allostasis, homeostasis, and the costs of physiological adaptation.* New York: Cambridge University Press.

Schulte-Ruether, M., Markowitsch, H. J., Fink, G. R., & Piefke, M. (2007). Mirror neuron and theory of mind mechanisms involved in face-to-face interactions: A functional magnetic resonance imaging approach to empathy. *Journal of Cognitive Neuroscience, 19*(8), 1354–1372.

Schulze-Bonhage, A., Trippel, M., Wagner, K., Bast, T., Deimling, F. V., Ebner, A., et al. (2008). Outcome and predictors of interstitial radiosurgery in the treatment of gelastic epilepsy. *Neurology, 71*(4), 277–282.

Schwartz, A. R., Gerin, W., Davidson, K. W., Pickering, T. G., Brosschot, J. F., Thayer, J. F., et al. (2003). Toward a causal model of cardiovascular responses to stress and the development of cardiovascular disease. *Psychosomatic Medicine, 65*, 22–35.

Schwartz, L., Taylor, H. G., Drotar, D., Yeates, K. O., Wade, S. L., & Stancin, T. (2003). Long-term behavior problems following pediatric traumatic brain injury: Prevalence, predictors, and correlates. *Journal of Pediatric Psychology, 28*(4), 251–263.

Segerstrom, S. C., & Miller, G. E. (2004). Psychological stress and the human immune system: A meta-analytic study of 30 years of inquiry. *Psychological Bulletin, 130*, 601–630.

Seidman, L. J. (2006). Neuropsychological functioning in people with ADHD across the lifespan. *Clinical Psychology Review, 26*(4), 466–485.

Seignourel, P. J., Kunik, M. E., Snow, L., Wilson, N., & Stanley, M. (2008). Anxiety in dementia: A critical review. *Clinical Psychology Review, 28*(7), 1071–1082.

Sekimoto, M., Kato, M., Kaneko, Y., & Onuma, T. (2007). Ictal nausea with vomiting as the major symptom of simple partial seizures: Electroencephalographic and magnetoencephalographic analysis. *Epilepsy and Behavior, 11*(4), 582–587.

Self, D. W. (1998). Neural substrates of drug craving and relapse in drug addiction. *Annals of Medicine, 30*(4), 379–389.

Seligman, M. E., & Maier, S. F. (1967). Failure to escale a traumatic shock. *Journal of Experimental Psychology, 74*(1), 1–9.

Sen, S., Burmeister, M., & Ghosh, D. (2004). Meta-analysis of the association between a serotonin transporter promoter polymorphism (5-HTTLPR) and anxiety-related personality traits. *American Journal of Medical Genetics: Part B, Neuropsychiatric Genetics, 127B*(1), 85–89.

Sergerie, K., Lepage, M., & Armony, J. L. (2006). A process-specific gunctional fissociation of the smygdala in rmotional memory. *Journal of Cognitive Neuroscience, 18*(8), 1359–1367.

Serota, H. M. (1939). Temperature changes in the cortex and hypothalamus during sleep. *Journal of Neurophysiology, 2*, 42–47.

Shamay-Tsoory, S. G., Aharon-Peretz, J., & Perry, D. (2009). Two systems for empathy: A double dissociation between emotional and cognitive empathy in inferior frontal gyrus versus ventromedial prefrontal lesions. *Brain: A Journal of Neurology, 132*(3), 617–627.

Shamay-Tsoory, S. G., Harari, H., Aharon-Peretz, J., & Levkovitz, Y. (2010). The role of the orbitofrontal cortex in affective theory of mind deficits in criminal offenders with psychopathic tendencies. *Cortex, 46*(5), 668–677.

Shamay-Tsoory, S. G., Harari, H., Szepsenwol, O., & Levkovitz, Y. (2009). Neuropsychological evidence of impaired cognitive empathy in euthymic bipolar disorder. *Journal of Neuropsychiatry and Clinical Neurosciences, 21*(1), 59–67.

Shamay-Tsoory, S. G., Shur, S., Harari, H., & Levkovitz, Y. (2007). Neurocognitive basis of impaired empathy in schizophrenia. *Neuropsychology, 21*(4), 431–438.

Shamay-Tsoory, S. G., Tomer, R., Goldsher, D., Berger, B. D., & Aharon-Peretz, J. (2004). Impairment in cognitive and affective empathy in patients with brain lesions: Anatomical and cognitive correlates. *Journal of Clinical and Experimental Neuropsychology, 26*(8), 1113–1127.

Shamay-Tsoory, S. G., Tomer, R., Yaniv, S., & Aharon-Peretz, J. (2002). Empathy deficits in Asperger syndrome: A cognitive profile. *Neurocase, 8*(3), 245–252.

Shapiro, B. E., & Danly, M. (1985). The role of the right hemisphere in the control of speech prosody in propositional and affective contexts. *Brain and Language, 25*(1), 19–36.

Sheldon, W. H., & Stevens, S. S. (1942). *The varieties of temperament: A psychology of constitutional differences.* Oxford, UK: Harper.

Sheline, Y. I., Barch, D. M., Garcia, K., Gersing, K., Pieper, C., Welsh-Bohmer, K., et al. (2006). Cognitive function in late life depression: Relationships to depression severity, cerebrovascular risk factors and processing speed. *Biological Psychiatry, 60*(1), 58–65.

Sherratt, S. (2007). Right brain damage and the verbal expression of emotion: A preliminary investigation. *Aphasiology, 21*(3), 320–339.

Shimokawa, A., Yatomi, N., Anamizu, S., Ashikari, I., Kohno, M., Maki, Y., et al. (2000). Comprehension of emotions: Comparison between Alzheimer type and vascular type dementias. *Dementia and Geriatric Cognitive Disorders, 11*(5), 268–274.

Shimokawa, A., Yatomi, N., Anamizu, S., Torii, S., Isono, H., & Sugai, Y. (2003). Recognition of facial expressions and emotional situations in patients with dementia of the Alzheimer and vascular type. *Dementia and Geriatric Cognitive Disorders, 15*(3), 163–168.

Shinagawa, S., Toyota, Y., Ishikawa, T., Fukuhara, R., Hokoishi, K., Komori, K., et al. (2008). Cognitive function and psychiatric symptoms in early- and late-onset frontotemporal dementia. *Dementia and Geriatric Cognitive Disorders, 25*(5), 439–444.

Shiner, R., & Caspi, A. (2003). Personality differences in childhood and adolescence: Measurement, development, and consequences. *Journal of Child Psychology and Psychiatry, 44*, 2–32.

Shippenberg, T. S., Herz, A., Spanagel, R., Bals-Kubik, R., Stein, C., Kalivas, P. W., et al. (1992). Conditioning of opioid reinforcement: Neuroanatomical and neurochemical substrates. In P. W. Kalivas & H. H. Samson (Eds.), *The neurobiology of drug and alcohol addiction* (pp. 347–356). New York: New York Academy of Sciences.

Siebert, M., Markowitsch, H. J., & Bartel, P. (2003). Amygdala, affect, and cognition: Evidence from 10 patients with Urbach–Wiethe disease. *Brain: A Journal of Neurology, 126*(12), 2627–2637.

Siegel, A., & Shaikh, M. B. (1997). A neural bases of aggression and rage in the cat. *Aggression and Violent Behavior, 2*(3), 241–271.

Signer, S. F. (1992). Capgras symptom and delusions of reduplication in neurologic disorders. *Neuropsychiatry, Neuropsychology, and Behavioral Neurology, 5*(2), 138–143.

Simard, M., van Reekum, R., & Cohen, T. (2000). A review of the cognitive and behavioral symptoms in dementia with Lewy bodies. *Journal of Neuropsychiatry and Clinical Neurosciences, 12*(4), 425–450.

Simon, D., Craig, K. D., Miltner, W. H. R., & Rainville, P. (2006). Brain responses to dynamic facial expressions of pain. *Pain, 126*(1), 309–318.

Simonsson-Sarnecki, M., Lundh, L.-G., Toerestad, B., Bagby, R. M., Taylor, G. J., & Parker, J. D. A. (2000). A Swedish translation of the 20-item Toronto Alexithymia Scale: Cross-validation of the factor structure. *Scandinavian Journal of Psychology, 41*(1), 25–30.

Singh, M., & Woods, S. A. (2008). Predicting general well-being from emotional intelligence and three broad personality traits. *Journal of Applied Social Psychology, 38*(3), 635–646.

Sirotkina, I. (2007). V. M. Bekhterev and the beginnings of experimental psychology in Russia. *Revista de Historia de la Psicologia, 28*(2–3), 315–320.

Skeem, J., Johansson, P., Andershed, H., Kerr, M., & Louden, J. E. (2007). Two subtypes of psychopathic violent offenders that parallel primary and secondary variants. *Journal of Abnormal Psychology, 116*(2), 395–409.

Skuse, D. H., Morris, J. S., & Dolan, R. J. (2005). Functional dissociation of amygdala-modulated arousal and cognitive appraisal in Turner syndrome. *Brain: A Journal of Neurology, 128*(9), 2084–2096.

Slaughter, J., Bobo, W., & Childers, M. K. (1999). Selective serotonin reuptake inhibitor treatment of post-traumatic Kluever–Bucy syndrome. *Brain Injury, 13*(1), 59–62.

Slomkowski, C. L., Nelson, K., Dunn, J., & Plomin, R. (1992). Temperament and language: Relations from toddlerhood to middle childhood. *Developmental Psychology, 28*(6), 1090–1095.

Smith, A. (2006). Cognitive empathy and emotional empathy in human behavior and evolution. *Psychological Record, 56*(1), 3–21.

Smith, A. (2009). The empathy imbalance hypothesis of autism: A theoretical approach to cognitive and emotional empathy in autistic development. *Psychological Record, 59*(2), 273–294.

Smith, A. B., Taylor, E., Brammer, M., Halari, R., & Rubia, K. (2008). Reduced activation in right lateral prefrontal cortex and anterior cingulate gyrus in medication-naive adolescents with attention deficit hyperactivity disorder during time discrimination. *Journal of Child Psychology and Psychiatry, 49*(9), 977–985.

Smith, K. S., & Berridge, K. C. (2007). Opioid limbic circuit for reward: Interaction between hedonic hotspots of nucleus accumbens and ventral pallidum. *Journal of Neuroscience, 27*(7), 1594–1605.

Smith, L., Ciarrochi, J., & Heaven, P. C. L. (2008). The stability and change of trait emotional intelligence, conflict communication patterns, and relationship satisfaction: A one-year longitudinal study. *Personality and Individual Differences, 45*(8), 738–743.

Smith, L., Heaven, P. C. L., & Ciarrochi, J. (2008). Trait emotional intelligence, conflict communication patterns, and relationship satisfaction. *Personality and Individual Differences, 44*(6), 1314–1325.

Smith, S. S. (2006). *The relationship between alexithymia and lower socioeconomic status African Americans.* Ann Arbor, MI: ProQuest Information & Learning.

Snaith, R. P., Hamilton, M., Morley, S., & Humayan, A. (1995). A scale for the assessment of the hedonic tone: The Snaith–Hamilton Pleasure Scale. *British Journal of Psychiatry, 167*(1), 99–103.

Snowden, J. S., Austin, N. A., Sembi, S., Thompson, J. C., Craufurd, D., & Neary, D. (2008). Emotion recognition in Huntington's disease and frontotemporal dementia. *Neuropsychologia, 46*(11), 2638–2649.

Sojka, P., Stalnacke, B.-M., Bjornstig, U., & Karlsson, K. (2006). One-year follow-up of patients with mild traumatic brain injury: Occurrence of post-traumatic stress-related symptoms at follow-up and serum levels of cortisol, S-100B and neuron-specific enolase in acute phase. *Brain Injury, 20*(6), 613–620.

Sondergaard, M. P., Jarden, J. O., Martiny, K., Andersen, G., & Bech, P. (2006). Dose response to adjunctive light therapy in citalopram-treated patients with post-stroke depression. *Psychotherapy and Psychosomatics, 75*(4), 244–248.

Sonino, N., & Fava, G. A. (2001). Psychiatric disorders associated with Cushing's syndrome: Epidemiology, pathophysiology, and treatment. *CNS Drugs, 15*(5), 361–373.

South, M. D., Ozonoff, S., Suchy, Y., Kesner, R. P., McMahon, W. M., & Lainhart, J. E. (2008). Intact emotion facilitation for non-social stimuli in autism: Is amygdala impairment in autism specific for social information? *Journal of International Neuropsychological Society, 14*, 42–54.

Spada, R. S., Cento, R. M., Proto, C., Roccasalva, G., Cosentino, F. I. I., Lanzone, A., et al. (2001). Twenty-four-hour urinary free cortisol levels in vascular dementia and in Alzheimer's disease. *Archives of Gerontology and Geriatrics, 7*, 363–367.

Spalletta, G., Serra, L., Fadda, L., Ripa, A., Bria, P., & Caltagirone, C. (2007). Unawareness of motor impairment and emotions in right hemispheric stroke: A preliminary investigation. *International Journal of Geriatric Psychiatry, 22*(12), 1241–1246.

Spence, S., Shapiro, D., & Zaidel, E. (1996). The role of the right hemisphere in the physiological and cognitive components of emotional processing. *Psychophysiology, 33*(2), 112–122.

Spencer, S. J., Steele, C. M., & Quinn, D. M. (1999). Stereotype threat and women's math performance. *Journal of Experimental Social Psychology, 35*(1), 4–28.

Speranza, M., Loas, G., Wallier, J., & Corcos, M. (2007). Predictive value of alexithymia in patients with eating disorders: A 3-year prospective study. *Journal of Psychosomatic Research, 63*(4), 365–371.

Spiegel, E. A., Wycis, H. T., Freed, H., & Orchinik, C. (1951). The central mechanism of the emotions (experiences with circumscribed thalamic lesions). *American Journal of Psychiatry, 108*, 426–432.

Spinella, M. (2007). Measuring the executive regulation of emotion with self-rating scales in a nonclinical population. *Journal of General Psychology, 134*(1), 101–111.

Spitzer, C., Vogel, M., Barnow, S., Freyberger, H. J., & Grabe, H. J. (2007). Psychopathology and alexithymia in severe mental illness: The impact of trauma and posttraumatic stress symptoms. *European Archives of Psychiatry and Clinical Neuroscience, 257*(4), 191–196.

Spoletini, I., Marra, C., Di Iulio, F., Gianni, W., Sancesario, G., Giubilei, F., et al. (2008). Facial emotion recognition deficit in amnestic mild cognitive impairment and Alzheimer's disease. *American Journal of Geriatric Psychiatry, 16*(5), 389–398.

Sprengelmeyer, R., Young, A. W., Mahn, K., Schroeder, U., Woitalla, D., Baettner, T., et al. (2003). Facial expression recognition in people with medicated and unmedicated Parkinson's disease. *Neuropsychologia, 41*(8), 1047–1057.

Stanfield, A. C., McIntosh, A. M., Spencer, M. D., Philip, R., Gaur, S., & Lawrie, S. M. (2008). Towards a neuroanatomy of autism: A systematic review and meta-analysis of structural magnetic resonance imaging studies. *European Psychiatry, 23*(4), 289–299.

Starkman, M. N., Giordani, B., Berent, S., Schork, A., & Schteingart, D. E. (2001). Elevated cortisol levels in Cushing's disease are associated with cognitive decrements. *Psychosomatic Medicine, 63*(6), 985–993.

Starkman, M. N., Wolkowitz, O. M., & Rothschild, A. J. (2003). Psychiatric manifestations of hyperadrenocorticism and hypoadrenocorticism (Cushing's and Addison's diseases). In O. M. Wolkowitz & A. J. Rothschild (Eds.), *Psychoneuroendocrinology: The scientific basis of clinical practice* (pp. 165–188). Arlington, VA: American Psychiatric Publishing.

Starkstein, S. E., Boston, J. D., & Robinson, R. G. (1988). Mechanisms of mania after brain injury: 12 case reports and review of the literature. *Journal of Nervous and Mental Disease, 176*(2), 87–100.

Starkstein, S. E., Federoff, J. P., Price, T. R., & Leiguarda, R. C. (1994). Neuropsychological and neuroradiologic correlates of emotional prosody comprehension. *Neurology, 44*(3), 515–522.

Starkstein, S. E., Jorge, R., & Mizrahi, R. (2006). The prevalence, clinical correlates and treatment of apathy in Alzheimer's disease. *European Journal of Psychiatry, 20*(2), 96–106.

Starkstein, S. E., Jorge, R., Mizrahi, R., & Robinson, R. G. (2005). The construct of minor and major depression in Alzheimer's disease. *American Journal of Psychiatry, 162*(11), 2086–2093.

Starkstein, S. E., & Lischinsky, A. (2002). Diagnosis, phenomenology and treatment of poststroke depression. *Revista Brasileira de Psiquiatria, 24*(1), 44–49.

Starkstein, S. E., & Migliorelli, R. (1993). ECT in a patient with a frontal craniotomy and residual meningioma. *Journal of Neuropsychiatry and Clinical Neurosciences, 5*(4), 428–430.

Starkstein, S. E., & Robinson, R. G. (1997). Mechanism of disinhibition after brain lesions. *Journal of Nervous and Mental Disease, 185*(2), 108–114.

Steele, C. M. (1997). A threat in the air: How stereotypes shape intellectual identity and performance. *American Psychologist, 52*(6), 613–629.

Steele, C. M., & Aronson, J. (1995). Stereotype threat and the intellectual test performance of African Americans. *Journal of Personality and Social Psychology, 69*(5), 797–811.

Steer, R. A., Clark, D. A., Kumar, G., & Beck, A. T. (2008). Common and specific dimensions of self-reported anxiety and depression in adolescent outpatients. *Journal of Psychopathology and Behavioral Assessment, 30*(3), 163–170.

Stefan, H., Pauli, E., Kerling, F., Schwarz, A., & Koebnick, C. (2002). Autonomic auras: Left hemispheric predominance of epileptic generators of cold shivers and goose bumps? *Epilepsia, 43*(1), 41–45.

Stegge, H., Terwogt, M. M., & Gross, J. J. (2007). Awareness and regulation of emotion in typical and atypical development. In J. J. Gross (Ed.), *Handbook of emotion regulation* (pp. 269–286). New York: Guilford Press.

Stevens, M. C., Kaplan, R. F., & Hesselbrock, V. M. (2003). Executive-cognitive functioning in the development of antisocial personality disorder. *Addictive Behavior, 28*, 285–300.

Stevenson, C. W., Marsden, C. A., & Mason, R. (2008). Early life stress causes FG-7142-induced corticolimbic dysfunction in adulthood. *Brain Research, 1193*, 43–50.

Stewart, J. C., Janicki, D. L., & Kamarck, T. W. (2006). Cardiovascular reactivity and recovery from psychological challenge as predictors of 3-year change in blood pressure. *Health Psychology, 25*, 111–118.

Stone, L. A., & Nielson, K. A. (2001). Intact physiological responses to arousal with impaired emotional recognition in alexithymia. *Psychotherapy and Psychosomatics, 70*(2), 92–102.

Storbeck, J., & Clore, G. L. (2008). The affective regulation of cognitive priming. *Emotion, 8*(2), 208–215.

Straube, T., Mentzel, H.-J., & Miltner, W. H. R. (2006). Neural mechanisms of automatic and direct processing of phobogenic stimuli in specific phobia. *Biological Psychiatry, 59*(2), 162–170.

Streb, J. M., & Smith, K. (1955). Frontal lobotomy and the elimination of conditioned anxiety in the rat. *Journal of Comparative and Physiological Psychology, 48*(2), 126–129.

Striano, S., Striano, P., Sarappa, C., & Boccella, P. (2005). The clinical spectrum and natural history of gelastic epilepsy–hypothalamic hamartoma syndrome. *Seizure, 14*(4), 232–239.

Strittmatter, M., Meyer, S., Fischer, C., Georg, T., & Schmitz, B. (2003). Location-dependent patterns in cardio-autonomic dysfunction in ischaemic stroke. *European Neurology, 50*(1), 30–38.

Strobel, A., Beauducel, A., Debener, S., & Brocke, B. (2001). Eine deutschsprachige Version des BIS/BAS-Fragebogens von Carver und White [The German-language version of the BIS/BAS-scales of Carver and White]. *Zeitschrift fuer Differentielle und Diagnostische Psychologie, 22*(3), 216–227.

Stroebel, C. F. (1998). Somatization and alexithymia as aspects of mind–body intelligence. *Advances in Mind–Body Medicine, 14*(2), 113–117.

Stuss, D. T. (1992). Biological and psychological development of executive functions. *Brain and Cognition, 20*(1), 8–23.

Stuss, D. T., Alexander, M. P., Floden, D., Binns, M. A., Levine, B., McIntosh, A. R., et al. (2002). Fractionation and localization of distinct frontal lobe processes: Evidence from focal lesions in humans. In D. T. Stuss & R. T. Knight (Eds.), *Principles of frontal lobe function* (pp. 392–407). London: Oxford University Press.

Suarez, G. A., Opfer-Gehrking, T. L., Offord, K. P., Atkinson, E. J., O'Brien, P. C., & Low, P. A. (1999). A new instrument to assess autonomic symptoms. *Neurology, 52*(3), 523–528.

Suchy, Y., Blint, A., & Osmon, D. S. (1997). Behavioral Dyscontrol Scale: Criterion and predictive validity in an inpatient rehabilitation unit population. *Clinical Neuropsychologist, 11*(3), 258–265.

Suchy, Y., & Chelune, G. (2001). Postsurgical changes in self-reported mood and composite IQ in a matched sample of patients with frontal lobe epilepsy. *Journal of Clinical and Experimental Neuropsychology, 23*(4), 413–423.

Suchy, Y., & Kosson, D. S. (2006). Forming, switching, and maintaining mental sets among psychopathic offenders during verbal and nonverbal tasks: Another look at the left-hemisphere activation hypothesis. *Journal of the International Neuropsychological Society, 12*(4), 538–548.

Suchy, Y., Kraybill, M., & Franchow, E. (2010). Instrumental activities of daily living among community-dwelling older adults: Discrepancies between self-report and performance are mediated by cognitive reserve. *Journal of Clinical and Experimental Neuropsychology.*

Suchy, Y., Rau, H., Whittaker, W. J., Eastvold, A., & Strassberg, D. S. (2009). Facial affect recognition as a predictor of performance on a reading comprehension test among criminal sex offenders. *Applied Psychology in Criminal Justice, 5*(1), 73–89.

Suchy, Y., Sands, K., & Chelune, G. J. (2003). Verbal and nonverbal fluency performance before and after seizure surgery. *Journal of Clinical and Experimental Neuropsychology, 25*(2), 190–200.

Suchy, Y., Whittaker, W. J., Strassberg, D., & Eastvold, A. (2009). Facial and prosodic affect recognition among pedophilic and non-pedophilic criminal child molesters. *Sexual Abuse: A Journal of Research and Treatment, 21*(1), 93–110.

Summers, M., Papadopoulou, K., Bruno, S., Cipolotti, L., & Ron, M. A. (2006). Bipolar I and bipolar II disorder: cognition and emotion processing. *Psychological Medicine, 36*, 1799–1809.

Sutton, S. K., & Davidson, R. J. (1997). Prefrontal brain asymmetry: A biological substrate of the behavioral approach and inhibition systems. *Psychological Science, 8*, 204–210.

Sutton, S. K., & Davidson, R. J. (2000). Prefrontal brain electrical asymmetry predicts the evaluation of affective stimuli. *Neuropsychologia, 38*(13), 1723–1733.

Sutton, S. K., Davidson, R. J., Donzella, B., & Irwin, W. (1997). Manipulating affective state using extended picture presentations. *Psychophysiology, 34*(2), 217–226.

Swanson, J., Oosterlaan, J., Murias, M., Schuck, S., Flodman, P., Spence, M. A., et al. (2000). Attention deficit/hyperactivity disorder children with a 7-repeat allele of the dopamine receptor D4 gene have extreme behavior but normal performance on critical neuropsychological tests of attention. *Proceedings of the National Academy of Sciences, 97*(9), 4754–4759.

Swinkels, W. A. M., van Emde Boas, W., Kuyk, J., van Dyck, R., & Spinhoven, P. (2006). Interictal depression, anxiety, personality traits, and psychological dissociation in patients with temporal lobe epilepsy (TLE) and extra-TLE. *Epilepsia, 47*(12), 2092–2103.

Sylvester, C.-Y., Wagner, T. D., Lacey, S. C., Hernandez, L., Nichols, T. E., Smith, E. E., et al. (2003). Switching attention and resolving interference: fMRI measures of executive functions. *Neuropsychologia, 41*, 357–370.

Tabbert, K., Stark, R., Kirsch, P., & Vaitl, D. (2005). Hemodynamic responses of the amygdala, the orbitofrontal cortex and the visual cortex during a fear conditioning paradigm. *International Journal of Psychophysiology, 57*(1), 15–23.

Tada, M., Kakita, A., Toyoshima, Y., Onodera, O., Ozawa, T., Morita, T., et al. (2009). Depletion of medullary serotonergic neurons in patients with multiple system atrophy who succumbed to sudden death. *Brain: A Journal of Neurology, 132*(7), 1810–1819.

Takahashi, T., Suzuki, M., Velakoulis, D., Lorenzetti, V., Soulsby, B., Zhou, S.-Y., et al. (2009). Increased pituitary volume in schizophrenia spectrum disorders. *Schizophrenia Research, 108*(1–3), 114–121.

Tamietto, M., & de Gelder, B. (2008). Affective blindsight in the intact brain: Neural interhemispheric summation for unseen fearful expressions. *Neuropsychologia, 46*(3), 820–828.

Tamm, L., Menon, V., & Reiss, A. L. (2003). Abnormal prefrontal cortex function during response inhibition in Turner syndrome: Functional magnetic resonance imaging evidence. *Biological Psychiatry, 53*(2), 107–111.

Tangney, J. P., Baumeister, R. F., & Boone, A. L. (2004). High self-control predicts good adjustment, less pathology, better grades, and interpersonal success. *Journal of Personality, 72*(2), 271–324.

Tang-Wai, D., Lewis, P., Boeve, B., Hutton, M., Golde, T., Baker, M., et al. (2002). Familial frontotemporal dementia associated with a novel presenilin-1 mutation. *Dementia and Geriatric Cognitive Disorders, 14*(1), 13–21.

Tate, R. L. (2003). Impact of pre-injury factors on outcome after severe traumatic brain injury: Does post-traumatic personality change represent an exacerbation of premorbid traits? *Neuropsychological Rehabilitation, 13*(1), 43–64.

Tateno, A., Jorge, R. E., & Robinson, R. G. (2004). Pathological laughing and crying following traumatic brain injury. *Journal of Neuropsychiatry and Clinical Neurosciences, 16*(4), 426–434.

Tatsch, M. F., Bottino, C. M., Azevedo, D., Hototian, S. R., Moscoso, M. A., Folquitto, J. C., et al. (2006). Neuropsychiatric symptoms in Alzheimer's disease and cognitively impaired, nondemented elderly from a community-based sample in Brazil: Prevalence and relationship with dementia severity. *American Journal of Geriatric Psychiatry, 14*(5), 438–445.

Taylor, A. N., Rahman, S. U., Sanders, N. C., Prolo, P., Sutton, R. L., & Tio, D. L. (2008). Injury severity differentially affects short- and long-term neuroendocrine outcomes of traumatic brain injury. *Journal of Neurotrauma, 25*(4), 311–323.

Taylor, G. J. (1984). Alexithymia: Concept, measurement, and implications for treatment. *American Journal of Psychiatry, 141*(6), 725–732.

Taylor, G. J., Bagby, R. M., & Parker, J. D. A. (2003). The 20-item Toronto Alexithymia Scale IV: Reliability and factorial validity in different languages and cultures. *Journal of Psychosomatic Research, 55*(3), 277–283.

Taylor, G. J., Parker, J. D. A., Bagby, R. M., & Bourke, M. P. (1996). Relationships between alexithymia and psychological characteristics associated with eating disorders. *Journal of Psychosomatic Research, 41*(6), 561–568.

Taylor, H. G., & Heilman, K. M. (1980). Left-hemisphere motor dominance in righthanders. *Cortex, 16*(4), 587–603.

Taylor, S. E., Way, B. M., Welch, W. T., Lehman, B. J., Eisenberger, N. I., & Hilmert, C. J. (2006). Early family environment, current adversity, the serotonin transporter promoter polymorphism, and depressive symptomatology. *Biological Psychiatry, 60*(7), 671–676.

Taylor, W. D., Steffens, D. C., Payne, M. E., Marchuk, D. A., Krishnan, K. R. R., Svenson, I. K., et al. (2005). Influence of serotonin transporter promoter region polymorphisms on hippocampal volumes in late-life depression. *Archives of General Psychiatry, 62*(5), 537–544.

Teitelbaum, P. (1964). Appetite. *Proceedings of the American Philosophical Society, 108*, 464–472.

Tellegen, A., Tuma, A. H., & Maser, J. D. (1985). Structures of mood and personality and their relevance to assessing anxiety, with an emphasis on self-report. In A. H. Tuma & J. D. Maser (Eds.), *Anxiety and the anxiety disorders* (pp. 681–706). Hillsdale, NJ: Erlbaum.

Tellegen, A., Watson, D., & Clark, L. A. (1999). On the dimensional and hierarchical structure of affect. *Psychological Science, 10*(4), 297–303.

Ter Horst, G. J., Hautvast, R. W. M., De Jongste, M. J. L., & Korf, J. (1996). Neuroanatomy of cardiac activity-regulating circuitry: A transneuronal retrograde viral labelling study in the rat. *European Journal of Neuroscience, 8*(10), 2029–2041.

Terraciano, A., McCrae, R. R., & Costa, P. T., Jr. (2003). Factorial and construct validity of the Italian Positive and Negative Affect Schedule (PANAS). *European Journal of Psychological Assessment, 19*(2), 131–141.

Tessitore, A., Hariri, A. R., Fera, F., Smith, W. G., Das, S., Weinberger, D. R., et al. (2005). Functional changes in the activity of brain regions underlying emotion processing in the elderly. *Psychiatry Research: Neuroimaging, 139*(1), 9–18.

Thayer, J. F., Hansen, A. L., Saus-Rose, E., & Johnsen, B. H. (2009). Heart rate variability, prefrontal neural function, and cognitive performance: The neurovisceral integration perspective on self-regulation, adaptation, and health. *Annals of Behavioral Medicine, 37*, 141–153.

Thayer, J. F., & Lane, R. D. (2007). The role of vagal function in the risk for cardiovascular disease and mortality. *Biological Psychology, 74*(2), 224–242.

Thomas, A. J., Kalaria, R. N., & O'Brien, J. T. (2004). Depression and vascular disease: What is the relationship? *Journal of Affective Disorders, 79*(1), 81–95.

Thompson, E. R. (2007). Development and validation of an internationally reliable short-form of the Positive and Negative Affect Schedule (PANAS). *Journal of Cross-Cultural Psychology, 38*(2), 227–242.

Thorberg, F. A., Young, R. M., Sullivan, K. A., & Lyvers, M. (2009). Alexithymia and alcohol use disorders: A critical review. *Addictive Behaviors, 34*(3), 237–245.

Thorpe, S., Fize, D., & Marlot, C. (1996). Speed of processing in the human visual system. *Nature, 381*, 520–522.

Timonen, M., Miettunen, J., Hakko, H., Zitting, P., Veijola, J., von Wendt, L., et al. (2002). The association of preceding traumatic brain injury with mental disorders, alcoholism and criminality: The Northern Finland 1966 Birth Cohort study. *Psychiatry Research, 113*(3), 217–226.

Titchener, E. B. (1914). A historical note on the James–Lange theory of emotions. *American Journal of Psychology, 25*(3), 427–447.

Tobin, R. M., Graziano, W. G., Vanman, E. J., & Tassinary, L. G. (2000). Personality, emotional experience, and efforts to control emotions. *Journal of Personality and Social Psychology, 79*(4), 656–669.

Todarello, O., Porcelli, P., Grilletti, F., & Bellomo, A. (2005). Is alexithymia related to negative symptoms of schizophrenia? *Psychopathology, 38*(6), 310–314.

Tomarken, A. J., Davidson, R. J., & Henriques, J. B. (1990). Resting frontal brain asymmetry predicts affective responses to films. *Journal of Personality and Social Psychology, 59*(4), 791–801.

Tomarken, A. J., Davidson, R. J., Wheeler, R. E., & Doss, R. C. (1992). Individual differences in anterior brain asymmetry and fundamental dimensions of emotion. *Journal of Personality and Social Psychology, 62*(4), 676–687.

Tomkins, S. S. (1962). *Affect, imagery, consciousness: Vol. 1. The positive affects.* Oxford, UK: Springer.

Tomkins, S. S. (1963). *Affect, imagery, consciousness: Vol. 2. The negative affects.* New York: Tavistock.

Tompkins, C. A., & Flowers, C. R. (1985). Perception of emotional intonation by brain-damaged adults: The influence of task processing levels. *Journal of Speech and Hearing Research, 28*(4), 527–538.

Tranel, D., Bechara, A., & Denburg, N. L. (2002). Asymmetric functional roles of right and left ventromedial prefrontal cortices in social conduct, decision making, and emotional processing. *Cortex, 38*(4), 589–612.

Tranel, D., & Damasio, A. R. (1988). Non-conscious face recognition in patients with face agnosia. *Behavioural Brain Research, 30*(3), 235–249.

Tranel, D., Damasio, H., & Damasio, A. R. (1995). Double dissociation between overt and covert face recognition. *Journal of Cognitive Neuroscience, 7*(4), 425–432.

Tranel, D., Gullickson, G., Koch, M., & Adolphs, R. (2006). Altered experience of emotion following bilateral amygdala damage. *Cognitive NeuroPsychiatry, 11*(3), 219–232.

Treadway, M. T., Buckholtz, J. W., Schwartzman, A. N., Lambert, W. E., & Zald, D. H. (2009). Worth the "EefRT"(tm)?: The effort expenditure for rewards task as an objective measure of motivation and anhedonia. *PLoS ONE, 4*(8), e6598.

Treiber, F. A., Kamarck, T., Schneiderman, N., Sheffield, D., Kapuku, G., & Taylor, T. (2003). Cardiovascular reactivity and development of preclinical and clinical disease states. *Psychosomatic Medicine, 65*, 46–62.

Tuccitto, D. E., Giacobbi, P. R., & Leite, W. L. (2010). The internal structure of positive and negative affect: A confirmatory factor analysis of the PANAS. *Educational and Psychological Measurement, 70*(1), 125–141.

Turk, J., & Cornish, K. (1998). Face recognition and emotion perception in boys with fragile-X syndrome. *Journal of Intellectual Disability Research, 42*(6), 490–499.

Turner-Stokes, L., & Hassan, N. (2002). Depression after stroke: A review of the evidence base to inform the development of an integrated care pathway. Part 2: Treatment alternatives. *Clinical Rehabilitation, 16*(3), 248–260.

Uchino, B. N., Smith, T. W., Holt-Lunstad, J., Campo, R., & Reblin, M. (2007). Stress and illness. In J. T. Cacioppo, L. G. Tassinary, & G. G. Bertson (Eds.), *Handbook of psychophysiology* (3rd ed., pp. 608–632). New York: Cambridge University Press.

Uekermann, J., Daum, I., Schlebusch, P., & Trenckmann, U. (2005). Processing of affective stimuli in alcoholism. *Cortex, 41*(2), 189–194.

Uno, H., Ross, T., Else, J., Suleman, M., & Sapolsky, R. (1989). Hippocampal damage associated with prolonged and fatal stress in primates. *Journal of Neuroscience, 9*, 1705–1711.

Urry, H. L., van Reekum, C. M., Johnstone, T., Kalin, N. H., Thurow, M. E., Schaefer, H. S., et al. (2006). Amygdala and ventromedial prefrontal cortex are inversely coupled during regulation of negative affect and predict the diurnal pattern of cortisol secretion among older adults. *Journal of Neuroscience, 26*(16), 4415–4425.

Ursu, S., & Carter, C. S. (2005). Outcome representations, counterfactual comparisons and the human orbitofrontal cortex: Implications for neuroimaging studies of decision-making. *Cognitive Brain Research, 23*(1), 51–60.

Uzunca, I., Utku, U., Asil, T., & Celik, Y. (2005). Four rire prodromique associated with simultaneous bilateral capsular genu infarction. *Journal of Clinical Neuroscience, 12*, 174–175.

Vaher, P. R., Luine, V. N., Gould, E., & McEwen, B. S. (1994). Effects of adrenalectomy on spatial memory performance and dentate gyrus morphology. *Brain Research, 656*(1), 71–78.

Valdes, M., Jodar, Ojuel, J., & Sureda, B. (2001). Alexitimia e inteligencia verbal: Un estudio psicometrico [Alexithymia and verbal intelligence: A psychometric study]. *Actas Espanolas de Psiquiatria, 29*(5), 338–342.

van den Heuvel, O. A., Groenewegen, H. J., Witter, M. P., Veltman, D. J., & Sanfelippo, A. J. (2005). Neuroimaging in panic disorder. In A. J. Sanfelippo (Ed.), *Panic disorders: New research* (pp. 83–111). Hauppauge, NY: Nova Biomedical Books.

van den Heuvel, O. A., Veltman, D. J., Groenewegen, H. J., Witter, M. P., Merkelbach, J., Cath, D. C., et al. (2005). Disorder-specific neuroanatomical correlates of attentional bias in obsessive–compulsive disorder, panic disorder, and hypochondriasis. *Archives of General Psychiatry, 62*(8), 922–933.

van de Putte, E. M., Engelbert, R. H., Kuis, W., Kimpen, J. L., & Uiterwaal, C. S. (2007). Alexithymia in adolescents with chronic fatigue syndrome. *Journal of Psychosomatic Research, 63*(4), 377–380.

van der Gaag, C., Minderaa, R. B., & Keysers, C. (2007). Facial expressions: What the mirror neuron system can and cannot tell us. *Social Neuroscience, 2*(3), 179–222.

Van Dongen, H. P. A., Maislin, G., Mullington, J. M., & Dinges, D. F. (2003). The cumulative cost of additional wakefulness: Dose–response effects on neurobehavioral functions and sleep physiology from chronic sleep restriction and total sleep deprivation. *Sleep, 26*(2), 117–126.

van Duijvenvoorde, A. C., Zanolie, K., Rombouts, S. A, Raijmakers, M. E., & Crone, E. A. (2008). Evaluating the negative or valuing the positive?: Neural mechanisms supporting feedback-based learning across development. *Journal of Neuroscience, 28*, 9495–9503.

van Furth, W. R., & van Ree, J. M. (1996). Sexual motivation: Involvement of endogenous opioids in the ventral tegmental area. *Brain Research, 729*(1), 20–28.

van Heck, G. L., den Oudsten, B. L., Vingerhoets, A., Nykicek, I., & Denollet, J. (2008). Emotional intelligence: Relationships to stress, health, and well-being. In A Vingerhoets, I. Nyklicek, & J. Denollet (Eds.), *Emotion regulation: Conceptual and clinical issues* (pp. 97–121). New York: Springer Science+Business Media.

van Honk, J., Schutter, D. J., Hermans, E. J., Putman, P., Tuiten, A., & Koppeschaar, H. (2004). Testosterone shifts the balance between sensitivity for punishment and reward in healthy young women. *Psychoneuroendocrinology, 29*(7), 937–943.

Van Lancker, D., & Sidtis, J. J. (1992). The identification of affective-prosodic stimuli by left- and right-hemisphere-damaged subjects: All errors are not created equal. *Journal of Speech and Hearing Research, 35*(5), 963–970.

Vanman, E. J., Dawson, M. E., & Brennan, P. A. (1998). Affective reactions in the blink of an eye: Individual differences in subjective experience and physiological responses to emotional stimuli. *Personality and Social Psychology Bulletin, 24*(9), 994–1005.

Van't Wout, M., Aleman, A., Bermond, B., & Kahn, R. S. (2007). No words for feelings: Alexithymia in schizophrenia patients and first-degree relatives. *Comprehensive Psychiatry, 48*(1), 27–33.

Vasa, R. A., Grados, M., Slomine, B., Herskovits, E. H., Thompson, R. E., Salorio, C., et al. (2004). Neuroimaging correlates of anxiety after pediatric traumatic brain injury. *Biological Psychiatry, 55*(3), 208–216.

Vasic, N., Walter, H., Hoese, A., & Wolf, R. C. (2008). Gray matter reduction associated with psychopathology and cognitive dysfunction in unipolar depression: A voxel-based morphometry study. *Journal of Affective Disorders, 109*(1–2), 107–116.

Vataja, R., Leppaevuori, A., Pohjasvaara, T., Maentylae, R., Aronen, H. J., Salonen, O., et al. (2004). Poststroke depression and lesion location revisited. *Journal of Neuropsychiatry and Clinical Neurosciences, 16*(2), 156–162.

Vataja, R., Pohjasvaara, T., Maentylae, R., Ylikoski, R., Kalska, H., Leskelae, M., et al. (2005). Depression-executive dysfunction syndrome in stroke patients. *American Journal of Geriatric Psychiatry, 13*(2), 99–107.

Veiel, H. O. F. (1997). A preliminary profile of neuropsychological deficits associated with major depression. *Journal of Clinical and Experimental Neuropsychology, 19*(4), 587–603.

Vendrell, P., Junque, C., Pujol, J., Jurado, M. A., Molet, J., & Grafman, J. (1995). The role of prefrontal regions in the Stroop task. *Neuropsychologia, 33*, 341–352..

Verissimo, R., Mota-Cardoso, R., & Taylor, G. (1998). Relationships between alexithymia, emotional control, and quality of life in patients with inflammatory bowel disease. *Psychotherapy and Psychosomatics, 67*(2), 75–80.

Vermeulen, N., & Luminet, O. (2009). Alexithymia factors and memory performances for neutral and emotional words. *Personality and Individual Differences, 47*(4), 305–309.

Vervoort, L., Wolters, L. H., Hogendoorn, S. M., de Haan, E., Boer, F., & Prins, P. J. M. (2010). Sensitivity of Gray's behavioral inhibition system in clinically anxious and non-anxious children and adolescents. *Personality and Individual Differences, 48*(5), 629–633.

Viding, E., Blair, R. J. R., Moffitt, T. E., & Plomin, R. (2005). Evidence for substantial genetic risk for psychopathy in 7-year-olds. *Journal of Child Psychology and Psychiatry, 46*(6), 592–597.

Voelm, B., Richardson, P., McKie, S., Elliott, R., Dolan, M., & Deakin, B. (2007). Neuronal correlates of reward and loss in Cluster B personality disorders: A functional magnetic resonance imaging study. *Psychiatry Research: Neuroimaging, 156*(2), 151–167.

Voigt, D. C., Dillard, J. P., Braddock, K. H., Anderson, J. W., Sopory, P., & Stephenson, M. T. (2009). Carver and White's (1994) BIS/BAS scales and their relationship to risky health behaviours. *Personality and Individual Differences, 47*(2), 89–93.

von Hippel, W. (2007). Aging, executive functioning, and social control. *Current Directions in Psychological Science, 16*(5), 240–244.

von Hippel, W., & Dunlop, S. M. (2005). Aging, inhibition, and social inappropriateness. *Psychology and Aging, 20*(3), 519–523.

von Hippel, W., & Gonsalkorale, K. (2005). "That is bloody revolting!": Inhibitory control of thoughts better left unsaid. *Psychological Science, 16*(7), 497–500.

Vuilleumier, P., & Pourtois, G. (2007). Distributed and interactive brain mechanisms during emotion face perception: Evidence from functional neuroimaging. *Neuropsychologia, 45*(1), 174–194.

Vyas, A., Mitra, R., Rao, B. S. S., & Chattarji, S. (2002). Chronic stress induces contrasting patterns of dendritic remodeling in hippocampal and amygdaloid neurons. *Journal of Neuroscience, 22*(15), 6810–6818.

Wacker, J., Dillon, D. G., & Pizzagalli, D. A. (2009). The role of the nucleus accumbens and rostral anterior cingulate cortex in anhedonia: Integration of resting EEG, fMRI, and volumetric techniques. *NeuroImage, 46*(1), 327–337.

Wainwright, M. A., Wright, M. J., Luciano, M., Geffen, G. M., & Martin, N. G. (2008). Genetic covariation among facets of openness to experience and general cognitive ability. *Twin Research and Human Genetics, 11*(3), 275–286.

Waldstein, S. R., & Katzel, L. I. (2005). Stress-induced blood pressure reactivity and cognitive function. *Neurology, 64*, 1746–1749.

Walker, E. F., Mittal, V., & Tessner, K. (2008). Stress and the hypothalamic pituitary adrenal axis in the developmental course of schizophrenia. *Annual Review of Clinical Psychology, 4*, 189–216.

Walker, E. F., Lewis, N., Loewy, R., & Palyo, S. (1999). Motor dysfunction and risk for schizophrenia. *Development and Psychopathology, 11*(3), 509–523.

Walker, E. F., Savoie, T., & Davis, D. (1994). Neuromotor precursors of schizophrenia. *Schizophrenia Bulletin, 20*(3), 441–451.

Wallentin, M. (2009). Putative sex differences in verbal abilities and language cortex: A critical review. *Brain and Language, 108*(3), 175–183.

Wallner, U., Schmitz-Habsch, T., Antony, G., Fimmers, R., Spottke, A., Oertel, W. H., et al. (2007). Autonomic dysfunction in 3414 Parkinson's disease patients enrolled in the German network on Parkinson's disease (KNP e.V.): The effect of ageing. *European Journal of Neurology, 14*(12), 1405–1408.

Wang, H. X., Karp, A., Herlitz, A., Kareholt, I., Fratiglioni, L., Winblad, B., et al. (2009). Personality and lifestyle in relation to dementia incidence. *Neurology, 72*(3), 253–256.

Wang, L., Li, Z.-Q., Liu, H.-C., & Du, W. (2007). Factor structure of general dimension scales of PANAS-xin Chinese people. *Chinese Journal of Clinical Psychology, 15*(6), 565–568.

Wang, Y.-H., Zhu, Z.-H., Wang, P., & Wang, Z.-H. (2008). The effect of rewards and punishment on affective decision-making in children with two subtypes of ADHD. *Acta Psychologica Sinica, 40*(9), 975–986.

Warnes, H. (1986). Alexithymia: Clinical and therapeutic aspects. *Psychotherapy and Psychosomatics, 46*(1), 96–104.

Watkins, E., & Brown, R. G. (2002). Rumination and executive function in depression: An experimental study. *Journal of Neurological and Neurosurgical Psychiatry, 72*, 400–402.

Watson, C., Hoeft, F., Garrett, A. S., Hall, S. S., & Reiss, A. L. (2008). Aberrant brain activation during gaze processing in boys with fragile X syndrome. *Archives of General Psychiatry, 65*(11), 1315–1323.

Watson, D. (1988). Intraindividual and interindividual analyses of positive and negative affect: Their relation to health complaints, perceived stress, and daily activities. *Journal of Personality and Social Psychology, 54*(6), 1020–1030.

Watson, D., Clark, L. A., & Tellegen, A. (1988). Development and validation of brief measures of positive and negative affect: The PANAS scales. *Journal of Personality and Social Psychology, 54*(6), 1063–1070.

Watson, D., & Tellegen, A. (1985). Toward a consensual structure of mood. *Psychological Bulletin, 98*(2), 219–235.

Watson, E. B. (2008). *Emotion regulation in affluent adolescents: Investigating the relationship between regulation and functioning*. Ann Arbor, MI: ProQuest Information & Learning.

Weber, S., Habel, U., Amunts, K., & Schneider, F. (2008). Structural brain abnormalities in psychopaths: A review. *Behavioral Sciences and the Law, 26*(1), 7–28.

Wechsler, D. (2008). *Wechsler Adult Intelligence Scale—Fourth Edition*. San Antonio, TX: Pearson.

Weddell, R. A. (1994). Effects of subcortical lesion site on human emotional behavior. *Brain and Cognition, 25*(2), 161–193.

Weiskrantz, L. (1956). Behavioral changes associated with ablation of the amygdaloid complex in monkeys. *Journal of Comparative and Physiological Psychology, 49*(4), 381–391.

Weiss, E. M., Siedentopf, C., Golaszewski, S., Mottaghy, F. M., Hofer, A., Kremser, C., et al. (2007). Brain activation patterns during a selective attention test: A functional MRI study in healthy volunteers and unmedicated patients during an acute episode of schizophrenia. *Psychiatry Research: Neuroimaging, 154*(1), 31–40.

Weiss, U., Salloum, J. B., & Schneider, F. (1999). Correspondence of emotional self-rating with facial expression. *Psychiatry Research, 86*(2), 175–184.

Weller, J. A. (2007). *The role of affect in decisions under varying levels of uncertainty: Converging evidence from neurological and temperament perspectives*. Ann Arbor, MI: ProQuest Information & Learning.

Welsh, M. C., Pennington, B. F., & Groisser, D. B. (1991). A normative-developmental study of executive function: A window on prefrontal function in children. *Developmental Neuropsychology, 7*(2), 131–149.

Weniger, G., Lange, C., Rather, E., & Irle, E. (2004). Differential impairments of facial affect recognition in schizophrenia subtypes and major depression. *Psychiatry Research, 128*(2), 135–146.

Wertz, R. T., Henschel, C. R., Auther, L. L., Ashford, J. R., & Kirshner, H. S. (1998). Affective prosodic disturbance subsequent to right hemisphere stroke: A clinical application. *Journal of Neurolinguistics, 11*(1), 89–102.

West, C. H., & Michael, R. P. (1990). Responses of units in the mesolimbic system to olfactory and somatosensory stimuli: Modulation of sensory input by ventral tegmental stimulation. *Brain Research, 532*(1), 307–316.

Whalen, P. J., & Phelps, E. A. (Eds.). (2009). *The human amygdala*. New York: Guilford Press.

Whitaker, H. A., Stemmer, B., Joanette, Y., Code, C., Wallesch, C.-W., & Lecours, A. R. (1996). A psychosurgical chapter in the history of cerebral localisation: The six cases of Gottlieb Burckhardt (1891). In C. Code, C.-W. Wallesch, Y. Joanette, & A. R. Lecours (Eds.), *Classic cases in neuropsychology* (pp. 275–304). Hove, UK: Psychology Press/Erlbaum.

Whitmer, A. J., & Banich, M. T. (2007). Inhibition versus switching deficits in different forms of rumination. *Psychological Science, 18*, 546–553.

Whittaker, J. F., Deakin, J. F. W., & Tomenson, B. (2001). Face processing in schizophrenia: Defining the deficit. *Psychological Medicine, 31*(3), 499–507.

Widen, S. (2005). *Preschoolers' use of emotion labels and understanding of emotion categories*. Ann Arbor, MI: ProQuest Information & Learning.

Wiest, G., Lehner-Baumgartner, E., & Baumgartner, C. (2006). Panic attacks in an individual with bilateral selective lesions of the amygdala. *Archives of Neurology, 63*(12), 1798–1801.

Wild, B., Erb, M., & Bartels, M. (2001). Are emotions contagious?: Evoked emotions while viewing emotionally expressive faces—quality, quantity, time course and gender differences. *Psychiatry Research, 102*(2), 109–124.

Wild, B., Rodden, F. A., Grodd, W., & Ruch, W. (2003). Neural correlates of laughter and humour. *Brain: A Journal of Neurology, 126*(10), 2121–2138.

Wilde, E. A., Bigler, E. D., Haider, J. M., Chu, Z., Levin, H. S., Li, X., et al. (2006). Vulnerability of the anterior commissure in moderate to severe pediatric traumatic brain injury. *Journal of Child Neurology, 21*(9), 769–776.

Williams, G. H., & Dluhy, R. C. (2008). Disorders of the adrenal cortex. In E. Braunwald (Ed.), *Harrison's principles of internal medicine* (17th ed.). New York: McGraw-Hill.

Williams, K. R., Galas, J., Light, D., Pepper, C., Ryan, C., Kleinmann, A. E., et al. (2001). Head injury and alexithymia: Implications for family practice care. *Brain Injury, 15*(4), 349–356.

Williams, L. M., Das, P., Liddell, B., Olivieri, G., Peduto, A., Brammer, M. J., et al. (2005). BOLD, sweat and fears: fMRI and skin conductance distinguish facial fear signals. *NeuroReport, 16*(1), 49–52.

Williams, L. M., Hermens, D. F., Palmer, D., Kohn, M., Clarke, S., Keage, H., et al. (2008). Misinterpreting emotional expressions in attention-deficit/hyperactivity disorder: Evidence for a neural marker and stimulant effects. *Biological Psychiatry, 63*(10), 917–926.

Williams, L. S., Ghose, S. S., & Swindle, R. W. (2004). Depression and other mental health diagnoses increase mortality risk after ischemic stroke. *American Journal of Psychiatry, 161*(6), 1090–1095.

Williams, P. G., Smith, T. W., Gunn, H. E., & Uchino, B. N. (in press). Personality and stress: Individual differences in exposure, reactivity, recovery, and restoration. In R. Contrada & A. Baum (Eds.), *Handbook of stress science: Biology, psychology, and health.* New York: Springer.

Williams, P. G., Suchy, Y., & Kraybill, M. (2010). Five factor model personality traits and executive functioning among older adults. *Journal of Research in Personality, 44*, 485–491.

Williams, P. G., Suchy, Y., & Rau, H. (2009). Individual differences in executive functioning: Implications for stress regulation. *Annals of Behavioral Medicine, 37*, 126–140.

Williams, W. H., & Evans, J. J. (2003). Brain injury and emotion: An overview to a special issue on biopsychosocial approaches in neurorehabilitation. *Neuropsychological Rehabilitation, 13*(1), 1–11.

Willner, P., Lappas, S., Cheeta, S., & Muscat, R. (1994). Reversal of stress-induced anhedonia by the dopamine receptor agonist, pramipexole. *Psychopharmacology, 115*(4), 454–462.

Wilson, R. (1998). Mania associated with dialysis: A literature review and new patient report. *Psychosomatics: Journal of Consultation Liaison Psychiatry, 39*(6), 543–546.

Wilson, R. S., Arnold, S. E., Beck, T. L., Bienias, J. L., & Bennett, D. A. (2008). Change in depressive symptoms during the prodromal phase of Alzheimer's disease. *Archives of General Psychiatry, 65*(4), 439–446.

Wilson, R. S., Buchman, A. S., Arnold, S. E., Shah, R. C., Tang, Y., & Bennett, D. A. (2006). Harm avoidance and disability in old age. *Experimental Aging Research, 32*(3), 243–261.

Wilson, R. S., Fleischman, D. A., Myers, R. A., Bennett, D. A., Bienias, J. L., Gilley, D. W., et al. (2004). Premorbid proneness to distress and episodic memory impairment in Alzheimer's disease. *Journal of Neurology, Neurosurgery, and Psychiatry, 75*(2), 191–195.

Windmann, S., Kirsch, P., Mier, D., Stark, R., Walter, B., Guentuerkuen, O., et al. (2006). On framing effects in decision making: Linking lateral versus medial orbitofrontal cortex activation to choice outcome processing. *Journal of Cognitive Neuroscience, 18*(7), 1198–1211.

Winston, J. S., Dolan, R. J., Manstead, A. S. R., Frijda, N., & Fischer, A. (2004). Feeling states in emotion: Functional imaging evidence. In A. S. R. Manstead, N. Frijda, & A. Fischer (Eds.), *Feelings and emotions: The Amsterdam symposium* (pp. 204–220). New York: Cambridge University Press.

Wise, T. N., Mann, L. S., Mitchell, J. D., & Hryvniak, M. (1990). Secondary alexithymia: An empirical validation. *Comprehensive Psychiatry, 31*(4), 284–288.

Wise, T. N., Mann, L. S., & Shay, L. (1992). Alexithymia and the five-factor model of personality. *Comprehensive Psychiatry, 33*(3), 147–151.

Wishart, J. G., Cebula, K. R., Willis, D. S., & Pitcairn, T. K. (2007). Understanding of facial expressions of emotion by children with intellectual disabilities of differing aetiology. *Journal of Intellectual Disability Research, 51*(7), 551–563.

Wittig, R. M., Crockford, C., Lehmann, J., Seyfarth, R. M., Cheney, D. L., & Whitten, P. L. (2008). Focused grooming networks and stress alleviation in wild female baboons. *Hormones and Behavior, 54*(1), 170–177.

Wittling, W. (1997). Brain asymmetry and autonomic control of the heart. *European Psychologist, 2*(4), 313–327.

Wittling, W., Block, A., Schweiger, E., & Genzel, S. (1998). Hemisphere asymmetry in sympathetic control of the human myocardium. *Brain and Cognition, 38*(1), 17–35.

Wolff, J. C., & Ollendick, T. H. (2006). The comorbidity of conduct problems and depression in childhood and adolescence. *Clinical Child and Family Psychology Review, 9*(3), 201–220.

Wood, R. L. L., & Williams, C. (2007). Neuropsychological correlates of organic alexithymia. *Journal of the International Neuropsychological Society, 13*(3), 471–479.

Wood, R. L. L., Williams, C., & Kalyani, T. (2009). The impact of alexithymia on somatization after traumatic brain injury. *Brain Injury, 23*(7–8), 649–654.

Woods, D. L., Kovach, C. R., Raff, H., Basmadjian, A., Hegadoren, K. M., & Joosse, L. (2008). Using saliva to measure endogenous cortisol in nursing home residents with advanced dementia. *Research in Nursing and Health, 31*(3), 283–294.

Woodworth, R. S., & Sherrington, C. S. (1904). A pseudoaffective reflex and its spinal path. *Journal of Physiology, 31*, 234–243.

Worling, D. E., Humphries, T., & Tannock, R. (1999). Spatial and emotional aspects of language inferencing in nonverbal learning disabilities. *Brain and Language, 70*(2), 220–239.

Wright, P., He, G., Shapira, N. A., Goodman, W. K., & Liu, Y. (2004). Disgust and the insula: fMRI responses to pictures of mutilation and contamination. *NeuroReport, 15*(15), 2347–2351.

Wyvell, C. L., & Berridge, K. C. (2000). Intra-accumbens amphetamine increases the conditioned incentive salience of sucrose reward: Enhancement of reward "wanting" without enhanced "liking" or response reinforcement. *Journal of Neuroscience, 20*(21), 8122–8130.

Xiong-Zhao, Z., Xiao-Yan, W., & Ying, H. (2006). A comparative study of Wisconsin Card Sorting Test in individuals with different degrees of alexithymia. *Chinese Journal of Clinical Psychology, 14*(2), 132–133.

Yaka, R., Salomon, S., Matzner, H., & Weinstock, M. (2007). Effect of varied gestational stress on acquisition of spatial memory, hippocampal LTP and synaptic proteins in juvenile male rats. *Behavioural Brain Research, 179*(1), 126–132.

Yechiam, E., Goodnight, J., Bates, J. E., Busemeyer, J. R., Dodge, K. A., Pettit, G. S., et al. (2006). A formal cognitive model of the go/no-go discrimination task: Evaluation and implications. *Psychological Assessment, 18*(3), 239–249.

Yehuda, R., & McEwen, B. (2004). *Biobehavioral stress response: Protective and damaging effects.* New York: New York Academy of Sciences.

Yerkes, R. M., & Dodson, J. D. (1908). The relation of strength of stimulus to rapidity of habit formation. *Journal of Comparative Neurology and Psychology, 18*, 459–482.

Yeung, N., Cohen, J. D., & Botvinick, M. M. (2004). The neural basis of error detection: Conflict monitoring and the error-related negativity. *Psychological Review, 111*(4), 931–959.

Yoo, S., Gujar, N., Hu, P., Jolesz, F., & Walker, M. (2007). The human emotional brain without sleep: A prefrontal–amygdala disconnect? *Current Biology, 17*, R877–R878.

Yoon, B.-W., Morillo, C. A., Cechetto, D. F., & Hachinski, V. (1997). Cerebral hemispheric lateralization in cardiac autonomic control. *Archives of Neurology, 54*(6), 741–744.

Young, A. W., & Cleeremans, A. (2003). Face recognition with and without awareness. In A. Cleeremans (Ed.), *The unity of consciousness: Binding, integration, and dissociation* (pp. 233–250). New York: Oxford University Press.

Young, A. W., Hellawell, D. J., Van De Wal, C., & Johnson, M. (1996). Facial expression processing after amygdalotomy. *Neuropsychologia, 34*(1), 31–39.

Ysrraelit, M. C., Gaitan, M. I., Lopez, A. S., & Correale, J. (2008). Impaired hypothalamic–pituitary–adrenal axis activity in patients with multiple sclerosis. *Neurology, 71*(24), 1948–1954.

Ytterberg, C., Johansson, S., Holmqvist, L. W. N., & von Koch, L. (2008). Longitudinal variations and predictors of increased perceived impact of multiple sclerosis: A two-year study. *Journal of the Neurological Sciences, 270*(1–2), 53–59.

Yuen, K. S. L., & Lee, T. M. C. (2003). Could mood state affect risk-taking decisions? *Journal of Affective Disorders, 75*(1), 11–18.

Yuii, K., Suzuki, M., Kurachi, M., Sulyok, K., Csermely, P. T., & Korcsmaros, T. S. (2007). Stress sensitization in schizophrenia. In P. Csermely & T. Korscmáros (Eds.), *Stress responses in biology and medicine: Stress of life in molecules, organisms, and psychosocial communities* (pp. 276–290). Malden, MA: Blackwell.

Zaja, R. H., & Rojahn, J. (2008). Facial emotion recognition in intellectual disabilities. *Current Opinion in Psychiatry, 21*(5), 441–444.

Zeitlin, S. B., Lane, R. D., O'Leary, D. S., & Schrift, M. J. (1989). Interhemispheric transfer deficit and alexithymia. *American Journal of Psychiatry, 146*(11), 1434–1439.

Zajonc, R. B. (1968). Attitudinal effects of mere exposure. *Journal of Personality and Social Psychology, 9*(2), 1–27.

Zakzanis, K. K., Mraz, R., & Graham, S. J. (2005). An fMRI study of the Trail Making Test. *Neuropsychologia, 43*(13), 1878–1886.

Zamboni, G., Huey, E. D., Krueger, F., Nichelli, P. F., & Grafman, J. (2008). Apathy and disinhibition in frontotemporal dementia: Insights into their neural correlates. *Neurology, 71*(10), 736–742.

Zelkowitz, P., Guzder, J., Paris, J., Feldman, R., Roy, C., & Schiavetto, A. (2004). Borderline pathology of childhood: Implications of early Axis II diagnoses. *Canadian Child and Adolescent Psychiatry Review, 13*(3), 58–67.

Zhou, F.-C., & Xu, Z.-L. (2005). Quality of life and affect of lung cancer patients receiving chemotherapy. *Chinese Mental Health Journal, 19*(6), 402–405.

Zhu, J.-N., Yung, W.-H., Chow, B. K.-C., Chan, Y.-S., & Wang, J.-J. (2006). The cerebellar–hypothalamic circuits: Potential pathways underlying cerebellar involvement in somatic–visceral integration. *Brain Research Reviews, 52*(1), 93–106.

Ziemssen, T., & Reichmann, H. (2010). Cardiovascular autonomic dysfunction in Parkinson's disease. *Journal of the Neurological Sciences, 289*(1–2), 74–80.

Zimmerman, E. K., Eslinger, P. J., Simmons, Z., & Barrett, A. M. (2007). Emotional perception deficits in amyotrophic lateral sclerosis. *Cognitive and Behavioral Neurology, 20*(2), 79–82.

Zimmerman, J. M., Rabinak, C. A., McLachlan, I. G., & Maren, S. (2007). The central nucleus of the amygdala is essential for acquiring and expressing conditional fear after overtraining. *Learning and Memory, 14*(9), 634–644.

Index

Page numbers followed by *f* indicate figure; *n*, note; and *t*, table

Abulia
  clinical populations, 261
  incentive sensitivity and, 189–190, 189*f*
  overview, 254
Acquired brain injury, 127. *See also* Traumatic brain injury
Acquired sociopathy, 145, 146*t*. *See also* Psychopathy
Addiction
  dopaminergic system and, 202*n*
  extraversion and, 229–230
  incentive sensitivity and, 192*t*, 200
  overview, 253
  rewards and punishments and, 192*t*
  See also Substance abuse
Addison disease, 213
Adhedonia, 190
Adrenal gland
  autonomic nervous system and, 74*t*
  stress and, 209*f*
Adrenal insufficiency, 213
Adrenaline
  autonomic nervous system and, 74*t*
  stress and, 207–209
Adrenocorticotropic hormone (ACTH), 207–208
Advanced Clinical Solutions (ACS) supplement, 132–133
Affect, 236. *See also* Emotion regulation; Stress
Affect recognition, 253. *See* Receptive paralinguistic communication
Affect regulation, 254, 255, 257. *See* Emotion regulation
Affective aggression, 78. *See also* Aggression
Affective communication
  assessment and, 249, 263
  clinical populations, 260
  development of clinical tools and, 249
  overview, 254, 258

See Communication, emotional
Affective loading, 47
Affective style
  assessment measure for, 263
  overview, 156*f*, 163
Agenesis of corpus callosum
  awareness of emotional experience and, 107–108
  overview, 253
Aggression
  affective communication and, 127, 131
  approach–withdrawal dichotomy and, 166
  emotion regulation and, 146*t*
  incentive sensitivity and, 201
  lesion studies and, 140
  mesencephalon and, 78–79, 79*t*
Aging
  amygdala and, 65
  stress and, 210, 216–217
  See also Dementia
Agreeableness
  cognitive and neuroanatomic substrates for, 231–232
  overview, 224, 225, 225*t*, 226*t*
Akinetic mutism
  clinical populations, 261
  incentive sensitivity and, 189–190, 189*f*
  overview, 191, 254
Alexithymia
  assessment and, 106–107, 263
  clinical populations, 260
  functioning and, 105–106
  interoceptive awareness and, 98
  neuropsychiatric disorders, 109
  overview, 97, 97*f*, 99–100, 103–105, 104*t*, 253, 254, 256, 257, 258
Allostasis, 238
Alzheimer's disease
  adhedonia and, 190
  affective communication and, 128*t*
  mood and, 173
  overview, 253–254
  rewards and punishments and, 199
  stress and, 216–217
American Congress of Rehabilitation Medicine, 189–191, 189*f*
Amygdala
  awareness of emotional experience, 102*t*
  clinical populations, 63–67
  clinical signs and syndromes, 61–63
  damage to, 60–61
  functioning and, 60
  heritability of temperament and personality and, 228*t*
  incentive sensitivity and, 201
  localization of emotions within the brain and, 28–30
  memory and, 58
  neuroticism and, 229
  overactive trigger mechanisms and, 59
  overview, 40*n*, 68
  posttraumatic stress disorder (PTSD) and, 215–216
  stress and, 209*f*
  trigger mechanism and, 48–55, 49*f*, 52*t*, 54*f*, 56*t*, 68*n*–69*n*
Amyotrophic lateral sclerosis (ALS), 88, 253
Ancient history, 10–13, 10*t*, 13*t*
Anger
  affective communication and, 127, 131
  approach–withdrawal dichotomy and, 166
  awareness of emotional experience, 101, 102*t*
Anhedonia
  assessment and, 196–197, 197*t*, 263
  clinical populations, 261
  incentive sensitivity and, 192*t*
  overview, 160–161, 191, 254, 255, 256, 257, 259
  rewards and punishments and, 192*t*, 200
Antagonism, 225*t*
Anterior cingulate cortex
  awareness of emotional experience, 102*t*
  heritability of temperament and personality and, 228*t*
  motivation and, 167
  paralinguistic communication and, 120
  reflexive process and, 81
  thalamic networks and, 79*t*

Anterior hypothalamic area, 77*t*
Anterior pituitary, 209*f*
Anterior regions, 120
Anterior temporal lobe, 30
Antisocial behaviors
  affective communication and, 127, 131
  amygdala and, 66–67
  incentive sensitivity and, 200–201
Antisocial personality disorder, 127, 131
Anxiety
  alexithymia and, 106
  awareness of emotional experience and, 97*f*
  Cushing syndrome (CS) and, 212
  heritability of temperament and personality and, 228*t*
  incentive sensitivity and, 192*t*
  rewards and punishments and, 192*t*
  social anxiety, 206
  See also Anxiety disorders
Anxiety disorders
  amygdala and, 59, 67
  emotion regulation and, 145–147, 146*t*, 154*n*
  hemispheric asymmetry and, 165
  incentive sensitivity and, 192*t*
  rewards and punishments and, 192*t*
  See also Anxiety
Apathy
  assessment measure for, 263
  clinical populations, 261
  incentive sensitivity and, 189–190, 189*f*
  overview, 191, 254, 255, 256, 257, 258
  rewards and punishments and, 200
Apathy Evaluation Scale (AES), 196, 263
Approach, 156*f*
Approach–withdrawal dichotomy
  cognition and, 167–169
  hemispheric asymmetry and, 165–166
  overview, 163
  See also Approach; Withdrawal
Arcuate nucleus
  reflexive process and, 77*t*
  thalamic networks and, 79*t*
Area postrema, 79*t*
Aristotle, 12–13, 24
Arrector pili muscles, 74*t*
Asperger syndrome, 104, 104*t*
Assessment
  affective communication and, 131–133, 249
  awareness of emotional experience, 106–107
  development of clinical tools, 247–250
  diagnostic sensitivity and specificity and, 250–251
  emotion regulation and, 142–143, 248–249
  executive functioning and, 175*n*
  incentive sensitivity and, 192–198, 192*t*, 193*f*–194*f*, 197*t*, 249–250
  list of measures, 263–264
  mood and, 170–171
  motivation and, 171
  personality and, 233*n*
  reflexive process and, 91–92
  trigger mechanism and, 59–60
  See also specific measures
Attention
  amygdala and, 61
  Iowa Gambling Task (IGT) and, 188
  trigger mechanism and, 57
  See also Cognition
Attentional blink task, 57
Attentional Network Test (ANT)
  heritability of temperament and personality and, 228*t*
  overview, 226–227, 233, 233*n*
Attention-deficit/hyperactivity disorder (ADHD)
  affective communication and, 129*t*
  emotion regulation and, 147
  extraversion and, 229–230
  heritability of temperament and personality and, 228*t*
  incentive sensitivity and, 192*t*
  overview, 86–87, 87*t*, 253
  rewards and punishments and, 191–192, 192*t*
Auras
  clinical populations, 261
  overview, 257
  reflexive process and, 84–85
Autism
  affective communication and, 129*t*
  amygdala and, 63–64
  Asperger syndrome, 104, 104*t*
  rewards and punishments and, 195

Autoimmune autonomic neuropathy (AAN), 85
Autonomic activation, 163
Autonomic failure
  clinical populations, 261
  overview, 85, 254, 255, 256, 258
  reflexive process and, 90*t*
Autonomic hypoactivation, 253
Autonomic nervous system
  overview, 72–73, 74*t*
  seizure disorder and, 90–91
Autonomic regulation
  anterior cingulate cortex, 81
  hemispheric asymmetry and, 81–82
Autonomic seizures
  clinical populations, 261
  overview, 257
  reflexive process and, 84–85
Autonomic/endocrine response
  assessment measure for, 263
  overview, 72–75, 74*t*
  reflexive process and, 84–86
Aversion, 184
Avoidance
  emotion regulation and, 136*f*
  social anxiety and, 206
Awareness of emotional experience
  assessment and, 106–107
  clinical populations, 107–109
  clinical signs and syndromes, 103–105, 104*t*
  cognition and, 101, 103
  functioning and, 105–106
  integrating theory and practice, 103–109, 104*t*
  neuroanatomic substrates, 98–101
  overview, 94–95, 98–101, 110
  theoretical background, 95–103, 97*f*, 102*t*

B

Basal forebrain, 76*f*
Basal ganglia
  paralinguistic communication and, 120–121
  reflexive process and, 72
Behavior, 182
Behavior activation system (BAS)
  extraversion and, 230
  overview, 156*f*, 175*n*, 233*n*
  rewards and punishments and, 181, 197–198
Behavior inhibition system (BIS)
  neuroticism and, 229
  overview, 175*n*, 233*n*
  personality and, 225
  rewards and punishments and, 197–198
Behavioral regulation
  cognition and, 168
  lesion studies and, 140–141
Behavioristic theory, 177
Bilateral amygdalar damage, 60–61. *See also* Amygdala
Bilateral frontal poles, 121
Bipolar disorder
  affective communication and, 130*t*
  emotion regulation and, 144–145
BIS/BAS Scale, 198, 233*n*, 264
Bladder, urinary, 74*t*
Blood pressure, 237
Blood vessels, 74*t*
Bottom-up approach for using this book, 2–5, 5*f*
Brain
  as the center of emotions, 23–26
  localization of emotions within, 26–30
  See also Traumatic brain injury
Brain injury, 239–240. *See also* Traumatic brain injury
Broca area, 119
Bronchi, 74*t*

C

Cannon–Bard theory, 17–18, 17*f*
Capgras syndrome
  clinical populations, 261
  dementias and, 65
  overview, 62–63, 253, 254, 255, 259
Cardiovascular recovery, 244–245
Cat–dog paradigm, 27–28
Catecholamines, 208
Catechol-O-methyltransferase (COMT), 228*t*

Caudate nucleus, 102*t*
Central nervous system, 23
Cerebellum, 76*f*, 79*t*, 81
Cerebral cortex
overview, 33–39
reflexive process and, 76*f*, 81–82
See also Frontal lobes; Hemispheric asymmetry; Lower brainstem
Cerebral hemispheres, 120
Cerebral-vascular accidents
awareness of emotional experience, 109
overview, 149–152, 150*f*, 151*f*
reflexive process and, 91
Chapman Physical Anhedonia Scale (CPAS), 196–197, 197*t*, 263
Childhood depression, 147. *See also* Depression
Chronic fatigue syndrome, 109
Closed mindedness, 225*t*
Cognition
affective communication and, 125–126
awareness of emotional experience, 101, 103
emotion regulation and, 141–142
incentive sensitivity and, 188
motivation and, 167, 167–169
personality and, 227, 229–233
reflexive process and, 82
stress and, 209–211
stress regulation and, 239–242
trigger mechanism and, 57–58
Cognitive appraisal theory, 19–20
Cognitive empathy
affective communication and, 125–126
overview, 113, 118*f*, 122–124, 124*f*, 255
Cognitive flexibility. *See* Switching
Cognitive reappraisals
emotion regulation and, 136*f*
feedback responsiveness and, 142–143
overview, 137
stress regulation and, 237*t*
Cognitive-behavioral therapy (CBT), 150–151
Communication, emotional
assessment and, 131–133
cognition and, 125–126
direction of, 114–115
integrating theory and practice, 126–133, 128*t*–130*t*
neuroanatomic substrates, 117–124, 118*f*, 124*f*
overview, 111, 133
theoretical background, 112–126, 116*f*, 118*f*
Composite Autonomic Symptom Scale (COMPASS), 91–92, 263
Conduct disorders
affective communication and, 131
emotion regulation and, 147
Conscientiousness
cognitive and neuroanatomic substrates for, 232–233
overview, 224, 225, 225*t*, 226*t*
Contagion, emotional
affective communication and, 124
overview, 113
Containment, 208, 209*f*
Context conditioning, 51–53, 52*t*
Continuous Performance Test (CPT)
heritability of temperament and personality and, 226–227
overview, 91–92
Coping strategies, 136*f*
Corpus callosum, 107–108, 253
Corticosterone, 207–208
Corticotropic pituitary adenomas, 218
Corticotropin-releasing hormone (CRH), 209*f*
Cortisol
adrenal insufficiency and, 213
Cushing syndrome (CS) and, 212
overview, 258
stress and, 207–208, 209*f*
Criminal offending
affective communication and, 127, 131
incentive sensitivity and, 201
Culture. *See* Openness to experience
Cushing syndrome (CS), 212, 218

D

Daily functioning. *See* Functioning
Davidson's theory
motivation and, 167
overview, 175*n*

Decision making
amygdala and, 61
assessment and, 195–196, 263
clinical populations, 261
functional imaging research, 202*n*
overview, 257, 258
rewards and punishments and, 181–182
Defensive aggression, 78, 79*t*. *See also* Aggression
Delusional misidentification syndrome. *See* Capgras syndrome
Dementia
adhedonia and, 190
affective communication and, 128*t*–130*t*
assessment and, 170–171
mood and, 173–174
motivation and, 173–174
of old age, 65, 147
stress and, 216–217
Dementia with Lewy bodies
adhedonia and, 190
overview, 255
rewards and punishments and, 199
Dendritic atrophy, 210
Depression
adhedonia and, 190
adrenal insufficiency and, 213
affective communication and, 130*t*
alexithymia and, 106
awareness of emotional experience and, 109
Cushing syndrome (CS) and, 212
dementias and, 173
emotion regulation and, 144, 147, 151–152
hemispheric asymmetry and, 165
mood and, 160–161
overview, 171–172, 254
stress and, 214–215, 219
Descartes, 21*n*
Development, stress and, 210–211
Developmental disorders. *See* Neurodevelopmental disorders
Diagnostic sensitivity and specificity, 250–251
Diastolic blood pressure, 237
Diathesis–stress model, 165
Diencephalon
localization of emotions within the brain and, 26–28
reflexive process and, 76*f*
Digest-and-repair processes, 72–73
Diminished motivation disorders
assessment and, 196
incentive sensitivity and, 189–191, 189*f*
Disgust, 101, 102*t*
Distancing
emotion regulation and, 136*f*
overview, 137, 139–140
Dopaminergic system
addiction and, 202*n*
adhedonia and, 190
heritability of temperament and personality and, 227, 228*t*
incentive sensitivity and, 182, 190
Dorsolateral-basal ganglia circuitry, 147
Dorsolateral prefrontal cortex
emotion regulation and, 139, 140
rewards and punishments and, 193*f*–194*f*
Dorsomedial nucleus, 77*t*
Down syndrome
affective communication and, 129*t*
overview, 255
Drive theory, 162. *See also* Motivation
Dual diagnosis, 109
Duchenne smile, 93*n*
Dysregulation, 140–141. *See also* Behavioral regulation; Emotion regulation

E

Effortful control, 226*t*
Ekman 60 Faces Test, 132
Electroconvulsive therapy (ECT), 41*n*
Emobodied emotions, 114
Emotion regulation
affective communication and, 124
assessment and, 142–143, 248–249, 263
clinical populations, 147–153, 150*f*, 151*f*, 261
clinical signs and syndromes, 143–147, 146*t*

cognition and, 141–142
development of clinical tools and, 248–249
integrating theory and practice, 142–147, 146*t*
neuroanatomic substrates, 138–141
overview, 135, 136*f*, 153, 236, 253, 254, 255, 256, 258, 259
stress regulation and, 236, 237*t*
theoretical background, 136–142, 136*f*
Emotion Regulation Questionnaire (ERQ), 143, 263
Emotional (in)stability, 224–225. *See also* Neuroticism
Emotional circuitry, 30–33, 31*f*
Emotional contagion
affective communication and, 124
overview, 113
Emotional decision making. *See* Decision making
Emotional deficits, 30
Emotional domains, 155
Emotional empathy, 113, 118*f*, 122–123, 124*f*
Emotional experience, 116*f*
Emotional intelligence, 105
Emotional learning circuitry. *See* Learning circuitry
Emotional stability, 225*t*
Emotional triggers. *See* Trigger mechanism
Emotions, historical origins and, 7–8
Empathy
affective communication and, 122–124, 124*f*, 125–126
alexithymia and, 104
clinical populations, 261
cognitive empathy, 113, 118*f*, 122–124, 124*f*
emotional empathy, 113, 118*f*, 122–123, 124*f*
overview, 255, 258
Endocrine response
overview, 258
reflexive process and, 72–75, 74*t*, 84–86
Endocrine system, 73
Environmental factors, 243*f*
Epilepsy
emotion regulation and, 152
Klüver–Bucy syndrome and, 61
reflexive process and, 84–85
seizure disorder and, 65–66
Epinephrine, 209*f*
Episodic memory, 58. *See also* Memory
Executive functioning
assessment and, 175*n*
cognition and, 168
cognitive and neuroanatomic substrates for, 227, 229–233
depression and, 171–172
emotion regulation and, 141–142
heritability of temperament and personality and, 226–227, 228*t*
overview, 235
stress regulation and, 239–242, 242–245, 243*f*
temperament and, 223
See also Functioning
Expressive affective communication, 114–115, 118*f*. *See also* Communication, emotional
Expressive linguistic communication, 118–119, 118*f*. *See also* Communication, emotional
Expressive paralinguistic communication, 118*f*, 122. *See also* Communication, emotional
Extraversion
cognitive and neuroanatomic substrates for, 229–230
overview, 224–225, 225*t*, 226*t*
Eyes, autonomic nervous system and, 74*t*

F

Facial affect
affective communication and, 114–115
expressive paralinguistic communication and, 122
Facial affect recognition
affective communication and, 125, 127, 133*n*–134*n*
overview, 254, 255, 256, 258, 259
Facial emotional paresis, 72, 84
Facial muscles, 116*f*

Facial processing
amygdala and, 54–55, *54f*
fear and, 127, 131
fragile X syndrome and, 64
smiles, *93n*
Facial symmetry, *116f*
Fawcett–Clark Pleasure Scale (FCPS), 197, *197t*, 263
Fear, 101, *102t*
Fear conditioning
amygdala and, 29
psychopathy and, 67
trigger mechanism and, 51–53, *52t*
Feedback mechanisms, 73, 75
Feedback responsiveness, 142–143
Feeding, *79t*
Feeling awareness
cognition and, 103
functioning and, 105–106
interoceptive awareness and, 96–98, *97f*
neuroanatomic substrates, 99–101
overview, 96
See also Awareness of emotional experience
Fetal alcohol syndrome
affective communication and, *129t*
overview, 255
Fight-or-flight response, 72–73, *79t*
Five-factor model of personality, 224–226, *225t*
fMRI (functional magnetic resonance imaging). *See* Functional magnetic resonance imaging (fMRI)
Foix–Chavany–Marie syndrome
clinical populations, 262
overview, 84, 254
Fou rire prodromique (FRP)
clinical populations, 262
overview, 84, 254, 256
Fragile X syndrome
amygdala and, 64
overview, 255
Fragile X–associated tremor/ataxia syndrome (FXTAS)
amygdala and, 65
overview, 255
Frontal lobes
overview, 34–39
paralinguistic communication and, 120
See also Cerebral cortex
Frontal lobotomies
motivation and, 167
overview, 36–39
Frontotemporal–lobar degeneration (FTD)
affective communication and, *128t*
amygdala and, 65
assessment and, 132
incentive sensitivity and, 198–199
overview, 255
Functional imaging research, *202n*. *See* Neuroimaging technologies
Functional magnetic resonance imaging (fMRI)
alexithymia and, 99–100
amygdala and, 29
awareness of emotional experience, *102t*
emotion regulation and, 138–139
heritability of temperament and personality and, *228t*
reflexive process and, 82
See also Neuroimaging technologies
Functioning
awareness of emotional experience and, 105–106
trigger mechanism and, 60–61
See also Executive functioning
Fusiform gyrus, *102t*
Future directions
development of clinical tools, 247–250
diagnostic sensitivity and specificity and, 250–251
interdisciplinary implications, 251–252
overview, 247

G

Gelastic seizures (GS)
clinical populations, 262
overview, 83–84, 257, 258
Genetic factors, 226–227, *228t*
Genotype, *243f*
Globus pallidus, *102t*
Glucocorticoids, 207–208, 242

Glycogen, 74*t*
Gray matter, 100
Gray matter, periaqueductal
  aggression and, 78–79, 79*t*
  reflexive process and, 76*f*
Greek philosophy, 10–12, 10*t*, 23–24

H

Habituation, 208–209, 209*f*
Harm avoidance, 175*n*
Heart, as the center of emotions, 24
Heart contraction, 74*t*
Heart rate
  autonomic nervous system and, 74*t*
  hemispheric asymmetry and, 81–82
  stress and, 208
Heartbeat perception paradigm, 98
Hedonic hotspots, 183–184
Helplessness, learned
  incentive sensitivity and, 192*t*
  rewards and punishments and, 192*t*
Hemispheric asymmetry
  amygdala and, 55, 56*t*
  autonomic regulation and, 81–82
  mood and, 163–167
  motivation and, 163–167
  overview, 33–34
  parasympathetic branch and, 93*n*
  See also Cerebral cortex
Heraclitus, 24
Heritability, 223, 226–227
High negative affect, 173–174
High-frequency heart rate variability (HF-HRV), 237
Hippocampus
  fragile X syndrome and, 64
  overactive trigger mechanisms and, 59
  posttraumatic stress disorder (PTSD) and, 215–216
  stress and, 209*f*, 210
  trigger mechanism and, 52–53
  Turner syndrome and, 64
Hippocrates, 11, 21*n*, 23–24
History
  19th and 20th centuries, 15–21, 16*f*, 17*f*
  ancient history, 10–13, 10*t*, 13*t*
  brain as center of emotions, 23–26
  cerebral cortex, 33–39
  emotional circuitry, 30–33, 31*f*
  localization of emotions within the brain, 26–30
  Middle Ages, 14–15
History of clinical neuropsychology, 1–2, 7–8
Homeostasis
  hypothalamus, 56
  trigger mechanism and, 56
Humors in ancient Greek philosophy, 10–12, 10*t*, 24
Huntington's dementia, 128*t*, 255
Hyperorality, 62
Hyperphasia, 62
Hypothalamic hamartoma (HH), 87–88
Hypothalamic–pituitary–adrenocortical (HPA) axis activation
  aging and dementia and, 216–217
  clinical populations, 262
  depression and, 214–215
  neuropsychiatric disorders and, 214–216
  overview, 205, 206*f*, 218–219, 254, 256, 257, 258, 259
  sensitization of, 211–212
  stress and, 207–209, 209–211, 209*f*
  stress regulation and, 237
Hypothalamus
  aggression and, 78–79, 79*t*
  homeostasis and, 56
  information processing and, 49*f*
  reflexive process and, 76*f*, 77–78, 77*t*
  trigger mechanism and, 56

I

Imposter syndrome. *See* Capgras syndrome
Impulsivity
  emotion regulation and, 146*t*
  overview, 234*n*
Incentive sensitivity
  assessment and, 192–198, 192*t*, 193*f*–194*f*, 197*t*, 249–250
  assessment measure for, 263
  clinical populations, 198–201, 262

Incentive sensitivity *(cont.)*
clinical signs and syndromes, 189–192, 189*f*, 192*t*
cognition and, 188
development of clinical tools and, 249–250
extraversion and, 230
integrating theory and practice, 189–201, 189*f*, 192*t*, 193*f*–194*f*, 197*t*
neuroanatomic substrates, 182–188
neuroticism and, 229
overview, 156*f*, 176, 201, 253, 254, 256, 257, 258
personality and, 225, 226
positive reinforcement, 202*n*
rewards and punishments, 176–182
theoretical background, 176–188
Individual differences
executive functioning and, 241–242
heritability of temperament and personality and, 226–227
rewards and punishments and, 193*f*–194*f*
Information processing, 48–50, 49*f*
Inherent affective loading, 47
Inhibition, 168
Initiation
overview, 168
stress and, 209*f*
Inquisitiveness, 225
Insula, 102*t*
Intellect. *See* Openness to experience
Intensity, 47
Interdisciplinary implications, 251–252
Interoceptive awareness
cognition and, 101, 103
feeling awareness and, 96–98, 97*f*
functioning and, 105
neuroanatomic substrates, 98–99
overview, 95–96
See also Awareness of emotional experience
Interpersonal relations, 104
Intestines, 74*t*
Introversion, 225*t*
Involuntary skeletal response, 71–72
Iowa Gambling Task (IGT), 264
decision making and, 195–196
functional imaging research, 202*n*
incentive sensitivity and, 249–250
overview, 187–188
Irritability
adrenal insufficiency and, 213
Cushing syndrome (CS) and, 212
lesion studies and, 140

J

James–Lange theory
awareness of emotional experience, 95
localization of emotions within the brain and, 27
overview, 15–16, 16*f*
Judgement, amygdala and, 61

K

Kidneys, autonomic nervous system and, 74*t*
Klüver–Bucy syndrome
clinical populations, 262
dementias and, 65
overview, 28–29, 61–62, 253, 255, 256, 257, 258
seizure disorder and, 66

L

Language, 169
Lateral hypothalamic area
reflexive process and, 77*t*
thalamic networks and, 79*t*
Lateral orbitofrontal cortex, 202*n*
Learned helplessness
incentive sensitivity and, 192*t*
rewards and punishments and, 192*t*
Learning
incentive sensitivity and, 184–188
Parkinson's disease (PD), 199–200
rewards and punishments and, 177, 178–179, 192*t*
Learning circuitry
information processing and, 49*f*
trigger mechanism and, 53
Left frontal lobe, 144

Left frontal operculum, 121
Lesions
  emotion regulation and, 140–141, 154*n*
  motivation and, 167
Limbic system, 31–33, 40*n*–41*n*
Linguistic mode of affective communication, 112, 117–119, 118*f*. *See also* Communication, emotional
Lipoid proteinsis. *See* Urbach–Wiethe disease (lipoid proteinosis)
Liver, autonomic nervous system and, 74*t*
Lobotomies, frontal
  motivation and, 167
  overview, 36–39
Localization of emotions within the brain, 26–30
Lower brainstem, 76*f*, 80–81. *See also* Cerebellum

M

Major depression
  affective communication and, 130*t*
  awareness of emotional experience and, 109
  overview, 171–172, 256
  stress and, 214–215
  See also Depression
Mammillary bodies, 77*t*
Mania
  Cushing syndrome (CS) and, 212
  emotion regulation and, 144–145
Medial prefrontal cortex
  functional imaging research, 202*n*
  stress regulation and, 242
Medial preoptic area
  reflexive process and, 77*t*
  thalamic networks and, 79*t*
Medulla oblongata, 76*f*, 80–81. *See also* Lower brainstem
Memory
  adrenal insufficiency and, 213
  amygdala and, 60–61
  heritability of temperament and personality and, 228*t*
  Iowa Gambling Task (IGT) and, 188
  overview, 58
  psychopathy and, 67
  stress and, 173
  trigger mechanism and, 60
Mental health
  overview, 156*f*, 235
  stress regulation and executive functioning and, 242–245, 243*f*
  See also Neuropsychiatric disorders
Mental retardation, 64
Mere exposure effect, 20–21
Mesencephalon
  aggression and, 79, 79*t*
  reflexive process and, 76*f*, 78–80, 79*t*
Mesolimbic dopaminergic system
  adhedonia and, 190
  incentive sensitivity and, 182, 185
  orbitofrontal cortex and, 185
Middle Ages, 14–15
Middle temporal gyrus, 102*t*
Mild cognitive impairment, 128*t*
Minnesota Multiphasic Personality Inventory (MMPI), 104
Mirror neuron system (MNS), 123
Modes of affective communication, 112. *See also* Communication, emotional
Monoamine oxidase A (MAOA) gene
  heritability of temperament and personality and, 228*t*
  incentive sensitivity and, 201
Mood
  assessment and, 170–171
  clinical signs and syndromes, 171–172
  integrating theory and practice, 169–174
  neuroanatomic substrates, 163–167
  overview, 156*f*, 159, 174–175
  as a stable trait, 172
  theoretical background, 159–169, 161*f*
Motivation
  adrenal insufficiency and, 213
  assessment and, 170–171, 196
  clinical signs and syndromes, 171–172
  cognition and, 167–169
  diminished motivation disorders, 189–191, 189*f*
  emotion regulation and, 146*t*
  incentive sensitivity and, 202*n*
  integrating theory and practice, 169–174

Motivation *(cont.)*
 neuroanatomic substrates, 163–167
 overview, 155, 157, 159, 174–175
 rewards and punishments and, 179–181, 192*t*
 stress and, 205–207
 theoretical background, 159–169, 161*f*
 See also Incentive sensitivity
Motor activity, 71
Motor cortex, 72
Motor system, 71–72, 71*f*
Multiple sclerosis
 awareness of emotional experience and, 108
 emotion regulation and, 148
 Klüver–Bucy syndrome and, 61
 overview, 174
 reflexive process and, 88–89
 stress and, 217
Multiple system atrophy (MSA), 89, 90*t*
Mutism, akinetic
 clinical populations, 261
 incentive sensitivity and, 189–190, 189*f*
 overview, 191, 254
Myocardial contractibility, 81–82

N

Negative affect
 dementias and, 173–174
 diagnostic sensitivity and specificity and, 251
 overview, 160–162, 161*t*, 254
 as a stable trait, 172
 See also Mood
Negative emotionality, 226*t*
NEO Personality Inventory
 alexithymia and, 104
 diagnostic sensitivity and specificity and, 251
NEO Personality Inventory—Revised (NEO PI-R), 224
Neuroanatomic substrates
 affective communication and, 117–124, 118*f*, 124*f*
 awareness of emotional experience and, 98–101
 emotion regulation and, 138–141
 incentive sensitivity and, 182–188
 mood and, 163–167
 motivation and, 163–167
 personality and, 227, 229–233
 reflexive process and, 75–82, 76*f*, 77*t*, 79*t*
 stress and, 207–209, 209*f*
 stress regulation and, 239–242
 trigger mechanism and, 47–56, 49*f*, 52*t*, 54*f*, 56*t*
Neurocognitive assessment, 106
Neurodegenerative disorders
 affective communication and, 126–127, 128*t*–130*t*
 amygdala and, 65
 awareness of emotional experience and, 108
 emotion regulation and, 147–148
 incentive sensitivity and, 198–199
 reflexive process and, 88–90
Neurodevelopmental disorders
 affective communication and, 126–127
 amygdala and, 63–64
 awareness of emotional experience, 107–108
 emotion regulation and, 147
 mood and, 173–174
 motivation and, 173–174
 reflexive process and, 86–88, 87*t*
Neuroimaging technologies
 alexithymia and, 99–100
 amygdala and, 29, 50–51, 55
 awareness of emotional experience, 102*t*
 emotion regulation and, 138–139
 hemispheric asymmetry, 55
 heritability of temperament and personality and, 228*t*
 incentive sensitivity and, 202*n*
 reflexive process and, 82
 stimuli and, 50–51
 trigger mechanism and, 50–51, 53
 valence hypothesis and, 185–186
Neuropsychiatric disorders
 affective communication and, 126–127
 amygdala and, 66–67
 awareness of emotional experience and, 109

emotion regulation and, 152–153
incentive sensitivity and, 200–201
stress and, 214–216
Neuroticism
cognitive and neuroanatomic substrates for, 229
overview, 224–225, 225*t*, 226*t*
Neurovisceral integration model, 240–241
New York Emotion Battery, 117
19th and 20th centuries, 15–21, 16*f*, 17*f*
Nonvolitional affective communication, 115–117, 116*f*. *See also* Communication, emotional
Norepinephrine, 209*f*
Nucleus accumbens
dopaminergic system and, 202*n*
incentive sensitivity and, 183
overview, 184
reflexive process and, 76*f*, 80
thalamic networks and, 79*t*
Nucleus paragigantocellularis, 79*t*

O

Obsessive–compulsive disorder (OCD), 109
Olfactory bulb, 79*t*
Openness to experience
cognitive and neuroanatomic substrates for, 230–231
overview, 224, 225, 225*t*
Orbitofrontal cortex
awareness of emotional experience, 102*t*
emotion regulation and, 146–147, 151*f*
emotional learning and, 53
incentive sensitivity and, 184–185, 201
paralinguistic communication and, 120
rewards and punishments and, 193*f*–194*f*
Organization of this book, 2–5, 3*t*, 4*f*, 5*f*
Overactive trigger mechanism
alexithymia and, 106
overview, 59
See also Trigger mechanism

P

Panic disorder, 67. *See also* Anxiety disorders
Papez circuit, 30–31, 31*f*, 40*n*–41*n*
Paralinguistic mode of affective communication, 112–113, 116*f*, 118*f*, 119–122. *See also* Communication, emotional
Parasympathetic branch, 81–82, 93*n*
Paraventricular nucleus
reflexive process and, 77*t*
stress and, 209*f*
thalamic networks and, 79*t*
Parkinson's disease (PD)
adhedonia and, 190
affective communication and, 128*t*
awareness of emotional experience and, 108
overview, 89–90, 90*t*
rewards and punishments and, 199–200
Paroxysmal autonomic instability with dystonia (PAID)
clinical populations, 262
overview, 85–86, 254, 258
Pathological Laughter and Crying Scale (PLACS), 91–92, 263
Patterns of emotional responses, 155
Performance-based assessments, 247–248. *See also* Assessment
Periaqueductal gray matter
aggression and, 78–79, 79*t*
reflexive process and, 76*f*
Perifornical nucleus, 77*t*
Periventricular zone, 77*t*
Personality
cognitive and neuroanatomic substrates for, 227, 229–233
mood and, 160
overview, 223, 224–226, 225*t*, 226*t*, 233
stress regulation and, 239–240
Personality traits
alexithymia and, 104–105
mood and, 161*t*
Philosophy, 23–24
Phrenology, 24–25

Physical health
coping strategies and, 137
overview, 156*f*, 235
stress regulation and executive functioning and, 242–245, 243*f*
Physiological arousal, 116*f*
Plato, 12–13, 13*t*
Pons, 80. *See also* Lower brainstem
Posed affective communication. *See* Volitional affective communication
Positive affect
diagnostic sensitivity and specificity and, 251
overview, 160–162, 161*t*, 258
See also Mood
Positive and Negative Affect Schedule (PANAS), 171, 263
Positive emotionality, 225–226, 226*t*
Positive reinforcement, 202*n*. *See also* Incentive sensitivity; Rewards and punishments
Positron emission tomography (PET), 164
Postconcussive syndrome, 239–240
Posterior hypothalamus, 77*t*
Posterior preoptic area, 77*t*
Poststroke depression (PSD), 149–150, 150*f*
Posttraumatic hypopituitarism (PTHP)
clinical populations, 262
overview, 213–214, 258
Posttraumatic stress disorder (PTSD)
amygdala and, 67
awareness of emotional experience and, 109
overview, 215–216, 257
stress and, 219
See also Anxiety disorders
Postural orthostatic tachycardia syndrome (POTS), 85
Predatory aggression, 78, 79*t*. *See also* Aggression
Prefrontal activation asymmetry, 165
Prefrontal cortex (PFC)
approach–withdrawal dichotomy and, 166
emotion regulation and, 140, 147
executive functioning and, 240–241
functional imaging research, 202*n*
hemispheric asymmetry and, 164
heritability of temperament and personality and, 228*t*
overview, 30
rewards and punishments and, 193*f*–194*f*
stress regulation and, 238, 242
Preifornical lateral, 79*t*
Presupplementary motor area, 202*n*
Primary adrenal insufficiency, 213
Proactive coping strategies
emotion regulation and, 136*f*
stress regulation and, 237*t*
See also Coping strategies
Prolonged cardiovascular activation, 238, 244–245
Prosodic affect recognition, 125
Prosodic messages, 114
Prosody
expressive paralinguistic communication and, 122
paralinguistic communication and, 120
Pseudoaffective reflexes, 27, 40*n*
Pseudobulbar affect (PBA)
overview, 83
reflexive process and, 91
Psuedobulbar affect (PBA)
assessment measure for, 263
clinical populations, 262
overview, 253, 254, 255, 256, 258
Psychiatric disorders. *See* Neuropsychiatric disorders
Psychological functioning, 137
Psychomotor speed, 58
Psychopathology, 165
Psychopathy
affective communication and, 127, 131
amygdala and, 66–67
emotion regulation and, 145, 146*t*
extraversion and, 229–230
incentive sensitivity and, 192*t*, 200–201
overview, 257
rewards and punishments and, 192*t*
Psychosis
adrenal insufficiency and, 213
Cushing syndrome (CS) and, 212
Psychosurgery, 36–39

Punishments. *See* Rewards and punishments
Pure autonomic failure (PAF)
 awareness of emotional experience, 95
 overview, 85
Putamen, 102*t*

Q

Quality of life, 106–107

R

Reactive coping strategies, 136*f*. *See also* Coping strategies
Reactive reappraisal, 237*t*
Reactive suppression, 237*t*
Reactivity, stress, 237–238. *See also* Stress
Reactivity hypothesis, 244
Reappraisals, cognitive
 emotion regulation and, 136*f*
 feedback responsiveness and, 142–143
 overview, 137
 stress regulation and, 237*t*
Reasoning skills, 61
Receptive affective communication, 114–115, 118–119, 118*f*. *See also* Communication, emotional
Receptive linguistic communication, 118, 118*f*
Receptive paralinguistic communication, 118*f*, 119–122
Receptive situational communication, 118*f*
Reflexive motor output, 71
Reflexive processes
 affective communication and, 115–117, 116*f*
 clinical populations, 86–92, 87*t*, 90*t*
 integrating theory and practice, 82–92, 87*t*, 90*t*
 neuroanatomic substrates and, 75–82, 76*f*, 77*t*, 79*t*
 overview, 70, 92–93
 theoretical background, 71–82, 71*f*, 74*t*, 76*f*, 77*t*, 79*t*
Regional cerebral blood flow (rCBF), 139
Regulation, emotion. *See* Emotion regulation
Reinforcement-based learning, 199–200. *See also* Learning; Rewards and punishments
Reinterpretation
 emotion regulation and, 136*f*
 overview, 137, 139–140
Relations, interpersonal. *See* Interpersonal relations
Repetitive transcranial magnetic stimulation (rTMS), 150–151
Reproductive system, 74*t*
Resiliency to stress. *See also* Stress
 overview, 156*f*
 stress regulation and, 242–245, 243*f*
Respiratory rate, 74*t*
Respiratory sinus arrhythmia (RSA), 237
Restorative processes
 executive functioning and, 241–242
 overview, 243*f*
 stress regulation and, 238, 245
Rewards and punishments
 assessment and, 249–250, 263
 development of clinical tools and, 249–250
 extraversion and, 230
 neuroticism and, 229
 overview, 176–182, 199–200, 201
 personality and, 225
 sensitivity to, 191–192, 192*t*
 See also Incentive sensitivity
Right anterior insula, 98–99
Right frontoparietal operculum, 121
Right temporal operculum, 121
Risk, 242–245, 243*f*
Rumination, 154*n*

S

Salivary glands, 74*t*
Schizophrenia
 affect recognition and, 125
 affective communication and, 130*t*
 awareness of emotional experience and, 109
 overview, 257

Schizophrenia *(cont.)*
  rewards and punishments and, 195, 196
  stress and, 216
Secondary adrenal insufficiency, 213
Secondary anxiety disorders, 145–147, 146*t*. *See also* Anxiety disorders
Secondary bipolar disorder, 144–145. *See also* Bipolar disorder
Secondary depression, 144. *See also* Depression
Secondary mania, 144–145. *See also* Mania
Secondary psychopathy, 145, 146*t*. *See also* Psychopathy
Seizure disorder
  amygdala and, 65–66
  clinical populations, 261
  overview, 257
  reflexive process and, 90–91
Selective serotonin reuptake inhibitors (SSRIs), 86
Self-assertion, 136*f*
Self-distraction, 136*f*
Self-regulation, 240–241. *See also* Behavioral regulation; Emotion regulation; Stress regulation
Self-report assessments, 247–248
Semantic dementia, 128*t*
Sensations
  incentive sensitivity and, 183–184
  rewards and punishments and, 177–178, 192*t*
Sensitivity to incentives. *See* Incentive sensitivity
Serotonin syndrome, 86
Serotonin transporter gene (5-HTTLPR), 227
Sexual behaviors
  Klüver–Bucy syndrome and, 62
  overview, 79*t*
Situational mode of affective communication, 113, 118*f*. *See also* Communication, emotional
Skeletal branch
  assessment and, 91–92
  reflexive process and, 83–84
Sleep disturbances
  Cushing syndrome (CS) and, 212
  stress regulation and, 245
Smiles, 93*n*
Snaith–Hamilton Pleasure Scale (SHAPS), 196–197, 197*t*, 263
Social anxiety, 206. *See also* Anxiety
Social Cognition Test, 132–133, 263
Social deficits, 30
Somatic marker hypothesis, 186–188
Somatization, 109
Somatoform illnesses, 106–107
Spontaneous emotional expressiveness, 117. *See also* Communication, emotional
Steadiness hypothesis, 185
Stereotype threat, 142
Stimulus
  amygdala and, 50–51
  compared to triggers, 46
  overview, 255, 258
Stomach, 74*t*
Stress
  aging and dementia and, 216–217
  alexithymia and, 105–106
  clinical populations, 214–218
  clinical signs and syndromes, 211–214
  cognition and, 209–211
  dementias and, 173
  integrating theory and practice, 211–218
  neuroanatomic substrates and, 207–209, 209*f*
  neuropsychiatric disorders, 214–216
  overview, 204, 218–219, 245*n*
  recovery, 238
  restoration, 238
  stress exposure, 236
  theoretical background, 204–211, 206*f*, 209*f*
  See also Stress regulation
Stress exposure
  executive functioning and, 240
  overview, 236, 243*f*
  See also Stress
Stress reactivity
  executive functioning and, 240–241
  overview, 237–238, 243*f*
  See also Stress
Stress recovery, 243*f*

Stress regulation
cognitive and neuroanatomic substrates for, 239–242
emotion regulation and, 237*t*
executive functioning and, 242–245, 243*f*
overview, 235, 236–238, 237*t*, 245
See also Stress
Stress response, 205. *See also* Stress
Striatum, 79*t*
Stroop task, 234*n*
Substance abuse
affective communication and, 131
extraversion and, 230
See also Addiction
Sudden unexplained death in epilepsy patients (SUDEP) syndrome, 85
Superior temporal sulcus, 102*t*
Suppression
cognition and, 141–142
emotion regulation and, 136*f*
overview, 137, 138
stress regulation and, 237*t*
Supraoptic nucleus, 77*t*
Surgency. *See* Positive emotionality
Sweat glands, 74*t*
Switching
incentive sensitivity and, 188
overview, 168
Sympathetic adrenomedullary (SAM) system activation
overview, 205, 206*f*
stress regulation and, 237
Sympathetic cardiac dysregulation (CVA), 91
Systolic blood pressure, 237

T

Tear glands, 74*t*
Temperament, 223–224, 233
Temporal cortex, 79*t*
Temporal lobe, 40*n*
Temporal lobe epilepsy
emotion regulation and, 152
reflexive process and, 84–85, 90–91
See also Epilepsy
Temporoparietal cortex, 121
Test performance
emotion regulation and, 142–143
functional imaging research, 202*n*
Testosterone, 201
Thalamic networks, 79*t*
Thalamus
localization of emotions within the brain and, 26
paralinguistic communication and, 120–121
reflexive process and, 76*f*
The Awareness of Social Inference Test (TASIT), 132, 263
Theory of mind (ToM)
cognitive empathy and, 123, 124*f*, 125–126
overview, 133*n*
Theory of the 16 basic desires, 162, 175*n*. *See also* Motivation
Top-down approach for using this book, 2–5, 5*f*
Toronto Alexithymia Scale–20 (TAS-20), 107, 110, 263
Trait anxiety, 224–225. *See also* Neuroticism
Trait negative affectivity, 224–225. *See also* Neuroticism
Trait positive affectivity, 224–225
Traumatic brain injury
affective communication and, 127
awareness of emotional experience and, 108–109
emotion regulation and, 146–147, 148–149
extraversion and, 230
Klüver–Bucy syndrome and, 61–62
overview, 258
rewards and punishments and, 196, 200
stress and, 217–218, 219, 239–240
Trigger mechanism
amygdala and, 48–55, 49*f*, 52*t*, 54*f*, 56*t*, 68*n*–69*n*
assessment and, 59–60
clinical populations, 63–67
clinical signs and syndromes, 61–63
cognition and, 57–58
defining, 46–47
functioning and, 60–61

Trigger mechanism *(cont.)*
  incentive sensitivity and, 250
  integrating theory and practice, 59–67
  neuroanatomic substrates, 47–56, 49*f*, 52*t*, 54*f*, 56*t*
  overview, 45–46, 68
  theoretical background, 46–58, 49*f*, 52*t*, 54*f*, 56*t*
  volitional control and, 115
Triune brain, 41*n*
Tumors
  overview, 258
  stress and, 218
Turner syndrome
  amygdala and, 64
  overview, 258
20th centuries, 15–21, 16*f*, 17*f*
Twin studies, 226–227
Two-factor theory, 18–19

U

Underactive trigger mechanism, 59. *See also* Trigger mechanism
Unreliability, 225*t*
Urbach–Wiethe disease (lipoid proteinosis)
  amygdala and, 66
  overview, 258
Urinary bladder, 74*t*

V

Valence, 47
Valence hypothesis, 185–186
Valence of stimuli, 53–55, 54*f*
Vascular dementia
  adhedonia and, 190
  overview, 259
Vasopressin, 209*f*
Ventral pallidum
  reflexive process and, 80
  thalamic networks and, 79*t*
Ventral prefrontal cortex
  emotion regulation and, 154*n*
  reflexive process and, 80
Ventral tegmental area
  aggression and, 78–79, 79*t*
  reflexive process and, 76*f*
Ventromedial dorsal premammillary, 79*t*
Ventromedial nucleus, 77*t*
Ventromedial prefronal cortex
  affective communication and, 131
  functional imaging research, 202*n*
  thalamic networks and, 79*t*
Violence, 127, 131
Visceral functions, 32
Visual agnosia
  Klüver–Bucy syndrome and, 62
  overview, 40*n*
Volitional affective communication, 115–117, 116*f*. *See also* Communication, emotional
Volitional control, 115–117, 116*f*
Vulnerability, 156*f*

W

Wechsler series for assessment of intelligence and memory, 132–133
Wernicke area, 119, 133*n*
White matter, 100
Wisconsini Card Sorting Test (WCST)
  heritability of temperament and personality and, 226–227, 233*n*
  incentive sensitivity and, 192–195, 193*f*–194*f*
  overview, 185
  stress regulation and, 241
Withdrawal, 156*f*
Working memory, 228*t*. *See also* Memory

Y

Yerkes–Dodson law, 82